The Other Milk

The Other Milk

REINVENTING SOY IN REPUBLICAN CHINA

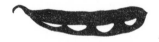

Jia-Chen Fu

UNIVERSITY OF WASHINGTON PRESS

Seattle

The Other Milk was made possible in part by grants from the Association for Asian Studies First Book Subvention Program and the Chiang Ching-kuo Foundation for International Scholarly Exchange. Additional support was provided by the Emory College of Arts and Sciences and the Emory Laney Graduate School.

A Study of the Weatherhead East Asian Institute of Columbia University
The Studies of the Weatherhead East Asian Institute of Columbia University were inaugurated in 1962 to bring to a wider public the results of significant new research on modern and contemporary East Asia.

UNIVERSITY OF WASHINGTON PRESS
www.washington.edu/uwpress

Cover illustration by LovetheWind, iStockphoto

LIBRARY OF CONGRESS CATALOGING-IN-PUBLICATION DATA
Names: Fu, Jia-Chen, author.
Title: The other milk : reinventing soy in Republican China / Jia-Chen Fu.
Description: Seattle : University of Washington Press, [2018] | Includes
    bibliographical references and index. |
Identifiers: LCCN 2018011125 (print) | LCCN 2018017624 (ebook) |
    ISBN 9780295744056 (ebook) | ISBN 9780295744049 (hardcover : alk. paper) |
    ISBN 9780295744032 (paperback : alk. paper)
Subjects: LCSH: Soymilk—Nutrition—China. | Soymilk—China. | Dairy
    substitutes.
Classification: LCC TX401.2.S69 (ebook) | LCC TX401.2.S69 F85 2018 (print) |
    DDC 641.3/097—dc23
LC record available at https://lccn.loc.gov/2018011125

For Zelda and JZ

Contents

Acknowledgments

I have benefited enormously from the patience and kindness of many. I would like to thank Jonathan Spence, Beatrice Bartlett, Annping Chin, Paul Gilroy, Susan Lederer, Mary Ting Yi Lui, and Peter Perdue for their steadfast support of my research. Judith Farquhar made some crucial suggestions that steered me toward (new-to-me) anthropological scholarship and challenged my thinking on the interplay between the material and human worlds. I have been fortunate to be able to present this research in a variety of formats, where people asked unexpected questions and suggested fruitful leads.

I especially want to thank Bride Andrews, Ina Asim, Nicole Barnes, Josep Barona, Alexander Bay, Morris Bian, Liping Bu, Daniel Buck, Janet Chen, Robert J. Culp, Katarzyna Cwierka, Lorraine Daston, Fa-ti Fan, David Gentilcore, Ian Hacking, Charles Hayford, Christian Henriot, Danian Hu, Michelle T. King, Chunghao Pio Kuo, Tong Lam, Seung-joon Lee, Victoria Lee, Sean Hsiang-lin Lei, Angela Ki Che Leung, Xun Liu, Rana Mitter, Rebecca Nedostup, Margaret Ng, Caroline Reeves, Naomi Rogers, Françoise Sabban, Jordan Sand, Volker Scheid, Helen Schneider, Grace Shen, Shen Xiaoyun, Nathan Sivin, William Summers, Mark Swislocki, Joanna Waley-Cohen, Shellen Wu, Yi-li Wu, and Michelle Yeh. My former colleagues at Case Western Reserve University, Molly Berger, Ananya Dasgupta, David Hammack, Ken Ledford, Miriam Levin, Alan Rocke, Renee Sentilles, Peter Shulman, Jonathan Sadowsky, and Gillian Weiss, were a boundless source of inspiration and erudition. They fielded many a question and provided astute feedback on my writing. My colleagues at Emory University, Tonio Andrade, Jeffery Lesser, Meredith Schweig, and Maria Sibau, helped and advised me through the final stages and kept my spirits up. Rachel Laudan, David Luesink, and Tom Mullaney read and commented on portions of the manuscript that were probably not ready to be read; I'm grateful for their good humor and sharp eye. Cheryl Beredo graciously helped me obtain a copy of Leonard A. Maynard's 1947 interview when getting to Ithaca, New York, wasn't practical. Audra Wolfe of The Outside Reader helped me identify the primary story I wanted to tell. Eric Karchmer and Hilary A. Smith, my steadfast writing companions, read many drafts of various chapters and always gave me smart ideas and suggestions for improvements.

I am grateful to the libraries and research institutions I visited over the years. My thanks goes out to the staff of the National Library of China, the Shanghai Municipal Library Republican Reading Room, the Shanghai Municipal Archives, the Second Historical Archives of China in Nanjing, the Jiangsu Provincial Archives, the Chongqing Municipal Archives, the Institute of Modern History Archives and Library at Academia Sinica, Academia Sinica in Taipei, the Harvard-Yenching Library, the Hoover Institution Archives, the New York Public Library's Manuscript and Archives Division, the Mudd Manuscript Library at Princeton University, the Rockefeller Archive Center, the Wellcome Library in London, the National Archives at Kew, and SOAS University of London Library's Special Collections. I would especially like to acknowledge the assistance of Martha Smalley and Joan Duffy at the Yale Divinity School Library's Special Collections; William Shurtleff of the Soyinfo Center in Lafayette, California; Ye Li for helping me navigate the Chongqing Municipal Archives; and John Moffett at the Needham Research Institute for allowing me to show up uninvited and work in the library.

A number of institutions and organizations supported the research and writing of this book. Research in China and elsewhere was supported by a Fulbright, travel grants from Yale University's Council on East Asian Studies and the Baker-Nord Center for Humanities at Case Western Reserve University, the W. P. Jones Presidential Faculty Fund, and a Flora Stone Mather fellowship from the Case Western Reserve University Department of History. I am grateful to the Association for Asian Studies and the Chiang Ching-kuo Foundation for International Scholarly Exchange for providing first-book subventions. Emory University's College of Arts and Sciences and Laney Graduate School defrayed publication costs.

I thank the University of Hawai'i Press for permission to reuse, in chapter 4, portions of my article "Confronting the Cow: Soybean Milk and the Fashioning of a Chinese Dairy Alternative," in Moral Foods: The Construction of Nutrition and Health in Modern Asia, edited by Angela Ki Che Leung and Melissa L. Caldwell (forthcoming), and I also thank Koninklijke Brill NV for permission to reuse, in chapters 5 and 6, portions of my article "Scientizing

Relief: Nutritional Activism from Shanghai to the Southwest, 1937–1945" (*European Journal of East Asian Studies* 11 [2012]: 259–82).

The manuscript found a warm home at the University of Washington Press, whose editor and staff have guided me through the publishing process. I especially thank Lorri Hagman for sensing the potential in my work, as well as Niccole Coggins, Beth Fuget, Richard Isaac, and Susan Stone for helping me get all the details right. Eugenia Lean and Ross Yesley of Columbia University's Weatherhead East Asian Institute publication series helped make sure this project came to fruition. The anonymous reviewers for the Weatherhead program and for the University of Washington Press made critical suggestions that vastly improved the book.

Last but never least, I want to thank my family—my wonderfully silly and clever family that has grown in number over the years. Despite our individual peregrinations, Michael, Linsey, and I keep coming back to a rambling red house lovingly lined with Christmas trees and a neighborhood grocery store just a few blocks from the state capitol building. Who could have guessed we would each find so much intellectual fodder in the union—and disunion—of food, medicine, and business? I cannot thank my parents enough for their love and support, and knowing when not to ask me how the book was going. And to John, who has generously given me a mountain of mathematical terms I have yet to incorporate into my own writing, thank you for sharing this path with me.

The Other Milk

Introduction

I N a short, elegant piece written in 1933, the modern essayist Zhu Ziqing (1899–1948) described bright, white parcels of tofu bubbling to the surface in a pot around which the writer, his father, and his brothers all huddled eagerly. The warmth that radiated from the gas burner drew them in on a cold winter's night, but it was not the warmth alone that animated Zhu's recollection.[1] The essay sought to capture the anticipation and delight that came with waiting for his father to pluck morsels of tofu, one by one, from the pot and place them in a dish of soy sauce. Although the boys could have easily undertaken this task themselves, they preferred to hover with anticipation, enjoying the full sensory experience of the meal. As Zhu explains, "This was not eating [*chi fan*] per se, but playing."[2]

For many of Zhu's contemporaries, however, eating—let alone eating tofu—could hardly be deemed play. Indeed, in a country whose international reputation and domestic self-image had been sealed by the moniker "the Land of Famine," eating—or the lack of eating or not eating correctly—was very serious business indeed.[3] It was likely the seriousness of food that led a writer for *Shenbao*, Shanghai's largest, longest-running, and most important newspaper, to appropriate Zhu Ziqing's essay in an unexpected manner. Zhu was surely not thinking about tofu as an ideal and tasty vehicle for conveying lots of good-for-you proteins, but that is how a *Shenbao* writer introduced the health benefits of the soybean to his audience in January 1939.[4] Having referenced Zhu's story, the piece continued, "Tofu! Tofu! Everyone loves to eat tofu, but no one understands why." To appreciate why tofu—as well as its "age-old friend," *doujiang* (soybean milk)—was so beloved, the author invoked the expertise of the "nutrition scientist" (*yingyang yanjiuzhe*) and catalogued the many and varied nutritive characteristics distinguishing tofu: it was high in protein, and "other important nutrients, like vitamins A, B, C, and all the way up to X (even though some [vitamins] have yet to be discovered), are all included."[5]

This literary moment of nostalgia and belonging was all the more striking given the immediate subtext of war and daily hardship. By January 1939, much of the eastern seaboard was under Japanese occupation. Despite several valiant attempts to counter Japan's military assault in 1937, the Nationalist government was forced to retreat multiple times before finally settling inland, in Chongqing, in October 1938. That soybeans and soybean-derived foods should figure at all in this conflict might seem surprising, but soybeans, and especially soybean milk, appeared again and again in newspaper articles, popular journal essays, government committee deliberations, and relief campaigns for the growing number of Chinese refugees. Soybeans were perceived as a common food with a long-standing and recognized place in local foodways, and in wartime, a more modern form of soybean milk, it was argued, could nurture and save China's young. Indeed, throughout the winter of 1937–38, soybean milk fortified with calcium and vitamins came to the rescue of starving, malnourished children in Shanghai's refugee camps. In tin bowls grasped by little fingers, soybean milk symbolized how a beleaguered China could struggle forward and protect its future.

As a fortified food designed and distributed for the express purpose of combating malnutrition, soybean milk had traversed ontological distance from its former incarnation as a tonic for aging, ailing bodies. We see inklings of these past lives in a 1920 poem by the traditional-style poet Chen Sanli (1853–1937) that appeared in the pages of *Eastern Miscellany* sporting the title "Playfully Composed while Drinking *Doujiang*" (Yin doujiang xi cheng). Both the form and thematic focus of this piece suggest a sense of fidelity with tradition.[6] Written in the form of a *jueju*, a poem of four lines, each containing seven characters, that adheres to a strict tonal pattern and rhyme scheme, it ruminates upon the effects of age and the techniques for stemming its tide. With allusions to the poet Su Shi (1037–1101) and perhaps *The Book of Changes* (Yijing), a rough translation would be as follows:

> Though I seek to preserve my peace of mind so as to dispel sickness,
>> I am afraid this is not effective.
> I chant long and continuously, like the tiger overtaking the wind.

Yet this is not as effective as soybean milk or astragalus root congee for
nourishing one's qi and pulse, which make old Su grateful.[7]

Chen's invocation of *doujiang* as a drink for the aged would likely have resonated with his readers, who were familiar with the various tonics (*buyao*)
advertised in major newspapers like *Shenbao*.

How did *doujiang*, which invoked such diverse associations as fortifica-
tion, familial warmth, and protein richness, come to be seen as the nutritional
savior of Chinese children? Why was such stress laid upon the scientific characteristics of the drink—its standardized recipe for production, its high
protein content, and its positive spectrum of vitamins? The answer is both
simple and counterintuitive: soybean milk was reinvented as traditional,
modern, and scientific.

In this book, I explore the curious paths by which thinking about the Chinese diet evolved, how this diet was defined as an inadequate one that
imperiled the nation, and how a local foodstuff was reinterpreted, rediscov-
ered, and reassigned social and scientific meanings in an attempt to solve
the problem of inadequacy during the first half of the twentieth century. At
its heart, this is the history of modern Chinese nutrition science and nutritional activism, seen through their engagement with the soybean, and especially soybean milk.

Investigating the soybean's biochemical properties, devising new and
improved recipes with soybeans to address China's many and profound nutritional problems, and provoking questions about the relationship between
diet, health, and nation all were constituent elements in the formation of
nutrition science in China. These activities were performed by many diverse
historical players, who can be subsumed under the heading of "nutritional
activists." In contrast to other subdisciplines of science and technology, nutrition science allows scientific experts to be knowledge producers and activists simultaneously. That nutrition science attracts a variety of historical
actors is a phenomenon not specific to China, and in the early twentieth
century, the indistinct, variable nature of the borders of nutrition as a scientific discipline enabled European and American scientists and industrialists
to seize upon the soybean as a kind of miracle plant with which to build
modern economies and healthy nations. In grappling with these global
currents, Chinese nutritional activists worked and reworked the familiar
and the foreign into everyday repertoires about food and health. Their
actions demonstrate how important the circulation, mutual implication,

and convergence of scientific ideas and practices were to the modern project of science-building in China.

Today, the soybean has traveled far beyond its Chinese roots, becoming one of the predominant commodities of the twentieth and twenty-first centuries. By tracing the emergence of the soybean in the form of soybean milk, as an object of scientific inquiry and a commodity in transition, this book examines the growth of Chinese nutrition science and how that science framed soybeans as the answer to China's many and profound nutritional and developmental problems. This process of self-definition and reinvention reveals the layered and transnational dimensions of the history of modern Chinese science. Moreover, it illuminates the conditions under which Chinese actors such as nutrition scientists, public health activists, and industrialists strategically decided which ways of knowing and engaging with the material world were modern and scientific. The role of food in Chinese modernity exemplifies the vexed ways in which China engaged with the new global discourses on food and security (what the historian Nick Cullather has described as "the governmentality of the calorie") as both a consumer and producer of scientific knowledge about the country's nutritional needs.

NURTURING MODERN NUTRITION

Histories of food and diet in China have typically presented the history of nutrition science in one of two ways: either as a Western import or as a modern manifestation of older dietetic knowledge. The latter pattern can be seen in Lu Gwei-djen and Joseph Needham's 1951 essay "A Contribution to the History of Chinese Dietetics," in which the long-time collaborators excavated citations from a handful of classical medical and dietary texts to demonstrate that Chinese "empirical knowledge of diet, especially in relation to certain deficiency diseases, is much older than commonly supposed."[8] In contrast, in 1953, when the biochemist Zheng Ji presented his historical evaluation of nutrition science to China, he avoided all mention of individuals and activities prior to 1913. Instead, he identified four periods of growth and development, all in the twentieth century: the 1913–24 "sprouts period," the 1925–37 "growth period," the 1938–49 "bitter struggle period," and the post-1949 "new life period." In a curious way, these two approaches function as a mirror of the same conceit, namely that modern nutritional knowledge represented a form of rupture whose place in Chinese society demanded either acceptance or cultural suturing. In other words, we remain firmly rooted in interpretations that emphasize Chinese appropriation and reception without a sense of how nutrition science was grafted onto existing epistemological regimes and practices while also creating new ones, let alone the specific worlds of relationality made by the scientists themselves.

More contemporary studies have refined and problematized these two approaches by challenging the ahistoricity implicitly underlining the attempts to find antecedents of modern nutritional knowledge in China's past.[9] The eminent historian of food and diet in China Ji Hongkun once observed that popular insistence on pitting two-hundred-year-old Western nutritional knowledge against the thousands of years of Chinese traditional nutritional knowledge was neither scientific nor in keeping with historical facts.[10] The juxtaposition was conceptually faulty, because it obliterated any sense of the traditional dietetic culture that had shaped European societies from antiquity through at least the eighteenth century, and it blurred differences between those older ideas and practices and the emergence of scientific nutrition after the eighteenth century.[11] Indeed, while one could not reasonably claim that the history of diet and nutrition was a mere two hundred years old in the West—without displaying an immodest amount of cultural chauvinism—one could narrow the parameters. The history of scientific nutrition was roughly two hundred years old, and its influence in China only slightly less. After all, as Ji writes, "Modern nutrition (*jindai yingyangxue*) in China was neither locally born nor bred (*bushi tushengtuzhang*). It came from the West, as a part of the 'spread of Western learning' (*xixue dongjian*), and it came together with the introduction of modern chemistry, physics, and medicine."[12]

For Ji, rearticulating the temporal framework allows one to consider the role played by Jesuit and Protestant missionaries in the transmission of Western science and medicine to China. While commendable, this alignment of modern nutrition in China as the natural consequence of Western science and medicine is nonetheless disconcerting—not because it is matter-of-factly incorrect but because it obscures how and why Chinese might have been attracted to Western physiological and dietary ideas. Understanding gastric digestion, for example, as a chemical reaction, as demonstrated by J. R. Young in 1803, may be more accurate than the explication provided in the famous classical Chinese medical treatise *The Yellow Emperor's Inner Canon* (Huangdi neijing), in which food enters the stomach and its essential qi is forwarded upward to the pulmonary tract, where it is transformed into blood (*xue*) that can be supplied to vivify the whole body.[13] But to assume the explanatory power of one or another explanation is more real, and therefore true, is to fall prey to presentist preoccupations. John Fryer (1839–1928), a Protestant missionary turned government translator, and his longtime collaborator Xu Shou (1818–1884) introduced the idea that human digestion was a chemical reaction in their scientific journal *Compendium for Investigating Things and Extending Knowledge* (Gezhi huibian).[14] But knowing this does not explain how a discerning, educated Chinese person familiar with Chinese medical concepts yet curious about Western learning would have understood this idea and why it might have resonated. Indeed, we need to grapple with the complexity of Chinese desires for nutrition science and its particular knowledge regime, because, as Grace Shen has emphasized in the case of geology, "Looking at those desires helps us to put progress and modernization in the context of other urgent motives, rather than in the realm of historical inevitability."[15] By examining the specific contexts of agency and mobilization in which nutrition science became embedded in Republican China, we can move away from simple descriptions of appropriation and reception.

A further consideration left unexamined in accounts of modern nutrition in China as the natural consequence of Western science and medicine lies in the very processes of scientific inquiry and exploration, and how such processes take root in different temporal and spatial settings. Nutrition science in the late nineteenth and early twentieth centuries did not just introduce new ideas to a willing (or unwilling), receptive (or unreceptive) Chinese audience; it attempted to forge a particular kind of ontological stability for the concept of "food" and the biological stability of the "eating body."[16] As scholars working on the history of nutrition in the United States and Europe have shown, nineteenth-century scientific investigations on the physiology of digestion and twentieth-century public health initiatives in the United States and Europe cooperated in naturalizing the aphorism "we are what we eat" through what Gyorgy Scrinis has described an ideology of "nutritionism" and what Jessica Mudry analyzes as "a discourse of quantification."[17] Nutrition science created an epistemological model for framing the body in terms of nutritional requirements—one that carried alongside it a disciplinary regime for materializing that body. Ideas that seem unquestionably obvious from a contemporary perspective—amino acids are our bodies' "building blocks," calcium and vitamin D "build strong bones," and calories are necessary "fuel" burned by metabolism to "run" bodies—obscure the on-the-ground processes of differentiation, amalgamation, and acculturation that might enable these ideas and scientific objects to travel cross-culturally or transhistorically.[18]

Thus, even while it became increasingly fashionable and compelling by the 1930s for Chinese scientists and science popularizers to speak of the human body as a steam engine, to delineate the nutritional composition of foods in terms of calories and vitamins, or even espouse the importance of increasing the protein content of Chinese diets, it is not clear that nutrition science in early twentieth-century China achieved this same kind ideological hegemony over the ways in which Chinese people thought about food and eating.[19] This is not to deny or diminish the strong didactic tone with which nutrition science has expressed itself in twentieth-century China. But the persistence of popular expressions of the tonifying value of soybean milk, like Chen Sanli's poem and popular advertisements for soybean milk, nonetheless attests to this history of incompleteness, even as the desire expressed and the activities undertaken to make calories, vitamins, and proteins real and significantly meaningful for the Chinese public dominated how Chinese scientists articulated and practiced modern science. The question that persists remains identical to the one first posed by the historian Mark Swislocki, who blazed a path forward by arguing in 2001 that the history of nutrition science in China must be linked to world history: How did nutrition science become "an authoritative idiom in China for understanding the relationship between food and health"?[20]

This book provides one answer. Building on recent historical scholarship that has sought to foreground the reciprocal, mutually constitutive—if nonetheless unequal—interactions among Chinese medicine, Western medicine, and Chinese actors, it shows how Chinese adoption, synthesis, and adaptation of nutrition science from the late nineteenth century through the first half of the twentieth occurred as a result of specific circumstances in which China found itself.[21] Moreover, the extent to which nutrition science helped construct and substantiate Chinese fears about the Chinese diet served to mobilize strikingly local and highly specific strategies for managing such fears.

As the role of science in imperialism became increasingly entangled with the wealth and power of the West, Chinese interest in nutrition science arose in conjunction with a vision of a modern China defined by technological and industrial development. The increasing urgency felt by many Chinese that both the nation and its people needed to be physically stronger was coupled with a growing sense that strength could be engineered through scientific foods and rational dietary practices. In this, China was not alone, but its path of convergence with these global ideas of science, technology, and power reflected a series of decisions and contingencies specific to a struggling empire and an emergent nation under real and perceived assault from foreign powers.[22]

The very word for "nutrition" in Chinese reflects this complex set of global dynamics informing and shaping Chinese strategies linking science to the formation of a patriotic and productive society and nation. The term *yingyang* as a referent for nutrition can also obscure the extent to which it was grafted onto late-imperial conceptualizations of nutrition that emphasized the personal or familial dimensions of self-care and the medical concerns of the wealthy and elite, as opposed to the poor or the general populace.[23] That Fryer and Xu did not use the modern term *yingyang* in their description of digestion is a telling sign that should challenge the impulse to see the transmission of Western science and medicine as a unidirectional exchange. The appearance of the term *yingyang* came later, and it came by way of Japan. When Fryer and Xu began publishing the *Compendium for Investigating Things and Extending Knowledge*, the Qing dynasty had survived a series of mid-century cataclysms, including a massive civil war with the Taiping rebels; armed and persistent rebellions in the north, northwest, and southwest; and two military defeats at the hands of both the British and the French. As foreign powers vied to obtain territorial and economic concessions from an ever-weakening Chinese imperial court, a complex and variegated effort by Chinese literati inside and outside the imperial bureaucracy to explore the bounds of Western learning—within which science was prioritized—emerged and shaped late Qing political life.[24] The hope was to glean the scientific and technological secrets that might enable the Qing state to modernize and deflect further foreign aggression. Much of this scientific popularization and translation, as well as Qing experimentations with arsenals, navy yards, and factories, was denigrated by later Chinese revolutionaries and reformers as foolhardy and insubstantial when, counter to all expectations, the Qing were defeated by Japan in the First Sino-Japanese War (1894–95).

Early twentieth-century Chinese reformers and revolutionaries condemned these Qing efforts to the dustbin of history and derided them as misguided and backward attempts to mimic rather than develop the country's scientific potential.[25] The military loss and the sudden crisis of identity that erupted among the literati spurred Chinese interest in Meiji Japan and its successful transformation into a modern imperial power. Japan quickly joined England, France, and Germany as a beacon of science and technology.

Between 1902 and 1907, over ten thousand Chinese traveled to Japan to study, and of the foreign-trained students who joined the Qing civil service after 1905, some 90 percent of them graduated from Japanese schools.[26]

As Shellen Wu has shown for the development of modern geology in China, this pre-1895 period of scientific translation and popularization was important for fostering awareness of a global culture of science and industrialization—that sense of the "giddy promise of science as the key to the West's wealth and power."[27] This global culture also nurtured the development of Chinese nutrition science and predated the formal institutionalization of the scientific discipline at Chinese universities and various research institutes, which occurred in the 1920s through the efforts of reformers such as Wu Xian (Wu Hsien, 1893–1959), who had returned from study overseas. The power and seduction of this culture extended deep into the fabric of daily life and encapsulated reimaginings of what it meant to be a Chinese person eating certain foods and engaged in certain activities (chapter 2). Nutrition scientists such as Wu Xian engaged in an epistemological project of self-invention with the concept of the Chinese diet, which conceived of food as analyzable units serving specific physiological needs in service of a higher national purpose. Their scientific investigations into Chinese foodstuffs and dietary values formed the basis of modern knowledge of Chinese nutrition and helped reconceptualize the diversity of local foodways into a generalizable, if not national, rubric that became "the Chinese diet." Without this shift in worldview—made all the more poignant and urgent by Japan's seemingly successful transformation into a modern nation—the rise of nutrition science in China could not have unfolded as it did.

Given the prominent position afforded Japan's own experiences with global science, it may be less surprising to learn that the modern Chinese term for nutrition, *yingyang*, came from the kanji term *eiyō*, which was a loanword from modern Japanese that had been created using Chinese classical characters to translate the European original.[28] As a loanword that was introduced into China in the twentieth century by way of Chinese intellectuals who had studied in Japan, *yingyang* as "nutrition" was conceptually and historically framed by its translingual interactions. Zheng Zhenwen (1891–1969), the scientific editor at the Commercial Press in Shanghai, played a key role in ushering *yingyang* into the Chinese vernacular.[29] Zheng had learned both Japanese and English and graduated from the Northeastern Imperial University in Tokyo with a major in physical chemistry. Although he was not a professional scientist, his service as the scientific editor for the Commercial

Press provided him broad discretion and control over how modern scientific ideas were explained and introduced to a growing Chinese reading public.[30] He was the first to use *yingyang* to encapsulate the chemical and physiological study of human nutrition.

Zheng Zhenwen's role in popularizing *yingyang* flags the importance of the mutually constitutive ways in which science and social identities were formed. As a member of what Robert Culp has described as "petty intellectuals"—editors, teachers, and journalists—Zheng exerted tremendous influence through his professional endeavors on the repackaging of new currents of disciplinary learning for broad dissemination to a mass public.[31] He was not alone. While nutrition scientists like Wu Xian, Zheng Ji, and Hou Xiangchuan actively worked to bridge the professional and discursive divide through public lecture circuits and popular writings on the deficiency of the Chinese diet (chapters 2 and 3), the potency of modern nutrition science was derived from the on-the-ground translational efforts of knowledge workers who made the abstract concrete through popular advertisements, new commercial products, and dietary campaigns.

Individuals such as Nellie Lee, the young Chinese-American woman who strove to popularize soybean milk as a nutritional supplement throughout Southwest China during the war years, accepted and propagated the conviction that the future health of both the individual and the nation were inextricably tied (chapters 6 and 7). Modern nutrition science characterized this relationship as a technical one responsive to social engineering—an idea that had been gaining in circulation in Western social and scientific circles, and when translated into Chinese, cohered with other modern discourses about nationalism, self-determination, and anti-imperialism.[32] Although historically the Chinese imperial state had adopted the idea that among the state's various responsibilities "nourishing the people" (*yangmin*) was foremost, the nourishment in question did not entail any accompanying concern for the health of the recipient. *Yangmin* as a form of imperial governance involved a range of different administrative measures to ensure and facilitate access to grain in times of distress and hardship.[33] It was designed to manage famine. In contrast, modern nutrition science elevated the importance of the health of the individual as the unitary basis for the integrity of the nation and the key to its survival.[34] As one Chinese nutritional scientist explained, "Sound nutrition enables a body to receive all that it needs to grow. Those who are of sallow complexion, lacking muscle, and infirm beyond one's years (*weilao xianshuai*) are suffering from insufficient nourishment (*yingyang buzu*). For the individual, these [qualities] are [a sign of] misfortune; for a country, [a sign of] loss."[35]

As will become evident in the following chapters, modern nutrition science, with its linkage of the individual to the nation and the medicalization of the pursuit of wealth and power, was both the foundation and the tool for diagnosing and curing China's maladies. Modern nutrition science shifted attention away from the diets of the wealthy, the previous focal point of older dietetic thinking, toward the diets of the poor, and crucially, it furnished the empirical tools with which to study what people ate. Tools are empowering, but they are not necessarily predictive. How and why Chinese nutrition scientists conceived of the Chinese diet as they did reveals the deep imbrication of science, wealth, and power in the first half of the twentieth century.

Modern nutrition science recast the humble soybean as both intrinsically Chinese and modern. Although Chinese nutrition science explored a wide range of foodstuffs in its broader enterprise to understand the organic requirements of the Chinese body and the most economical method of consumption from the standpoint of physiology, soybean research functioned as a bridge between the needs of the individual and the demands of the nation (chapter 3). Scientific investigation and experimentation enabled Chinese scientists to characterize the Chinese diet as inadequate and potentially harmful to China's development into a modern nation. Translating economic concerns about China's national development into a biochemical language of power and energy, Chinese scientists emphasized the need for more protein to compensate for the nutritional inadequacy of the Chinese diet. The soybean provided a homegrown answer.

Spurred by the propagation of a nutritional paradigm that identified dairy as an essential food category in the human diet and milk especially as a critical protective food whose consumption ensured both individual and national fitness, Chinese entrepreneurs and scientists in the 1910s and 1920s began experimenting with ways in which to refashion a common food, *doujiang*, into a modern food that we know as soybean milk (chapter 4). Such experimentation drew together several scientific strands of interest in Republican China: physiological research on metabolism and growth; the establishment of new academic disciplines dedicated to understanding children, childhood, and child development; and the growing conviction that national wealth and progress was inextricably tied to the health and well-being of Chinese children.

Although Chen Sanli and Zhu Ziqing incorporated references to soybean-derived foods in their respective works, there were no indications that the reader was expected to interpret the soybean as a metonymic symbol for Chineseness. For Chen, *doujiang* evoked popular remedies for fortifying an aging body and long-standing literary tropes about aging; for Zhu, tofu summoned the slipperiness between materiality and memory and projected one back into the affective landscape of comfort and warmth. In neither instance did the soybean (or its related foods) connote some essential quality of Chineseness.

In contrast, for nutritional activists seeking to stem the tide of malnutrition in war-torn China, the soybean was inherently, proprietarily both modern and Chinese. Its nutritional profile and adaptability in the service of a modern diet made it an ideal base upon which to construct a scientific campaign for social relief. For Chinese industrialists and entrepreneurs, the soybean's Chineseness was both self-evident and a selling point. And they were not alone in seeing its representative force. Western commentators too found it difficult not to highlight the soybean's Chinese origins, as is apparent in the opening lines of the following ditty written in 1956 by a medical nutritionist and his wife:

"Little Soybean who are you
From far off China where you grew?"
"I am wheels to steer your cars,
I make cups that hold cigars.
I make doggies nice and fat
And glue the feathers to your hat.
I am very good to eat,
I am cheese and milk and meat.
I am soap to wash your dishes,
I am oil to fry your fishes,
I am paint to trim your houses,
I am buttons on your blouses.
You can eat me from the pod,
I put pep back in the sod.
If by chance you're diabetic
The things I do are just prophetic.

I'm most everything you've seen
And still I'm just a little bean."[36]

Just a little bean with the magical power of transformation and a question mark behind its nativity! What had once been exotic from "far off China" could be domesticated in the forms of cars, cigars, milk, and meat. The soybean, ever humble, had made it. But like all suddenly famous interlopers, could the soybean remain true to its Chinese origins?

What Westerners saw as a geographical birthmark, early twentieth-century Chinese proponents of the soybean identified as adaptability, innovation, and the power of self-invention (chapter 1). Semantic cadences of the soybean shifted as global economic conditions reshaped Chinese scientific and medical enthusiasm for soybeans and soybean milk. Older associations as a famine crop, a base for fertilizer, and a source for cooking, lubrication, and lighting joined newer, techno-scientific visions of the soybean as a global industrial commodity and modern foodstuff. Chineseness as manifest in the humble bean evoked the power of transformation: an empire and civilization in decline could be reborn just like the soybean. This belief in the potential of the soybean to remake the Chinese diet, the Chinese body, and the Chinese nation has largely been lost, and though a variety of soybean-derived foods continue to grace the tables of families and restaurants throughout China, the cultural significance of the soybean as a form of modern alterity has transmuted as Chinese agriculture and eating habits have shifted since the country began liberalizing its markets in the early 1980s. Chinese today eat more meat and dairy than ever before, and soybean foods are increasingly esteemed as hallmarks of Chinese tradition—a veritable feast of local tastes and artisanal creativity.[37] But if we allow the soybean, and especially soybean milk, to claim our focus, we find that that food was integral to both the history of Chinese nutrition science and Chinese understandings of modernity. It was through the materiality of the soybean—the new and not-so-new ways in which the soybean could be materially transformed into a global commodity and health-enhancing superfood—that Chinese scientists, industrialists, and public health activists sought to instill and domesticate new practices and ideas about the proper relationship between food and health, and between food and nation.[38]

As twenty-first-century studies have shown, Nationalist concerns regarding food supply and consumption depended on the importance of other Chinese foods, especially rice, to local dietaries and notions of political legitimacy.[39] Republican statecraft tended to foreground new forms of economic calculus and statistical representation in an attempt to protect the economic integrity of the Chinese nation by limiting Chinese importation of rice, adopting protective tariffs for rice grown domestically, and promoting the consumption of national rice. This enthrallment with Western science and technology typified the Nationalists' forward-looking stance, even as local governments, like the Municipal Government of Greater Shanghai, deliberately rooted their approach to the city's rice supply problem in older, more traditional methods, such as granary policy, fixed price sales, and vilification of rice merchants.[40] Recognizing the variety of approaches to the rice supply problem, the Nationalist preoccupation with rice nonetheless functioned as a continuation of a longer history of imperial governance that understood the provision and/or protection of grain supplies as the hallmark of traditional authority.

To focus on soybeans instead of rice moves us outside of the direct ambit of political authority and into the margins of social and scientific world-making.[41] In particular, it forces us to consider the fragmented patchwork of intellectual communities engaged in redefining China's place within a modern capitalist economy and the extent to which their commitment to the soybean arose from a vision of the soybean as a scientifically tailored (or tailorable) instrument of development (chapters 6 and 7). The Nationalist government was not insensitive to this potential, but its role was distinctly secondary to the many and diverse ways in which non-state actors sought to articulate and disseminate the soybean's potential to change China.

Although in China the soybean has traditionally been considered one of the five staple grains (wugu)—along with wheat, rice, sorghum, and millet—its social, cultural, economic, and political significance over the centuries has been typically overshadowed by the "high degree of symbolic magnetism" that has defined rice's place in Chinese society.[42] And yet in the early twentieth century, the soybean as crop, as food, and as industrial commodity converged in ways that have not been fully explained. Part of this convergence derived from the intimate association of the soybean with the young field of modern chemistry.

The most thorough and detailed investigation of the history of the soybean in Chinese agriculture and foodways was conducted by H. T. Huang, whose work remains the authority on the history of food science in ancient China.[43] The earliest textual references to the soybean as food date from the Warring States period (480–221 BCE) and describe prolonged cooking in water to achieve edibility. This was a simple yet effective method for making soybeans edible. It did not, however, improve the soybean's culinary graces. Raw, mature soybeans can pose significant challenges to the human diet on account of the presence of trypsin (or protease) inhibitors that have to be inactivated or removed before the soybean is ready for human consumption. The use of fire in food preparation was a crucial step in unlocking the nutritive benefits of soybeans and facilitating their domestication. Other techniques—including fermentation, sprouting, and grinding—emerged by the end of the Han dynasty (206 BCE–220 CE) and rendered soybeans digestible and palatable.[44] Products such as soy sauce, bean curd (tofu), and soybean milk then spread throughout East Asia. The integration of these soyfoods into local dietaries was not, however, consistent. Soybean milk, for example, likely was invented during the early Han dynasty, but it did not become a part of the Chinese diet until the eighteenth or nineteenth century, when prolonged heating was found to make the milk both palatable and easily digestible.[45] Even so, it does not appear to have become popular among the Chinese public until the late nineteenth or early twentieth century. Why did the turn of the twentieth century generate such sudden, frenetic interest in soyfoods?

Recent scholarship has begun to address the global diffusion of the soybean in the twentieth century. The collection of essays contained in *The World of Soy* represents an important anthropological contribution to understanding the many diverse dietary practices associated with soyfoods in East and Southeast Asia, Africa, and the Americas.[46] Historians Ines Prodöhl and Wen Shuang have begun illuminating the intricate and unexpected ways in which the history of the soybean has been entwined with global networks of industrial capitalism by focusing on the political economy of the global soybean trade.[47] This growing body of scholarship has deepened our understanding of how critical a role the soybean has played in linking the histories of Africa and the Americas, Europe, and much of Asia. But there remains a Janus-like quality that seeks resolution, as soybeans are both ancient and modern: "On the one hand, they harken back to ancient practices, as in the manufacture of bean curd (tofu), soy sauce, and bean pastes. On the other hand, they involve highly modernized, industrialized processes for the extraction of the oil, the manufacture of animal feed (a use that ultimately leads to human food in the form of meat), the fabrication of extruded soy protein for use in new food analogues such as veggie burgers, the preparation of infant formula and health-promoting nutraceuticals, and so on."[48]

The soybean is thus marked by bipolar temporalities discernible by different, mutually divorced technological ecosystems. Among the various strengths imputed to the soybean, and soybean milk, was its adaptability to traditional and modern registers of significations. Being naturally rich in protein yet already incorporated into customary dietary practices represented the soybean's simultaneous occupation of the new and old. Long-standing practices involved in the production of soybean milk, for example, were not jettisoned so much as reinterpreted into a vision of industrial modernity that could be built on top of existing technologies. This was certainly Li Shizeng's contention when he called for the Chinese to take advantage and further develop Chinese technological expertise with the soybean (see chapter 1). Similarly, the commercial refashioning of *doujiang* as scientific soybean milk entailed less rejection than selective appropriation of the language of Chinese medicine and Daoist longevity to produce a polyphonic, hybrid modernity (see chapter 5). It was on account of the soybean's temporal doubleness that Chinese nutritional activists believed in the possibility of raising soybean consciousness in wartime China. Their efforts at translating a refugee relief program built around the distribution of scientific soybean milk into everyday life were predicated on the idea that Chinese people understood, or could be made to understand, the soybean's unique positioning as both traditional and modern. They argued that fortified soybean milk represented a rational, economical, scientifically supported, and already familiar solution to inadequacies of the Chinese diet. Their wartime experiences demonstrate how strong the will to change how the Chinese people ate was, and the challenges they encountered—the solutions they proposed—highlight how nutrition science was value laden and context specific.

The fungibility and temporal doubleness of the soybean mark out the tensions and contradictions of Chinese experiences of global capitalism and scientific modernity. As Chinese nutritional activists often insisted, the Chinese diet was never simply what the Chinese people ate. And yet what Chinese people ate mattered, and the desire for control over both the alimentary composition and semantic meanings of such foods represented critical components in the search for modern China.

CHAPTER 1

The Romance of the Bean

Rethinking the Soybean as Technology and Modern Commodity

I n February 1911, the *North-China Herald* reported that "the most up-to-date factory in France, and perhaps in Europe, has, states a Paris correspondent, just been established here by a Chinese, and all its employees are young Chinese."[1] The news, whether carried in an English-language newspaper in China or by American or European presses, was both surprising and unprecedented. At the time, "up-to-date" was perhaps not the first adjective to come to mind when referring to China. The *North-China Herald*, the most important and longest-running English-language newspaper in China, served a mixed readership of foreigners and elite Chinese literate in English. Its lead story in the same issue concerned Japan's increasingly intimate friendship with Russia as the two empires sought mutual support and justification for their presence in Manchuria. The newspaper, which was also the official journal for British consular notifications and the British-led Shanghai Municipal Council,[2] patronizingly suggested, "A frank and clear-cut statement in regard to her continental policy, could, if Japan harbors no ulterior designs, do her not the slightest harm, while it would relieve China of anxiety and other countries interested in the Far East of doubt."[3] The second lead item concerned the spread of the plague in northern Chinese provinces, also in contrast to China's association with an "up-to-date factory."

In addition to this factory's modernness, its specialization in the production of foods made from soybeans signaled a world turned upside down and counter to popular perceptions. As an editorialist for the *Christian Science Monitor* had pointedly observed, "Oriental cooking has not so far inspired the celebrated chefs of the world centers. For famous recipes, the epicures would hardly look to China."[4] And yet, the *Monitor* went on to report, a young Chinese man who had studied agricultural science in France dared to do the unimaginable: "What then, shall be said of Li Yu Ying, home address Peking, who has established himself in Paris and believes he has something of value in the cooking line for even the surfeited Parisians? This, assuredly, is blazing a new trail where it must have required considerable courage to venture. China teaching France how to cook! Here, to say the least, is a gastronomical novelty."[5]

The man in question, Li Yuying, more commonly known as Li Shizeng (1881–1973), was the son of a former grand councilor of the Qing dynasty and tutor of the Tongzhi Emperor in the 1860s. Li arrived in Paris in 1902 as one of two embassy students in the entourage of the newly appointed Chinese minister to France. He enrolled in the École Pratique d'Agriculture in Montargis and after graduating in 1905, studied chemistry and biology at the Pasteur Institute. The factory, Usine Caséo-Sojaïne, or "soybean foods factory", which Li established in the Parisian suburb of Colombe, produced a variety of food products, all derived from soybeans.[6] In making common, everyday Western foodstuffs—milk, jams, breads, condiments—Li's soybean foods factory marked a significant shift in how young, modernizing Chinese intellectuals understood the social and economic value of soybeans.

Soybeans, which had long been recognized by the Chinese as an important famine crop, base for fertilizer, and source of oil for cooking, lubrication, and lighting, became globally esteemed as an agro-industrial commodity of tremendous economic importance in the early twentieth century. Chinese reassessment of the indigenous plant and crop occurred in conjunction with and as a response to changes in the global commodity markets. Japanese and Western interest in Chinese soybeans reframed the social and economic importance of soybeans such that Chinese scientists and entrepreneurs increasingly saw soybeans and especially soybean-derived products as critical components for Chinese progress and modernization.

A TIME OF DEARTH

Although soybeans had been grown and sold on a commercial scale in East Asia for more than a thousand years, the early twentieth century marked a radical shift in both scale and content for the soybean trade. Its introduction onto a world stage was so sudden that Western commentators repeatedly invoked refrains of fantasy and fairy tale when speaking of the soybean. As *The Times* (London) observed in July 1910, "The history of the growth of the bean trade in Manchuria is as captivating as the story of the rise of Jack's famous beanstalk of our nursery days. It reads more like a fairy tale than a page from the Board of Trade Returns."[7] The Japanese-American journalist Kinnosuke Adachi waxed poetic in calling it a "miracle bean," whose history in the West was a "wonder tale."[8] For many, these evocations of the fantastical only skirted the boundary between truth and exaggeration. The "little bean" from China was wondrous precisely because it could be used to make plastics, tires, soaps, and oils, as well as serve as the basis for everyday food-stuffs like flour and milk.

That such a humble legume could stir the imaginative fancies of so many in the early twentieth century could not have been predicted by its more pro-saic and well established role in traditional Chinese agriculture and dietar-ies. Archeological evidence indicates that by 1000 BCE, the soybean was already being cultivated, and textual references to the soybean in the *The Book of Odes* (Shijing), a collection of folk songs and ceremonial odes that dates from the eleventh to the seventh centuries BCE, identify both the seedlings and the leaves as edible vegetables.[9] Considered one of the five staple grains (*wugu*) of ancient China, the soybean was likely boiled and then steamed to produce cooked granules (*doufan*). This method resulted in a coarse product that gave the taint of inferiority to the soybean. Like wheat, which could also be boiled and then steamed to produce *maifan*, the soybean was regarded as an inferior grain. The biochemist turned historian of science, H. T. Huang recounted a passage from the "Contract between a Servant and His Master" (59 BCE) stating that one of the hardships the servant had to accept was "to eat only cooked soybeans (*fan dou*), and drink only water." When confronted with this and other indignities to be borne as part of his employment, the poor man broke down and cried.[10] Soybeans could assuage hunger, but they signified a humbleness of circumstance. When, for example, local irrigation works broke down in Anhui during the first century BCE, local people com-posed a song complaining that all they had to eat were soybeans and yams.[11] Thus, prior to the development of the technology to ferment and process them, soybeans occupied a relatively unappealing place in local foodscapes.

Knowledge of the nutritional disadvantages of eating unprocessed soy-beans goes back to very early times. Apart from the immature beans (now known internationally by the Japanese term *edamame*), which can be eaten directly as a vegetable, mature beans require substantial processing to enable proper digestion, because they suffer from three serious defects when cooked as food. Soy proteins are difficult to digest. The carbohydrate component in soybeans, if not properly hydrolyzed by human digestive enzymes, will lead to the generation of gas and flatulence. Cooking the beans also produces an unpleasant beany flavor that results from the oxidation of polyunsaturated oils by the enzyme lipoxidase.[12] To make soybeans more palatable, ancient Chinese devised a variety of ways—fermentation, sprouting, and grinding—to convert soybeans into wholesome, attractive, digestible, and nutritious foods.

Fermentation, or exposing cooked beans to microbial action, was perhaps the first method employed by Chinese to make soybeans more digestible and palatable.[13] A fermented soy relish (*shi*) was found among the pottery jars and identified on bamboo slips discovered at Mawangdui, Changsha, Hunan, a burial site dating from the second century BCE. *Shi*, which arises from a two-step process in which cooked and cooled soybeans are first exposed to air (aerobic mold growth) and then salted and incubated anaerobically (anaerobic digestion), was a major trade commodity as well as a daily culinary necessity. Permutations of this process led to the development of a fermented soybean paste (*jiang*) and soy sauce (*jiangyou*). Tofu, the making of which does not involve fermentation, appeared significantly later, perhaps as late as the tenth or eleventh century.[14] The soybean's primary virtue over the many centuries of use in China was, as the anthropologist Francesca Bray has described, "that it produced good crops even on poor land, that it did not deplete the soil, and that it guaranteed good yields even in poor years, so that it made a useful famine crop."[15] Moreover, because soybeans fix nitrogen in the soil, local farmers did not need to leave land fallow if they included soybeans in their crop rotation.

Oil could also be extracted from soybeans and used for cooking, lubrication, and lighting. What remains after the extraction of oils from soybeans can be compressed into sixty-four-pound rounds, that is, beancakes, and used as nitrogen-rich fertilizer. The famed agronomist and inventor Wang Zhen wrote in the 14th century: "Black soybeans are a food for times of dearth; they can supplement [cereals] in poor years, and in good years they can be used as fodder for cattle and horses."[16] Shandong, Hebei, Shanxi, and Henan in China proper were major growers of soybeans, and they sold soybeans to other parts of China, and on a lesser scale to Korea and Japan, to be used as fertilizers.

Beginning in the late Ming dynasty, the use of beancake, as well as other cake fertilizers derived from other vegetable oils, became increasingly popular.[17] By the mid-eighteenth century, at least three macroregions—Lingnan, the Southeast Coast, and the Lower Yangzi—had become dependent on outside supplies of ecologically sensitive goods, namely food, timber, and beancake.[18] The Qing maintained a ban on the domestic exportation of grain and soybeans from Manchuria in order to protect the food supply for the bannermen residing there. The government lifted the ban in 1749, but due to restrictions on how much could be transported through the customs office at Shanhaiguan, the only exit for Manchurian exports, a full-scale trade in soybeans and beancake did not develop until after 1772, when the Qing eliminated all domestic restrictions on transporting soybeans and beancake by sea.[19]

For the Lower Yangzi, which was China's most agriculturally and commercially rich region, imported beancake from North China and Manchuria was crucial for sustainable agricultural growth and to ensure the fertility of the soil under a double-cropping system.[20] The precise magnitude of the domestic soybean trade between Manchuria and the Lower Yangzi region during the late eighteenth century and through the first half of the nineteenth remains a topic of debate, but it is apparent that there was a popular recognition of, and enthusiasm for, the soybean's agricultural and commercial benefits.[21]

Beancake fertilizer was especially important in relieving cotton-growing soil, a persistent problem for the Lower Yangzi region. It also became the fertilizer of choice for sugar growers in Zhejiang, Guangdong, and Fujian, who emerged as the biggest importers of northern soybeans after the 1840s.[22] According to a 1911 report issued by the Maritime Customs, "The sugar plantations in these sub-tropical regions had for centuries drawn upon northern beancake for fertilizing, and beans were needed also for the southern mills, where their oil was extracted and used as a substitute for ground-nut oil."[23] Chinese trading junks plied the waters from the coastal south to Manchuria, delivering imported beancake throughout the nineteenth century, but their share of the soybean trade diminished after the 1860s when the Qing lifted its ban against foreign ships carrying soybeans and beancake in 1862—a political bid to seek foreign support in its ongoing campaign to crush the

Taiping Rebellion. The opening of Yingkou in Manchuria as a treaty port—one of five new treaty ports stipulated by the Treaty of Tianjin, which Britain and France had forced the Qing to sign in 1859—also facilitated the rise of foreign steamships in the sea transport of soybean products. Although Chinese junks continued to play a role in the domestic soybean trade from Manchuria, foreign competition dominated the transport of Manchurian soybeans well into the early twentieth century.[24]

Knowledge of beancake fertilizer became more sophisticated from the late Ming dynasty through the nineteenth century. Although originally prescribed as a base fertilizer, and in large quantities, by the late Ming, agricultural treatises suggested pairing beancake with other fertilizers to enhance the fertilizing effects. The late Ming polymath Xu Guangxi, who is perhaps best known for his conversion to Christianity and intellectual collaborations with the Jesuit Matteo Ricci, but who also authored *The Complete Treatise on the Administration of Agriculture* (Nongzheng quanshu), recommended that beancake be used as additional fertilizer when ox manure was used as the base. In the early nineteenth century, agricultural treatises prescribed a more nuanced regime of application in which beancake fertilizer was used as a supplementary fertilizer and only after an earlier round of pig manure had been applied. The rationale behind such prescriptions reflected agricultural knowledge about the different efficacies of "slow fertilizers" and "quick fertilizers." Beancake, in contrast to river mud or ox manure, was considered to be a quick fertilizer that stimulated crop growth, especially during the final growing phases of the season.[25]

Famine crop, animal feed, fertilizer—the soybean served many purposes in addition to its role as the base constituent of everyday foods like tofu, soy sauce, and bean paste. But its importance as a major interregional agricultural commodity relied less upon its culinary transformations than its nutritive role in replenishing the fertility of soil. Moreover, like all other major agricultural crops or raw materials for trade, soybeans were traded primarily as whole beans or slightly processed products (soybean oil and beancake) as opposed to finished consumer goods.

By 1887, the southern sugar growers of Guangdong and Fujian who had been the primary importers of northern soybeans were superseded by Japanese buyers. Crop failures in Korea and an increased scarcity of herring along the coast motivated Japanese farmers to find other fertilizer alternatives to maintain their rice crop yields.[26] Japanese interest in soybeans, and with it the vast Manchurian plain, rerouted the Chinese domestic soybean trade away from the southern sugar-growing provinces toward the proto-industrialization of the Japanese economy.[27] The little bean from China had entered the industrial age.

The romance of the bean narrated a darker tale when viewed from China and its contested northeastern provinces.[28] The region referred to as Manchuria by Europeans and the Japanese since at least the eighteenth century, but known by the Chinese as Northeastern China, occupied a powerful place in the political imaginations of both imperial and Republican times. The Manchu emperors of the Qing dynasty had deliberately cultivated Manchuria as the traditional and untainted preserve of Manchu heritage.[29] It was the territorial home that nursed and nurtured the distinctiveness of Manchu identity, bound up as it was with such venerable customs and practices as archery, horsemanship, the Manchu language, and frugality. Early Manchu rulers banned Han migration and settlement to the region. Such bans were occasionally lifted in times of famine, but up until the eighteenth century, the region remained sparsely populated and undercultivated. For early twentieth-century Japanese commentators keen on celebrating the rise of modern industry and economy, Manchuria's former seclusion had "retarded the economic progress of the country."[30] Han migration opened the region to agriculture and trade.[31]

The rationale for relaxing migration bans into Manchuria reflected the tumultuous turns of political fortune for the Qing during the nineteenth century. As the Qing state struggled to meet a mounting debt brought on by midcentury rebellions in China proper and indemnities to Western powers for the Opium Wars, it found itself increasingly challenged by Russian expansion into the northeast. After 1850, the Qing state actively encouraged Han migration, settlement, and cultivation of the northeastern territories in order to colonize the region against other imperial powers.[32] The influx of Han settlers reconfigured the demographic makeup of the region and expanded the area of land under cultivation.[33] Between 1890 and 1942, approximately eight million Han from the North China provinces of Hebei and Shandong migrated to Manchuria—more than doubling its population of seven million at the turn of the twentieth century.[34] Although less well known than European immigration to the Americas over a comparable period, the flow of Chinese immigrants was of a similar magnitude and constituted one of the three long-distance migrations that redistributed the world's population and drove twentieth-century industrial development.[35] Han settlers from North China brought with them their seeds, tools, and trading networks. And while soybeans and wheat had been grown throughout the fertile Liao Valley in southern Manchuria, the scale of these agricultural operations during the second half of the nineteenth century and into the twentieth increased dramatically alongside the growth of the Han population. Trade between Manchuria and the markets of China proper had included a variety of natural products like ginseng, pearls, and furs, but by the end of the nineteenth century, agricultural products (cash crops) such as cotton, indigo, tobacco, grain, and especially soybeans eclipsed those earlier trades and brought to Manchuria the salt, sugar, cotton, and foreign manufactures it needed.

Between the late nineteenth and early twentieth centuries, soybeans and soybean products (beancake and bean oil) constituted 70 to 80 percent of Manchuria's exports.[36] Until 1891, China proper served as the primary importer of Manchurian soybeans and beancake; after 1891, Japan emerged as the leading importer, such that by 1903, nearly half of all soybean exports (including soybean-derived products) went to Japan.[37] Domestically, Japan allocated about 3.8 percent of its total area of cultivation for soybeans, which were grown not as separate fields but in rows along the edges of rice and wheat fields.[38] The Japanese considered domestically grown soybeans to be superior in quality to those of Manchuria and Chosen and therefore used such beans exclusively in the manufacture of food products such as soy sauce (shoyu), miso, tofu, and fermented beans (natto). In contrast, Manchurian soybeans were purchased specifically for the production of oil and beancake.[39]

Japanese occupation of southern Manchuria during the Sino-Japanese War of 1895 further intertwined the region's economic fortune with Japan. Manchuria's agricultural richness attracted Japanese businessmen and adventurous migrants, thereby creating unprecedented trade ties between the region and Japan.[40] The journalist Adachi Kinnosuke characterized Manchurian soybeans as "something much more serious than the Chinese forces" Japan battled during its yearlong advance during the war. Soybeans conquered "not only the Japanese army but the Japanese market and the Japanese rice-fields. . . . Japanese armies came back from Manchuria with a keen appreciation of the food value of the Manchurian beans."[41] Japanese farmers, who had traditionally used fish manure as fertilizer, found a more inexpensive and less pest-attractive alternative.[42]

Japan's economic interests in the region, as well as its imports of Manchurian soybeans, did not diminish in the decade after the Sino-Japanese war. Tensions between Japan and Russia escalated, and war broke out in 1904. The Japanese victory in the Russo-Japanese War of 1905 resulted in the transference of the Russian leasehold of the Liaodong Peninsula, as well as its associated privileges and concessions, to Japan.[43] Japan gained control and ownership of the Chinese Eastern Railway branch running south from Changchun to the Yellow Sea, which was renamed the South Manchurian Railway. After 1905, Japan completed unfinished Russian projects, like the construction of the port of Dairen, and repositioned itself as the regional military and economic hegemon by expanding its role in the Manchurian soybean economy.[44] Its steady and effective restructuring of the burgeoning global Manchurian soybean trade from the traditional river port of Yingkou to the rail-connected seaport of Dairen marked the decline of Chinese merchants who had previously dominated the trade.[45]

But for an international shortage of vegetable fats and oils, the soybean might have remained ignored and unimportant to the Western economic and political contests of the early twentieth century. In 1908 and 1909, low yields of American cotton and flaxseed, typical crops used for the production of margarine and soap, led to high commodity prices and a European search for alternative vegetable oils. Up until the early twentieth century, Europeans and Americans who knew of the soybean knew it only within the context of botanical gardens and agricultural experimentation.[46] In the United States, for example, soybeans had been introduced with limited success on several occasions by scientists, seed dealers, merchants, military expeditions, and private individuals. They were grown in small plantings and occasionally for commercial use as hay or a forage crop.[47] Agricultural and nutritional experimenters had by the 1880s identified many reasons to promote the nitrogen-fixing, high-protein legume. Medical physicians, for example, attempted to establish soybeans as a food for diabetics.[48] But despite its integration into the realm of agro-scientific research and certain strains of nutritional faddism, the soybean remained largely unknown by the general public in Europe and the United States.

The Russo-Japanese War of 1905 had stymied shipments of Manchurian soybeans to China proper, such that after the cessation of fighting, Russian and Japanese traders were keen to offload their surplus supplies to emerging soybean markets in Europe and North America.[49] Their commercial success in this venture proved breathtaking. According to a special report issued by the Imperial Maritime Customs Service in 1911, "It is only in the last three years that soya beans have become important in intercontinental commerce, and their rapid emergence has, indeed, been one of the most remarkable commercial events of recent times."[50]

The apparent suddenness of this new international trade magnified the soybean's allure as industrial interest in the soybean as an oil resource grew. Not only did European and American oil mills, which had been designed to obtain cottonseed oil, require little if any technical reconfiguration to press soybeans, they found they could use the by-products of the oil-making process in similar ways. In addition to its use as fertilizer, beancake, which contained higher amounts of protein (than the comparable "cake" obtained from cottonseed), could also be fed to animals and was cheaper, as Japanese suppliers priced Manchurian soybeans lower than American cottonseed.[51] Other industrial applications included the manufacture of toilet powders, paint oils, lubrication and lighting oils, and candles.[52] The immediate beneficiary of this burgeoning global trade in soybeans, however, was not China but Japan, whose improved transportation infrastructure and system of banking and credit undergirded the soybean trade from Manchuria to the rest of the world.[53]

A Divergence of Meaning

Chinese perception of the increasing economic and political importance of soybeans worldwide was influenced by the emerging geopolitical contests in the northeast, but it also predated these imperial rivalries and was linked to the reevaluation of Chinese epistemological values during the late nineteenth and early twentieth centuries. Japanese and Western interest in soybeans, especially as an agro-industrial crop, reaffirmed the growing sense among the Chinese elite that modern science was essential for modernization. Understandings of soybeans as famine food, animal feed, and fertilizer persisted, but within a heightened intellectual climate in which modern science increasingly became the arbiter of social and economic value.

Although a lively interest in Western sciences had already existed since the early nineteenth century, it was not until after the fall of the Taipings in 1865 that late Qing literati began systematically, and with great urgency, building conceptual bridges between post-industrial Western learning and the traditional Chinese sciences.[54] Late Qing intellectual life was rife with scientific exchange and experimentation that crisscrossed between the realms of private activities and public concern.[55] Journalists, translators, scientists, and diplomats emerged from the ranks of the Qing intellectual elite and knitted together a constellation of different institutions invested in the dissemination of Western learning, ranging from arsenals and new schools to museums and newspapers. With the support of key post-Taiping reformers like Zeng Guofan and Li Hongzhang, these new institutions served as important technological venues for experimental practice and scientific knowledge that served the goal of wealth and power (*fuqiang*).[56] Agriculture, which had held a key role in traditional Chinese writing on statecraft, ranked low among the intellectual priorities of these self-strengthening reformists, who emphasized the development of the military and hard industries.[57]

The growth of Western learning also exposed the Chinese to the limits of the traditional categories of scientific learning. Previously, Chinese scientific interests in the natural world, medicine, the arts and crafts, and commerce had been subsumed under the umbrella of "investigating and extending knowledge" (*gezhi*). Faced with China's disastrous defeat against Japan in the Sino-Japanese War of 1895 and keen to identify the sources of Japan's quick and successful modernization, young Chinese literati increasingly promoted the Japanese neologism *kagaku* (*kexue*, in Chinese, lit., "knowledge classified by field") as a less encumbered, more accurate translation for the modern sciences.[58] The shift in terminology reflected in part the intense period of self-recrimination that followed China's defeat. Not only was this earlier period of self-strengthening decried as a failure for not insuring Chinese victory by scientific and technological arms, elite and popular opinion extended this "failure narrative" to encapsulate the story of Chinese political decline and economic deterioration during the late empire.[59]

Japan's apparent success at modernization led many Chinese to recast Japan as a model to emulate as China pursued the dual goals of wealth and power. Interest in how the Japanese reorganized and modernized their economy, agriculture, and education boomed in the post-war period. The first Chinese overseas students arrived in Japan in 1896, only a year after the country's defeat. By the 1905–6 school year, there were reportedly 8,000 to 10,000 Chinese students in Japan.[60] Many of these students, while in Japan and especially after they returned to China, played a critical role as cultural mediators and translators of Japanese texts into Chinese.

Post-Boxer reforms undertaken by an embattled and struggling dynasty further facilitated the transformation of education in favor of Japanese-style science and technology. In 1904, the Qing abolished the civil service examination system, which had been based on the Confucian classics and preserved the Chinese-origins approach to Western learning. Within a year's time, the Qing Ministry of Education began to promote science education, and Japanese science texts became models for Chinese education at all levels of schooling.[61] Japanese scientific terms were adopted, new and updated Sino-Japanese dictionaries were compiled, Japanese faculty were invited to take up positions at the Imperial University in Beijing, and Chinese presses unleashed greater numbers of translations of Japanese texts.

Luo Zhenyu (1866–1940), in particular, played an essential role in the propagation of works on agriculture in the post-1895 period. A promising young scholar who had been recruited by the Qing government for his adeptness in promulgating new knowledge and a reputable figure in late Qing reform, Luo established the Society for Learning Agriculture (Nongxueshe) and the Agriculture Journal Publishing House (Nongbaoguan) in Shanghai in 1896.[62] As an organization, the Society for Learning Agriculture sought to reform Chinese agriculture by promoting land reclamation initiatives, the importation of new foreign agricultural equipment and technologies, the adoption of successful breeding practices that had been developed abroad, the establishment of industrial-agricultural enterprises (e.g., sugar refineries and alcohol distilleries), and the creation of agricultural schools. In the words of Luo's close friend and colleague, Zhang Jian (1853–1926), "All nations have been founded, not on the military or commerce but on industry and agriculture, with the latter being especially important. The recent establishment of the Society for Learning Agriculture for the specific purpose of translating Japanese and Western books and newspapers on agriculture marks a significant leap for Chinese agricultural administration."[63]

Luo's Society for Learning Agriculture was one of many such organizations being established in the post-1895 period. As a study society whose primary objective was to facilitate the dissemination and propagation of new agricultural technologies and scientific research, it depended on membership dues, as well as a substantial personal investment from Luo himself, to fund its publication and demonstration activities. In contrast, peasant associations, especially those established as part of the Xinzheng Reforms, bore closer and more direct affiliations with the Qing government, whose officials provided funding and supervision for their various activities.[64]

Luo's edited journal, *Agricultural News* (Nongxuebao), and book series, *Collectanea of Works on Agricultural Science* (Nongxue congshu), introduced and translated agriculture-related news and publications from Japan and the West with the objective of improving farming technology in China.[65] The late Qing reformer Zhang Zhidong was especially receptive to Luo's efforts. Zhang's enthusiasm for Japanese models of agricultural improvement seems to have burgeoned alongside his praise for Luo's agricultural journal, and he ordered every district and county under his jurisdiction to obtain a subscription. Large counties were designated ten copies, while smaller counties three, but for all areas, Zhang insisted that the paper should be distributed widely for all the gentry to read.[66] Luo, alongside other eminent intellectuals such as Fan Bingqing (1876–1931) and Wang Guowei (1877–1927), translated most of the material that appeared in *Agricultural News* and the *Collectanea of Works on Agricultural Science*.[67]

In the pages of *Agricultural News*, readers learned how to prevent and manage the spread of epidemic disease (should it occur) among livestock, about the latest farming machinery, and how to build corrals for mountain goats. They became acquainted with the idea that cow's milk was an essential component of health (*ru wei weisheng yao pin*), whose constituent ingredients could be presented in a table detailing water, fats, lactose (*rutang*), sugars, and ash. According to the 1892 Japanese text *New Treatise on Cow's Milk and Its Products* (Nyugyu oyobi seinyu shinsho) by Taizo Kawai, which had been translated by Shen Hong at the request of the Hubei Agricultural Office, cow's milk was not only an important food for health, it was a product of industrial innovation.[68] The section introducing the manufacture of condensed milk, for example, explained how it, in contrast to fresh milk, could travel long distances and not suffer any degradation of quality.[69]

This linkage between food and industry was evident throughout the pages of *Agricultural News*, such that when discussions turned to soybean and soybean-derived products, it was within the context of agricultural manufactures and their analysis according to nutrition science. Here too Japan's influence may be discerned. Two years after translating Taizo's book on cow's milk and milk products, Shen translated another Japanese study of agricultural manufactures that covered grain-based liquors, flours, sugars, and soybean products. The translation, published in *Agricultural News*, appeared in installments spread over three sequential issues in 1900.[70]

The products considered would not have been unfamiliar to the Chinese reader, but the discussion of soy sauce, for example, included not only general descriptions of regional differences in production but also technical explanations of its chemical constituents. The production of soy sauce, in

Shen's translation, required expertise in the scientific field of chemistry, because assessments of quality could be only achieved through chemical means: "The highest quality of soybeans comes from the yellow and white varieties, which have a lustrous appearance and plentiful kernels. They do not grow to a great height, nor are they especially wide/coarse. These varieties are rich in proteins and oils."[71] In contrast, soybeans imported from Niuzhuang [Manchuria], the Japanese report asserted, were demonstrably inferior in quality on account of their fibrousness and poorer protein and oil content. Agricultural manufactures in the service of food production required raw materials of the highest quality, which was ascertained through chemical assays, and the constituent elements to be measured were primarily macronutrients.

Amid these articles ascribing characteristics of industrial modernity to soybeans and other agricultural manufactures, a disjunction of meaning emerged. The extent to which the soybean offered a vision for technological modernity became increasingly intertwined, not with its agricultural export status but with the technologies involved in producing soybean-derived food products. Thus, even while late Qing intellectuals became inured to the idea of industrial modernity in the form of technologically sophisticated and scientifically nutritious agricultural manufactures, soybeans as an export moved further away from this vision.

The economic value of soybeans for the Chinese export trade lay in their unprocessed or minimally processed form as beancake and oil. Commercial interest in the soybean trade had increased dramatically as Japan's purchasing power came to dominate the entire soybean market. Chinese news reports on soybeans, especially those included in trade and commercial papers like the *Commercial News* (Shangwubao), *Hubei Business News* (Hubei shangwubao), and *Chinese Business News* (Huashang lianhebao), focused on the shifting dynamics of the expanding soybean trade. One report observed, "Shanghai's soybeans usually come from Niuzhuang. More recently, tens of thousands of *dan* of soybeans have been sent from Hankou and Jiujiang, with booming sales at Jiaxing in Zhejiang."[72] A later report enthused, "Exports of soybeans to Japan are high, with the bulk coming from Niuzhuang. But this year has yielded a poor harvest of Niuzhuang soybeans, while Hubei soybeans are enjoying a bumper crop. Consequently, many orders have been redirected to Hankou. With prices rising and based on early sales, profits look to be huge."[73] As Japanese demand for beancakes rose, news outlets increased their coverage by also translating and reprinting Japanese reporting of the increased sales of Chinese and Manchurian soybeans.[74]

But with so much emphasis on gross sales, the commercial discourse on soybeans for export tended to stress its traditional export forms as beancake and oil instead of its potential to improve agricultural industry.[75] For those Chinese most persuaded by the link now established between soybeans and industrial modernity, this narrowness of vision threatened to impinge upon the commercial and industrial benefits that might otherwise accrue from the expanding Manchurian soybean trade. In 1910, one Chinese observer under the nom de plume "Benevolent Cause" wrote, "Who could have known that the soybean market would have taken off as it has during these past three years? Soybeans have become one of China's most important commodities and a boon for the northeastern provinces. Is it any wonder that Japan should covet Manchuria?" The soybean was being used for its oil, but as the commentator pointed out, "the English have even begun to use it [in the manufacture] of medicinal drugs. . . . Europeans use soybeans for all manner of things. A large amount [of soybeans] serves as one of the base ingredients for soap. The extracted oil can be used to manufacture food products. Even the dregs can be used as feed for livestock or repurposed and added to foods."[76] An export crop whose sales rivaled China's traditional export strengths in tea and silk, soybeans heralded a new future, but one that required reeducation for everyone: officials, gentry, and the common man alike: "Agricultural science must be stressed. We must improve our soybean cultivation techniques in order to enhance the soybean's inherent qualities and strengths."[77]

MODERN FOOD, MODERN TECHNOLOGY

Enter a young Chinese man, raised in a house of privilege, learned in Western sciences, and a transplanted resident in the City of Light. His embrace of the soybean for its nutritional and technological advantages and his establishment of the first soybean processing plant (Usine Caséo-Sojaïne) on the outskirts of Paris blazed a path by which the soybean could help build a modern China (figure 1.1). In locating his factory in Paris, Li Shizeng also benefited from increased exports of Manchurian soybeans to Europe after 1909, but his interests lay primarily in soybean-derived foods, and the potential for industrialized food production to transform and modernize Chinese agriculture.

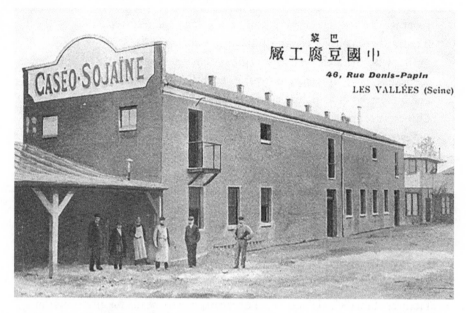

FIGURE 1.1. Paris Tofu Company (Usine Caséo Sojaïne, Bali Doufu Gongchang). Originally printed in Shijie She, *Lü Ou jianyu yundong* [1916].

In sharp contrast with older understandings that cast the soybean as food for the poor and the benighted or feed for livestock, Li celebrated the humbleness of the soybean for its hygienic, scientific, and technological characteristics.[78]

By the time Li had established his factory in 1909, his interest and promotion of the soybean had already been widely reported by the French press. As a student at the Pasteur Institute, Li had conducted research on "China's soybean problem" (*Zhongguo de dadou wenti*) and discovered for himself how the soybean plant exhibited some of the more curious characteristics of vegetable physiology.[79] In his own words, "From the perspective of agriculture, the soybean plant is a bit unusual and very productive. Its nitrogen-fixing properties surpass other more commonly used pulses. Finally, it must not be forgotten the number of industrial applications one can achieve with the oil and vegetable protein (*caséine de soja*) from soybeans."[80] Li's scientific investigations with the soybean focused in particular on soybean milk, which he called *caséosojaïne*, and its potential to serve as a dairy alternative. Li thought it may be possible through innovations in handling and fermentation techniques to produce soybean milk amenable to the Western palate.[81] His application for a British patent, dated December 30, 1910, indicated that his invention produced a "vegetable milk and its derivatives by means of soja grains (Chinese peas)." The resulting milk would have "the appearance, the color, and the taste of ordinary milk, its chemical composition greatly resembling the same. It has moreover approximately the same nutritive and alimentary properties."[82]

Li's growing passion for the soybean led him to propagate its virtues among France's scientific community. He spoke before the Société d'Agriculture de France, and perhaps to everyone's surprise, attended the International Dairy Congress in October of that year, where his presentation to the attendees attracted media attention.[83] Speaking before an audience of prominent men "in the dairy and general agricultural circles of Europe," Li spoke earnestly of the Chinese practice of producing "milk" from a plant.[84] The entire world, Li remarked, recognized the many advantages associated with animal milk. And yet, the Chinese drank little of it. To explain this curious situation, Li expostulated for ten minutes about the soybean and Chinese methods for producing soyfoods, which not only looked similar in appearance to dairy products but were comparable in chemical composition. China, with its vast and varied regions and its humid soil and climate, was largely ill suited to the raising of cattle and livestock. Excluding areas to the far north and east, which Li identified as "dairy regions" (régions laitières), most parts of China depended on soybeans, which could be made into a "vegetal milk, rich in proteins and fats," for its dairy needs.[85]

At the International Dairy Congress and later again at expositions and trade shows, Li celebrated the remarkable versatility of the soybean in satisfying the nutritional needs of the Chinese population. "When cooked, then forcefully pressed, soybeans, which are rich in nitrogenous materials and fats, are transformed into a thick paste that dissolves in lukewarm water and becomes a vegetal milk, comparable in nutritional value to cow's milk."[86] Possessing a high proportion of legume or vegetal casein, Li explained, the vegetal milk, if allowed to coagulate, becomes a kind of "cheese" (called "tofou"), which plays an important role in Chinese and Japanese diets. But the uses to which the soybean might be applied were not limited to vegetal milk. Li emphasized the versatility of the soybean, and reporters, persuaded by his scientific arguments or swayed by the romance of this unusual plant, conveyed his message with enthusiasm. In the words of one French journalist, the soybean—as livestock feed, fertilizer for crops, and many other food products achieved by means of fermentation or smoking—was a plant that could benefit French agriculture, even in limited capacity as a forage crop.[87]

But there was a further advantage to soybean milk, according to Li. Ever sensitive to the economic stratification associated with food consumption, Li had argued before the International Dairy Congress in 1905 that the spread of soybean culture (*la culture du* soja hispida) in Europe would enable the poor, who would otherwise be unable to afford even base-quality cow's milk, to nonetheless receive the nutritive benefits of soybean milk. Moreover, because soybean milk was more uniform, more hygienic to produce, and less prone to fraud and manipulation, it represented a boon to public health and the purses of the poor.[88]

By the end of 1909, Li had moved on to producing food products (e.g., "cheeses," sauces, noodles, biscuits, cakes, oils, breads, and spreads) from his factory at Les Vallées, a suburb fifteen minutes by train from Paris.[89] Reporters described the bread as "excellent" and the biscuits as "marvels of lightness." If there was anything unusual to be discerned in the taste as a consequence of the use of soybeans, it was the "meaty taste, which is peculiar, but agreeable and very satisfying."[90]

Li's education and training in the sciences had afforded him an unexpected opportunity to reconsider a domestic agricultural crop. According to Li, "China's land is vast, and its products many, making for a wide variety of agricultural goods. The soybean is one among many Chinese agricultural products, but it is special, because of the development of specialized technologies [entailed in the preparation of soybeans]."[91] His identification of the commercial prospects of soybeans reflected a larger preoccupation with Chinese science and technology. "China's soybean technology emerged early, and the products [it produces] are excellent. But its scientific basis is murky, the specific techniques unrefined. With even a little bit of effort, [however,] one cannot fail to exhaust the inherent strengths/advantages of the soybean."[92]

Li presented his case for celebrating and modernizing traditional soybean processing technologies in a lengthy article published in 1910 in the pages of *Eastern Miscellany* (Dongfang zazhi), one of the oldest and most influential journals in China. Published by the Commercial Press, Shanghai's largest publishing company, *Eastern Miscellany* served as an open forum for the discussion of politics, national economy, foreign policy, education, and other public issues.[93] Although not the first time in which Li had sought to engage the Chinese reading public on the value and virtues of the soybean, this article represents his most sustained and thoughtful engagement with the topic of Chinese technology, its place within a global history of science and technology, and how soybean technologies could uplift the country.[94]

The central question he tackled was "How does a country's technology change?" In Li's assessment, Chinese technology could be broadly classified into two categories: native handiwork or craftsmen technologies, and imitative technologies that had been imported from the West. Native technologies produced a variety of goods that ranged from trinkets to everyday essentials like textiles, and yet they could not compete in terms of quality against similar goods produced by Western technologies (be they imported as finished goods or made domestically). The unfortunate consequence of this technological differential was a vicious cycle in which native technologies producing inferior goods lost profits to better-quality products produced by foreign technologies. Calls to boycott foreign goods were, Li insisted, correspondingly myopic and self-defeating, since China could not make enough of even its daily necessities and was still reliant on foreign resources.

For native technologies to compete with Western technologies, the key was not simply to appropriate and imitate. The more effective strategy entailed identifying the technological features and spaces undeveloped and unexplored by the West. Li saw no advantages in preserving native technologies as they were. Instead, he argued that what the Chinese needed was to adopt and adapt Western technologies with great sophistication and discrimination by looking at individual strengths and advantages. For example, sometimes the strength [to develop] lay in the material used, sometimes the technique employed, sometimes the two working in conjunction. The point was to identify and exploit those areas and strengths that others lacked and had not yet developed. For Chinese technology to reach world standard, it was essential to search out material and technical advantages that others did not possess.[95]

The examples he cites were striking, especially as they were the same examples critics invoked to mark the imminent peril threatening Chinese commercial power in the world market: silk and tea. Li's point was that both of these traditional exports represented significant areas of Chinese technological expertise. Were it not for a failure to further refine and develop these areas, China would not have lost its technological preeminence with respect to silk and tea to other countries (e.g., Western silks and Indian teas). What China needed was to identify other sorts of technological expertise that Westerners lacked and develop those. Soybean technology was his primary example.[96]

Soybeans, Li argued, were one of China's domestic crops, and as an agricultural crop, soybeans possessed special traits unmatched in other crops. With scientific research, China's body of native technological knowledge could be advanced and developed, making soybean technology into an independent technology unbeholden to any country.[97] His examples of new soybean-made foods gestured to a world more familiar now than in the first decade of the twentieth century: soybean milk, bread, pasta and noodles, coffee, chocolate, and ice cream.

Conclusion

Li Shizeng's soybean foods factory continued to operate until 1921, when his anarchist-inspired work-study program that sought to bring Chinese students to France collapsed in the face of post–World War I economic depression.[98] The initial excitement and bemusement that had accompanied the introduction of his soybean-derived foods to a French consuming public had faded after a couple of years. Li, for his efforts, expended considerable energy ensuring that news of his soybean research and commercial work reached a Chinese reading public. In addition to his essays on the technological benefits of developing a soybean industry, Li wrote extended pieces introducing the botanical and agricultural history of soybeans in China and the various types of foods that could be made with soybeans. Throughout, he extolled their hygienic and economical virtues.[99]

His efforts were rewarded by the steady stream of Chinese commentary that appeared throughout the 1910s and 1920s. Some, like the late Qing literatus Huang Shirong, recapitulated Li's writings by emphasizing the many advantages associated with soybeans. "Soybean nutrients benefit health and economics. The development of its commercial industry deserves to be further promoted."[100] Others homed directly in on the competitive dimensions of the soybean for navigating the brave new social Darwinian world. In an unattributed 1910 piece that appeared in the *Journal of Chinese and Western Medicines* (Zhongxi yixuebao) under the title "A Comparison of Soybean Milk and Cow's Milk," the author high-lighted soybean milk's more advantageous nutritional profile, which had been demonstrated not only by chemical analysis but also in connection with the medical treatment of patients. Li's factory, which had been warmly received by the French, was, in the author's estimation, an example of the shifting winds of progress from East to West. "It is unavoidable that soybean milk will become one of cow's milk's most formidable adversaries."[101]

By the turn of the twentieth century, soybeans had accrued a variegated cast of meanings: famine food, fertilizer, animal feed, export commodity, and a base for industrial products such as soap and paint, as well as a modern superfood whose credentials were supported by science. Although these meanings were not mutually exclusive, the perception that soybeans could be both a food of famine and dearth as well as a potential generator of national wealth and power marked a significant shift in how Chinese intellectuals assessed their social world and the role played by traditional crops in a global capitalist order. Soybeans as they were extracted from local, and often traditional, networks during the late nineteenth and early twentieth centuries brought with them a host of meanings and associations that were reworked and upended but not necessarily erased in the process. Japan's growing interest in Chinese, especially Manchurian, soybeans during the late 1900s took an already traded domestic crop and turned it into a major export to service Japan's industrial and fertilizing needs. This expansion of trade did not undercut existing perceptions of soybeans as valuable for their oil and as fertilizer, but the volume of trade did recast the plant's potential and redirected attention to its food-related technologies. Japanese and Western enthusiasm in soybeans reframed how Chinese scientists and entrepreneurs understood the soybean and helped to articulate another path by which an indigenous crop could transform China's role on an international stage.

Li's soybean experiment in Paris proved short-lived, but his insistence that soybeans offered a key to a modern, industrial China did not fail to impress his compatriots. Popular accounts celebrated the soybean's many industrial and gastronomic uses and as late as 1920, highlighted Li's foresight and ingenuity in promoting an indigenous product, *doujiang* (soybean milk), as both more nutritious and sanitary than cow's milk, on the world stage.[102] If the soybean could signify modern, industrial development, could it also challenge perceptions of Chinese physical and nutritional precarity, of China as "the Sick Man of Asia"? When coupled with a newly emergent discursive concept of the Chinese diet as a thing scientists and social scientists could measure and adjust, the aspiration grew for soybeans to change not just Chinese industry but Chinese bodies.

CHAPTER 2

The Light of Modern Knowledge

Accountability and the Concept of the Chinese Diet

S PEAKING before a crowded auditorium of medical students and fellow scientists in 1926, the Chinese biochemist Wu Xian (Wu Hsien, 1893–1959) opened his lecture on the Chinese diet with a reference few in the room would have misunderstood: clothing, food, and shelter are life's necessities. The first president of the Chinese republic and elder statesman, Sun Yat-sen (Sun Zhongshan, 1866–1925) had affirmed their importance to his doctrine of the people's livelihood (*minsheng*) two decades previously, but in large part, his acknowledgment reflected what everyone already understood. Nations rise and fall on the backs on their people, and without food, there can be no people.[1] A veritable groundswell of concern had materialized in local newspapers and among government officials about China's food problem, as headlines rearranged "clothing, food, and shelter" to become "food, clothing, and shelter" to emphasize just how important food was. Growing popular interest in modern nutritional knowledge found expression in public gatherings and newly organized societies, such as Wu Tingfang's Society for Cautious Diet and Hygiene, established in 1910s Shanghai to promote new lifestyles and healthy dietary practices.[2]

As a biochemist and nutrition scientist, Wu Xian's concern for the Chinese diet could not have been better timed. He had been among the first class of sixty-two Boxer Fellows who sailed to the United States in 1911 for academic study.[3] A quiet, serious scholar, he graduated from MIT in 1917 and then joined the highly selective laboratory of Otto Folin at Harvard Medical School, where his dissertation research led to the development of a new system for analyzing the constituents of blood, a process that has since become routine in patient care. In 1920, he returned to China and joined the faculty of the Peking Union Medical College (PUMC), one of the leading research and medical educational institutions in Republican China. By 1926, his intellectual energies were increasingly directed toward a new field of interest: the Chinese diet. Together with a handful of Chinese and Western scientists, Wu Xian began generating a sizeable and compelling body of data that detailed everything from the monthly food expenses of working-class families in Beijing to the "fuel values" of local foods such as the green mung bean, steamed buns, and bean curd found throughout North and South China. Seeking to introduce to his audience this growing body of empirical data, Wu raised the following question: Was the Chinese diet adequate in the light of our modern knowledge of nutrition?[4]

His framing was deliberately provocative and very telling. His insistence that the Chinese diet should and ought to be evaluated in the light of modern science signaled the social and political stakes redefining the role of food in China's modernity. Wu challenged his audience to rethink what they knew about food and its purpose by homing in on the substance and value of the Chinese diet when evaluated against some universal measure—a challenge denoted by his use of the word "adequate." Wu had famously said, "Ordinary prudence suffices to judge the adequacy of shelter and clothing, but neither instinct nor common sense is a reliable guide in the choice of foods." He, perhaps more than anyone, popularized the idea that there was such a thing as the "Chinese diet," that it could be studied and evaluated for its optimality, and that it was a problem—a problem that, left unsolved, imperiled the nation.

For a diet to be adequate, Wu implied, it had to be accountable: it had to be answerable to the dictates of science and the demands of the modern age. Moreover, it had to be quantifiable.[5] The parts of the whole had to be investigated—each one tested and confirmed for its potential benefits; all adding up to one singular, unitary whole that was the Chinese diet. The construction of this new form of rationality, one that conceived of food as analyzable units addressing specific physiological needs in service of a higher national purpose, occurred through the convergence of three sets of discursive interests: Chinese scientific skepticism of older dietetic knowledge, Western desire for explicating dietary differences through the lens of race and ethnicity, and the Chinese impetus to fashion a nation from the disparate, dissonant crush of local foods and practices.

Although the phrase "Chinese diet" (*shanshi*) was often used interchangeably with "Chinese food" or "Chinese foodstuffs" (*shiwu* or *yinshi*) to refer to what the Chinese people ate, the concept of the Chinese diet was an artifact of the collective scientific interest of China's biochemical and nutritional science pioneers in constructing a cohesive, if not national, dietary pattern from customary local food practices. The extent to which the diet was necessarily circumscribed by the Chinese nation-state can be seen in the designations preceding "diet": China (Zhongguo), citizens (*guomin*), ethnonationals (*minzu*), masses (*minzhong*), and compatriots (*guoren*); while a culturalist understanding predicated on the social mores of the Han might also have been entailed, the emphasis was firmly rooted in the Chinese geopolitical body. This impulse to systematize and construct a sense of Chineseness through food can also be seen in the enduring appeal of "traditional" foodways, which emphasized the regional dimensions of Chinese cultural identity and shaped restaurant culture during this period.[6] For scientists such as Wu Xian, thinking about the Chinese diet mitigated the influence and persuasiveness of regional difference and instead served as a synecdoche of the nation and represented the unitary wholeness of Chinese people.

This is not to suggest that there is either fallacy or fancy in talking about the various foods that have comprised daily eating practices over the centuries. Soybeans, for example, have had a long and well-established role in traditional Chinese agriculture and dietaries. Considered one of the five staple grains (*wugu*) of ancient China, soybeans had become a domesticated crop in North China and Korea by 1000 BC.[7] Ancient Chinese expended significant effort to find ways of transforming soybeans into processed foods like tofu, soy sauce, and fermented bean paste.[8] This long history of customary production and consumption cannot, however, explain the sudden burst of interest in the nutritional and industrial potential of the soybean at the turn of the twentieth century. Chinese fascination with the soybean highlighted a shift in conceptual thinking about food and diet and elevated the role a single foodstuff could play in ensuring the nutritional health and optimality of the Chinese people. Chinese scientific interest in dietary habits developed in tension with both a presumed past dominated by the apparent eclecticism and lack of accountability in older, traditional forms of dietetic knowledge and a purported past described by late nineteenth-century Anglo-American commentators in which the foods eaten, or not, exposed inherent qualities of being Chinese. For nutrition scientists, the concept of the Chinese diet could be mobilized as an index of the nation and a site for Chinese agency.

A DISCERNING STOMACH

Chinese thinking about food has been a long-standing, if not perennial, facet of social and cultural life over the centuries.[9] Food, beyond the immediate, practical needs of sustenance, has played many roles in Chinese political, social, and cultural life. Writings about food, cooking, banqueting, and diet were central to the social, political, and ritual structure of imperial and Republican-period China, because culinary activity not only governed human relationships—that is, the arts of government and social relationships operated through the exchange, acceptance, or refusal of food gifts and the social interplay and etiquette during banquets and feasts—it also enabled communication between humans and the spirit world.[10] Ritual behavior, including alimentary offerings to ancestors, who also needed nourishment in the afterlife, and folk songs contrasting festival and daily foods were enduring features of daily life. Chinese philosophers and moralists regularly invoked food as a yardstick to measure a person's character or moral aptitude, and metaphors about cooking abounded in political and philosophical discourse. Confucius is said to have demonstrated propriety in receiving food and tasting it, did not allow himself to be overcome by drink during periods of intensive sacrificial activity, possessed a sensitive palate, and always knew the correct proportioning of sauces or condiments.[11] Early ritual texts construed cooking with civilization, such that civilized people were as seen as "cooked" while the uncivilized were distinguished as much by their "rawness" as their failure to eat grains or use fire to cook their meat.[12]

Chinese medical authors were no less loquacious about the importance of food for health and well-being. Culinary thinking was directly related to medical knowledge and concepts of health and the body, all of which were derived from the traditional notion of the cosmos. Indeed, the body itself was understood as a microcosm of the cosmos, both of which were animated by a life force, or qi. Food too possessed different kinds of qi, and in general, the goal of eating was to achieve and maintain a perfect equilibrium between strengthening and weakening foods.[13] To achieve this goal, one sought to balance the yin and yang forces within the body through a sensitive calculus of the thermostatic qualities attributed to foods themselves (e.g., hot, warm, neutral, cool, and cold). By the third century BCE, a pentic system of correspondences, known as the "five phases" (*wuxing*) came to dominate treatises on ritual and technical thought. All food exhibited one of the "five flavors/sapors" (*wu wei*), whose various properties possessed the power to stimulate and influence the movement of qi that animated and invigorated the body. The five flavors extended the pentic correspondence into the realm of nutrition.[14]

By the late medieval period, Chinese *materia dietetica* had established a complex nutritional world in which every foodstuff had a flavor, which was associated with a qi that was further associated with the healing of different parts of the body.[15] Since each of the five flavors also corresponded with one of the body's main organ systems—bitter to the heart system, sour to the liver, sweet to the spleen, pungent to the lungs, and salty to the kidneys—a correct diet had to harmonize these various notes (table 2.1). Illness could arise from disruptions and imbalances resulting from improper dietary arrangements. In the words of the seventh-century CE scholar-physician Sun Simiao (fl. ca. 581–682), "If the qi of different foods are incompatible, the *essence* will be damaged. The body achieves completion from the flavors that nourish it. If the different flavors of foods are not harmonized, the body becomes impure. This is why the sage starts off by obeying the alimentary prohibitions in order to preserve his nature; if that proves ineffective, he has recourse to remedies for sustaining life."[16] For Sun, correct patterns of eating protected the body's essences, such that the deployment of medical or nutritional remedies should be reserved for instances in which food combinations and prohibitions have failed. While later medical authors may have disputed Sun's approach, they nonetheless accepted the presumption of nutrition as an integral part of a larger framework of medical knowledge and thereby helped establish what became an enormous and influential tradition of food combinations and prohibitions.[17]

How such a rationale built upon food qualities and dietary prohibitions diffused through Chinese society at any one time remains an area for further historical investigation. It is clear, however, that for Republican-period

TABLE 2.1. Pentic correspondences

Earth	Metal	Water	Wood	Fire
Sweet	Pungent/acrid	Salty	Sour	Bitter
Late Summer	Autumn	Winter	Spring	Summer
Panicled Millet	Sorghum	Millet	Millet	Beans
Beef	Dog	Pork	Mutton	Fowl

medical physicians and researchers who had been trained in scientific medicine, these ideas encapsulated the backwardness and ignorance of traditional Chinese medicine on matters of diet and nutrition. While aspects of this tradition could be salvaged, modified, and elaborated upon, the tradition as a whole had to be replaced by modern science. The problem most Chinese nutrition scientists had with this older body of dietetic understandings concerned the apparent hypersensitivity to specific food qualities, even specific foods, that could not be justified by reference to the chemical sciences, physiology, or germ theory. Of particular consternation was the extensive and detailed attention traditional Chinese medical authors paid to nutritional prohibitions or interdictions (*shijin*).

Consider the assessment of Hou Xiangchuan (H. C. Hou, 1899–1982), a biochemist in the employ of the Henry Lester Institute of Medical Research located in Shanghai. As a graduate of St. John's University Medical School in Shanghai who had also studied in the United States and Canada before returning to China in 1929, Hou held attitudes toward traditional Chinese dietetics that were shaped by his educational training. In evaluating the dietary principles to be extracted from ancient Chinese medicine, Hou made light of the many recommendations found in Hu Sihui's fourteenth-century text, *Yinshan zhengyao* (Propriety and Essentials of Food and Drink), a *materia dietetica* and cookbook that had been presented to the Mongol court.[18] Hou argued that too much emphasis had been placed "upon the necessity of restricted diets under various conditions, . . . and for which we find no sound reason." Why should pork not be eaten with beef? Or mutton with liver? Did eating pork with coriander actually lead to an ulceration of the intestines? Would consuming rabbit meat with ginger really result in cholera? Such proscriptions evidenced neither rhyme nor reason and could only be described as "absurd."[19] Hou's befuddlement at the apparent logical contortions of proscribing certain pairings of food did not, however, prevent him from recognizing some redeemable value in ancient dietary principles. A call for moderation in eating, the importance of seasonality (which he interpreted as a recommendation for a varied diet), and the application of wild green amaranth juice or a seaweed preparation for the treatment of beriberi and goiter, respectively, were all commendable and in concurrence with modern scientific thinking.

Not all nutrition scientists were as disparaging as Hou, but the general attitude reflected more skepticism than appreciation. The biochemist and molecular biologist Shen Tong (1911–1992) framed the distinction in terms of expertise versus experience. Shen had graduated from Tsinghua University before receiving his doctorate in biochemistry from Cornell University. "Nutrition," Shen insisted, "is a discipline that is at once newly emerged and scientific as well as an ancient art (*gulao de yishu*). Although most people are familiar with the contributions [made by nutrition science] on vitamins in the past three decades, even before the discovery of vitamins, mankind had from an early date figured out how to nourish itself—hence, [our characterization of this form of nutrition] as an ancient art."[20] This body of accumulated experience was valuable, but it alone did not constitute the substance of nutrition science. For Shen, the main difference between nutrition as art and nutrition as science retraced the distinctions between theory and practice. Nutrition as art derived from accumulated experience. It was what many, many people over a long period of time had determined to be successful through trial and error. Nutrition as science, however, explained the function and rationale undergirding such experiences. But for nutrition science to advance the interests of the Chinese people and achieve the greatest potential for the Chinese diet, raw accumulated experience needed to be translated, refined, and explained.

For the many young patriotic Chinese who had studied science in Japan, the United States, and/or Europe, their collective sense of shame over perceived national weaknesses and their desire to transform the society around them led them to promote the study of science at home in popular and professional media. Although not among the first generation of the "returned students," whose education had begun with the Confucian classics and ended with a degree from some of the world's most preeminent institutions of the time period (Oxford, Yale, Tokyo University, etc.), nutrition scientists like Hou Xiangchuan, Shen Tong, and Zheng Ji (1900–2010) were a part of what the historian Mary Bullock has described as the second generation of medical scientists.[21] These young men and women received modern educations, for the most part in China, and gave voice to a vision of social cohesion that arose from the criticism of China and the Chinese from a perspective of complicity.

Zheng, who graduated from National Nanjing University (Guoli Nanjing Daxue) in 1924 and wrote extensively for both specialist and lay audiences, did not so much disparage older dietetic knowledge and practices as seek a more rational, scientifically demonstrable path by which individual Chinese could fix their food problems. Zheng observed that although nutritional knowledge, by which he meant scientific nutritional knowledge, had been absent in China, the general populace was not unaccustomed to thinking about the nutritional value of food. But popular understanding of nutrition tended to be colored by the expertise of cooks who preoccupied themselves with issues of palatability, visual appeal, and the technical arts of cooking, or guided by social and economic concerns. The wealthy insisted upon etiquette, the poor upon satiation. Questions about how to pair food, or which foods complemented each other, did not originate from established scientific principles but instead revolved around concerns that might be counterproductive to the goals of nutrition science. In the words of one commentator, "When the Chinese speak of food, it has been in every possible way. There are the grand banquets of yore—'fried dragon and roasted phoenix'—and when a mere 'half bowl of lamb stew' can satisfy hunger. But for most people, judging food means judging its aesthetic and gustatory qualities, as well as the expensiveness of its price. Few consider its 'essential substances' or 'ingredients.'"[22] Zheng's basic criticism lay not with the potential advantages one might derive from such culinary knowledge but rather with its fixed observance of superficial food qualities, as opposed to scientific principle. As he explained in a lecture to the Nanjing Biological Research Center (Nanjing Shengwu Yanjiusuo) in 1934, food was nothing more nor less than "that which gave the body motility, furnished material for its construction, and regulated normal physiological function."[23] Without this basic definition, the food combinations and proscriptions of the past could not be rendered accountable to the needs of the Chinese nation.

Zheng Ji recognized some value in Chinese culinary knowledge. He believed that the traditional emphasis upon cooked foods, as opposed to raw foods, was beneficial, because it aided digestion and was more hygienic. He also praised the sophisticated use of spices, because when done appropriately, proper flavoring increased one's appetite and furthered digestion. But if taken to extremes, such practices might contravene the nutritional value of the foods being prepared. For example, heavy-handed spicing not only spoils food but may also result in a loss of nutrition.[24] Whatever merits one identified with traditional knowledge, the fundamental problem, which nutrition scientists like Zheng Ji repeatedly invoked, lay in the apparent consequences wrought from accrued experience and a long tradition of food combinations and prohibitions: the Chinese body was weak. "When it comes to us Chinese, the poor don't have much to eat, and the rich don't know how to eat [properly]. As a result, the physique of the Chinese people grows progressively worse and worse. With each generation, our heights and weights decline."[25] In a modern industrial world, such weakness could not be countenanced.

An Unscrupulous Stomach

The sense of shame that Chinese weakness may have been the unintended consequence of long-established practices and misperceptions was aggravated by persistent Western criticism that Chinese eating habits revealed inherent qualities about the people themselves. The celebrated Chinese bilingual Anglophone writer Lin Yutang once pronounced seriousness about food, above religion or learning, to be one of the defining characteristics of Chinese culture, but his insistence arose from the perceived need to explain who the Chinese were to his American audience and why they do what they do. "We are," Lin wrote in his 1937 book *My Country and My People*, "unashamed of our eating." Lack of shame, and in its place a penchant to anticipate, discuss, eat, and comment upon food, distinguished the Chinese, for whom eating was one of life's few joys.[26] Economic necessity may have determined what the Chinese ate in some gross sense, but the zeal with which they savored each morsel and extemporized about the glories of Shanghai honey nectar peach or a real Nanjing salted duck, Lin insisted, was what made the Chinese true connoisseurs of living. Appealing to a longer tradition of literati gourmets such as Su Dongpo, Yuan Mei, and Li Liweng (Li Yu), Lin Yutang embraced the catholicity of Chinese culinary practices as demonstrative of a kind of cosmopolitanism that the West increasingly lacked.[27]

Lin's celebration of the Chinese lack of shame with respect to eating inverted, if not reappropriated, a prominent nineteenth-century trope that the Chinese had, in the words of Walter H. Medhurst (1796–1857), an early nineteenth-century Protestant missionary, "the most unscrupulous stomachs imaginable." What Lin described as a culture that was "catholic in our tastes," Medhurst described as a palate that included "every thing [sic] animal from hide to the entrails,—and almost every thing [sic] vegetable, from the leaves to the roots."[28] And Medhurst was not alone. The historian J. A. G. Roberts has argued that the attitudes of Westerners encountering Chinese food in China from the thirteenth century forward shifted from curiosity and exoticism to contempt and suspicion.[29] Early travelers like Marco Polo or Odoric of Pordenone, a Franciscan friar who spent three years in China in the 1320s, also remarked upon the Chinese propensity to eat everything.

Referring to residents of Hangzhou, Marco Polo wrote, "They eat all sorts of flesh, including that of dogs and other brute beasts and animals of every kind which Christians would not touch for anything in the world."[30] His insistence may have planted the seed of Western stereotypes of Chinese eating, and while hardly complimentary, Marco Polo's descriptions of Chinese flesh-eating were nonetheless interspersed with more admiring statements about the magnificence of Chinese feasts, the deliciousness of the black-fleshed fowl of Fujian, and the variety of Chinese beverages. The focus on the exotic aspects of Chinese food did not fade over time, but Western descriptions from the late eighteenth century onward increasingly became more overtly hostile to such differences. Indeed, for many nineteenth-century Anglo-American observers like Medhurst, Chinese dietary practices elicited a mix of fascination and revulsion, because such practices ostensibly revealed hidden truths of the Chinese character.

Although not a topic to which they would dedicate an entire book, observations about Chinese food habits peppered nineteenth-century Anglo-American writings of China. Their pronouncements upon such matters as the "Chinese dinner" or the agricultural productivity of the Chinese people ranged from such incredibly detailed accounts as one finds in S. W. Williams's *The Middle Kingdom* (1848 and revised in 1883) to more anecdotal ones, as in John L. Stoddard's *China* (1897). Decrying the Chinese for eating everything, including dogs and cats, vegetables lacking English names, and even aquatic plants like nelumbium (lotus), functioned as an easy rhetorical device for flagging both the moral character and the strangeness of the Chinese as a people.[31] Eating everything under the sun was deemed to be either a necessary strategy for survival (and therefore an indication of the backwardness of the society and economy) or a sign of moral weakness—neither rationale being particularly flattering.

Like others in this first generation of Protestant missionaries who began their careers hovering at the periphery in places like Malacca, Batavia, Singapore, and Penang, Medhurst wrote from a position of learned, but mediated, observation. He learned Chinese as an adult, and though he published thirty-four works in Chinese and some sixty-two Malay volumes, including a new translation of the Bible, he depended on his Chinese collaborators to polish the translations.[32] Strong and independent minded, Medhurst opened the first London Missionary Society mission in Shanghai in 1842, just after the town, along with four other ports, was opened to British merchants by the provisions of the Treaty of Nanking (Nanjing).[33] His keen sense of opportunity was justly rewarded. The Qing defeat by the British in the First Opium War transformed not just merchants' lives but missionaries' as well. After 1842, missionaries were legally permitted to rent properties to serve as hospitals, churches, and cemeteries. They were permitted residence in the cities and their immediate suburbs that had been designated by treaty and protected from the Chinese legal system through extraterritoriality. After the signing of the Treaty of Tianjin in 1858, the Qing government guaranteed that Christianity could be openly taught and practiced. Missionaries, and all other foreigners, could travel anywhere, purchase property, and spread their message as they saw fit.[34]

Greater access to different parts of China did not modulate the increasingly negative Western depictions of Chinese dietary habits. Anglo-American missionaries like Medhurst discussed the Chinese diet as a curious custom or habit, one among many that differentiated the Chinese from Westerners. When the Chinese were not eating everything under the sun, they appeared to eat very little that shared common affinity with the diets of Anglo-American China experts, or so-called "China hands." Beef and dairy lacked pride of place—a particularly damning point of difference as Anglo imperial power spread over the course of the nineteenth century.[35] The basic Chinese diet, according to Medhurst, comprised "a little rice and salt fish, or salted vegetable; a species of *brassica* being commonly used for this purpose, which being thoroughly impregnated with salt, helps to flavor the insipid rice, and enables them to relish their food."[36] Variation was achieved through "certain preparations of pulse or millet." On rare occasions, "a few ounces of pork are stewed down with the vegetable preparations, in the proportion of one to five." The poor ate mostly sweet potatoes or yams, and meat only on festival occasions.

A country teeming with people whose greatest strength lay in the extent of their practice of economy, the Chinese outpaced Europeans in their frugality. But such frugality arose from necessity, because life in China was miserable, squalid, poor, and godless: "The want of feeling generally apparent among the Chinese, argues their deep poverty; for where provisions are scarce and dear, the human heart, unsanctified by Divine grace, soon becomes closed against the cry of distress, and the sick poor are allowed to perish by the roadside, without a helping hand to relieve them. There is some charity manifested towards kindred, but none to strangers, who are left alike destitute of public provision and private benevolence."[37] Medhurst drew upon apparent differences in food to demarcate the line separating the heathen from the saved. The profound difference, the unscrupulousness of the Chinese stomach, necessitated Christian intervention, whose benefits included not just a greater sense of humanity toward one's fellow man but also a more sensitive and discerning stomach.[38]

The notion that the Chinese willingly ate anything and everything was a recurring trope in Anglo-American writings, but explanations for why the Chinese diet should be so catholic varied. Interestingly, nineteenth-century speculations did not associate such gastronomic liberality with wealth nor did they perceive wealth as the precondition for eating well. The Victorian botanist Robert Fortune (1812–1880), who succeeded in smuggling tea plants to India in 1848 for the British East India Company, attributed the large numbers of diseased persons he encountered on his trips through the Chinese interior to their "peculiar diet" and "dirty habits."[39] But he also spoke admiringly of the bountifulness of food and its accessibility. When describing the vast array of fish, pork, fruit, and vegetables that "crowd the stands in front of the shops," Fortune suggested, "For a few cash (1000 or 1200 = one dollar) a Chinese can dine in a sumptuous manner upon his rice, fish, vegetables, and tea; and I fully believe, that in no country in the world is there less real misery and want than in China. The very beggars seem a kind of jolly crew."[40] By Fortune's estimation, the Scottish farm laborer fared much worse. The Chinese diet, composed as it was of the simplest kinds—"namely, rice, vegetables, and a small portion of animal food, such as fish or pork"—became "a number of very savory dishes, upon which [the Chinese laborer] breakfasts or dines most sumptuously." In contrast, "In Scotland, in former days—and I suppose it is much the same now—the harvest laborer's breakfast consisted of porridge and milk, his dinner of bread and beer, and porridge and milk again for supper. A Chinaman would starve upon such food."[41]

However varied the Chinese diet might have appeared to observers like Medhurst and Fortune, such plentitude was likely serendipitous rather than the honest rewards of providence or, as later observers like James Harrison Wilson suggested, progress. Wilson (1837–1925), an American topographic engineer and avid railroad enthusiast, traveled to China in 1885 to determine American prospects for railroad concessions. His account of his year traveling throughout the country, mostly on horseback and sometimes in the company of Li Hongzhang (1823–1901), repeated many of Medhurst's and Fortune's descriptions, while also stressing the importance of modern technology.[42] Wilson envisioned a future in which China and Korea, linked by railroads, became one huge market for US goods.[43] Guided by his commitment to progress and economic development, which railroads epitomized,

Wilson's travels convinced him that despite suggestions to the contrary, China was a growing country with a "remarkably strong, robust, and healthy" populace that was "specially free from consumption and all other forms of constitutional disease." Personal hygiene was in Wilson's estimation nearly nonexistent, but in general, the people "seem everywhere to be well fed and comfortably though cheaply clad."[44]

Wheat, Wilson observed, was grown and used extensively in the lands adjacent to the Yellow River. "It is ground into a coarse flour by the primitive means employed in all Oriental countries, and made into unleavened cakes, or into bread, which, owing to the scarcity of fuel, is boiled instead of baked." Cabbage of various kinds was plentiful and "boiled with seaweed, in order to increase the volume and season the cabbage with salt . . . Sweet-potatoes are grown and consumed in the greatest abundance. Radishes and pulse-foods of various sorts are cultivated; persimmons as large as tomatoes are common, but, generally speaking, the country is not rich in fruits." Wilson did not specify his point of comparison with regard to fruit, but he took time to mention the "excellent peaches" grown on the Yangzi; the more inferior apples and pears found further north; the grapes grown in the north and buried in the winter; and the oranges, wild plums, kumquats, loquats, lychees, and lemons grown in the south "and carried in small quantities by itinerant fruit-vendors to the principal cities of the country."[45]

Although beef was "practically unknown, except near the principal foreign settlements," mutton was much more common, especially in the north, where "the broad or fat-tailed Mongolian sheep are raised in sufficient numbers to supply the foreigners, and the richer Chinese, who use it sparingly." Pork made from the black Chinese hog was the "national flesh-food of the Chinese," but its primacy of place at feasts troubled the sensibility of "most [Western] travelers." The hog, as Wilson explained, was "a natural scavenger, and permitted to roam at large in the dirt and filth of every town and village." Other meaty delights abounded: ducks and common barnyard chickens; eggs; game birds like pheasants, partridges, ducks, and snipe; venison; hare: and even the "occasional bustard." The Chinese did not drink milk, and what milk was produced was only for foreigners. All and all, "food [in China] is cheap and good, and the natives appear to be well fed, while the foreigner can get practically everything he would find in the most favored regions of Europe or America."[46]

The riches of food resources that Wilson detailed did not obviate the harsh backdrop of famine or the danger of famine. Although not persuaded that the Chinese, "even in poorer districts of China," were in want or suffering, he nonetheless cautioned against drawing too rosy an assessment. "It is evident to even the casual observer that there is never any great surplus of food or clothing, and that the masses live literally from hand to mouth now, as they have always lived. They are a strictly agricultural people, and have neither mines, furnaces, rolling-mills, nor manufacturing establishments. They live in poor habitations, and have no grand buildings constructed of stone and iron. Even their largest temples and government offices are badly designed, built of perishable materials, and are poorly kept."[47] All this, however, would change with the introduction of the railways, mining, and other "appliances and varied industries of modern progress," and for the better, Wilson prophesized, as wages rose, bringing with it "increased comfort in clothing and habitation, as well as an increased demand for and a wider and more perfect distribution of food of all kinds now grown by the Chinese, and of the many kinds produced only by foreign nations."[48] Variety and plenty marched alongside the forces of progress, and Wilson doubted even China would find herself exempt.

Wilson's belief in the transformative powers of modern technology to uplift and "prevent national disgrace and humiliation" shared common intellectual ground with the famed American missionary Arthur Smith (1843–1932), whose influence extended well beyond missionary circles to include religious and secular audiences in Britain and Canada and throughout Asia.[49] But where Wilson argued for modern technology and industry as the essential means for bringing order, rationality, and progress, Smith argued for something more radical, if not divine. Like Medhurst, Smith prioritized the role of Christianity and insisted that China needed Christian civilization first and foremost, by which he meant a fundamental character transformation based on "a knowledge of God and a new conception of man, as well as of the relation of man to God."[50] In disposition, he shared his missionary forebears' Orientalist sentiment that recognized the possibility that China could become Christian and transform itself on the basis of its own ancient civilization without Europeanizing itself, but his experiences among the local people led him to advance a more radical argument for the transformation of China's inherited cultural and social characteristics along Anglo-European lines. As part of the first generation of Protestant missionaries to move inland and set up residences far from the treaty ports that dotted the eastern seaboard, Smith and his fellow missionaries pursued a strategy of living as "natives" in a village. They adopted local dress, followed local customs, and assumed obligations like paying for the repair of wells, roads, and bridges. They declined to support activities associated with temples or operas on account of their "heathen" character, but in general, they scrupulously, if selectively, followed village proprieties.[51]

Smith's *Chinese Characteristics* drew upon his experiences living in rural Shandong and became the most widely read and influential American work on China of its generation.[52] His characterization of China as a land without facts, which he vividly demonstrated through comical set pieces and anecdotes, became such a pervasive cultural stereotype that well into the twentieth century, Chinese and Western critics continued to cite the inability of the Chinese to understand and use facts properly in their daily lives as the raison d'être of China's myriad social, political, and economic problems.[53] In contrast to earlier China writers, whose descriptions of the "social life" of the Chinese often unfolded in an unsystematic way and without obvious or even explicit connection to an overarching rationale for why the Chinese were the way they were, Smith proposed a comprehensive, more sociological analysis that identified a myriad of instances of Chinese behavior as explicable results of human and historical factors. Food itself did not comprise a singular topic, but the manner in which the Chinese addressed food provided ample demonstration for two of Smith's thirty-nine general characteristics: eating and economy.[54]

Like Medhurst and Wilson, Smith regarded the Chinese diet as "extremely simple" and primarily vegetarian. "The vast bulk of the population seems to depend upon a few articles, such as rice, beans in various preparations, millet, garden vegetables, and fish." The Chinese ate meat only on special occasions, and for many, not even then. Yet "despite its coarseness, and its frequent lack of the requisite nutritive quality, it is eaten in a way, which is a silent admonition to the restless and over anxious foreigner, who is in too much haste, and who has his mind too full of a multitude of other subjects, to get the benefit of his food."[55] Smith's faint praise of the seriousness to which the Chinese applied themselves when eating bore the heavy impression of the suspicion he and his religious contemporaries displayed toward technology and its transformation of daily life in the United States. If the Chinese did not rush eating, they also did not recognize or practice the value of punctuality, accuracy, sympathy, or sincerity. What they did practice was economy to a fault. The thoroughness of their mode of preparation was such that a great variety of dishes might derive from only a few ingredients. They wasted little in preparation and ate everything. "Doubtless it will appear to some of our readers that economy is carried too far, when we mention that it is the general practice to eat *all* of these animals [e.g., fish, horse, mule, donkey, camel, cat, dog, etc.], as soon as they expire, no matter whether the cause of death be an accident, old age, or disease."[56]

The unscrupulousness of the Chinese stomach was, for Smith, a manifestation "that the Chinese are not as a race gifted with that extreme fastidiousness in regard to food which is frequently developed in Western lands."[57] This lack of "fastidiousness" was a function of the hypereconomy of the Chinese character and generated a somewhat contradictory appraisal, one that vacillated between degradation and discipline. On the one hand, a lack of culinary fastidiousness arose from necessity. What later writers on the Chinese diet owe to Smith can be captured in his insistence that blinding, pervasive poverty had made the Chinese gastronomically insensible: "The procurement of food in China is a serious matter; in fact it is the one serious matter of life, in presence of which all other matters fade into comparative insignificance. When one considers what a vast multitude of human beings are to be provided for, it does not seem strange that there are millions in China in any particular time, who do not know what it is to have a full meal, and who are actually in a condition of chronic starvation."[58] And yet, such poverty also illuminated how astounding and advantageous Chinese economy could be in meeting everyday concerns. The articles of food eaten were nonetheless physiologically nutritious and prepared with "a high degree of [culinary] skill." Contemporary Western concern for providing "nourishing food to the very poor, at a minimum cost," had largely been achieved by the Chinese, when in ordinary years it was "quite possible to furnish wholesome food in abundant quantity at a cost for each adult of not more than two cents a day."[59] With little waste and constant repurposing of all manner of material in Chinese food preparation, the Chinese diet satisfied the base needs of the general population—a feat worthy of commendation.

While earlier writers at least indicated some measure of health and well-being associated with eating Chinese foods, Smith mocked such a possibility. The vegetarian diet, whatever its "abstract merits," cannot "be admired in any respect." It was coarse, bulky, and lacking the requisite nutritive quality. The common Chinese people scrapped and saved on a less than full stomach—preeminently economical, and yet still suffering from chronic starvation. If they derived any nutritional merits from their diet, it was through "consumption of such quantity as would seem incredible if we were not daily witnesses of the fact."[60] Unscrupulousness, a lack of fastidiousness, a failure

of discernment—the Chinese diet, if not the foods themselves, was
and deficient, because it exacerbated the very characteristics the (
needed to change to achieve the modern social spirit.[61]

AN ACCOUNTABLE STOMACH

Smith's influence on Chinese intellectual elites was outsized—and not
because he was correct in his assessment of the Chinese national character.
As the historian Tong Lam has demonstrated, Chinese intellectual elites—
men like the novelist Lu Xun and the sociologist Li Jinghan—could continue
to claim ownership of their culture and history, but they could neither control
the meanings of their culture and history, nor how such meanings were produced.[62] Having directly experienced epistemic violence through which they
were made aware of their inability to challenge Western stereotypes on the
basis of a new knowledge framework predicated on the production of social
facts, Chinese intellectual elites transformed themselves into self-appointed
investigators (social, scientific, and literary) with the "heroic mission to
awaken and rescue what they considered the apathetic, muddleheaded, and
helpless masses. In so doing, they effectively turned themselves into active
agents rather than passive victims of the colonial civilizing mission."[63]

The impetus to produce social facts about Chinese society drove Chinese
interest in the Chinese diet in two arenas: social science and nutrition science, both of which strived to articulate universal parameters by which to
measure and gauge China's place within the wider world. As a secondary
topic of interest that emerged from social scientific studies undertaken as
part of the social survey movement, the Chinese diet assumed quantitative
shape when young Chinese investigators, often in collaboration with or at the
behest of more senior Western missionaries turned social scientists, began
to study the livelihood of poor and working-class communities in China's
major metropolitan centers.[64] Small in scale and with limited knowledge of
social science, the earliest surveys (*shehui diaocha*) undertaken by Chinese
intellectuals occurred in the 1910s. These early investigations were in part
prompted by the advent of social survey research in the United States, as
many Chinese social scientists were trained, directly or indirectly, by their
American colleagues.[65] The YMCA secretary John Burgess and Sidney Gamble,
an heir to the Procter & Gamble fortune, each played formative roles in
shaping this early phase of social survey research.[66] Like other evangelical
social science proponents, Burgess and Gamble believed that science and

reason had the power to awaken and lift the Chinese people out of their misery. For this to occur, they needed to help their Chinese students "discover the fundamental social conditions" of Chinese cities with the aim of developing viable social programs of redress.[67]

By the 1920s, this religion-driven social science approach had begun to lose traction due to secularization and professionalism. Moreover, the emergence of a veritable "army of liberal social scientists," composed of Chinese students who had studied in the United States and Europe in the 1920s and 1930s and those trained by mission colleges in China and later by Chinese universities, led to what Lam has called the indigenization of social survey research. Chinese social scientists retained the conviction that social science afforded a "universal" language for understanding social facts collected in China but comparable to conditions elsewhere, but they redirected the purpose of the social sciences away from religious salvation or the perfectibility of the human soul and toward the containment of the afflictions caused by industrialization and progress and their management in order to reduce the risk of social disruption.[68] A further shift away from American precedents occurred when Chinese social scientists began exploring the facets of rural, as opposed to urban, life in China.

The Chinese diet that emerged from urban surveys indicated the strengths and limitations of abstraction.[69] Motivated by the desire to obtain a fuller and more intimate knowledge of the living conditions of working communities in Beijing, Tao Menghe (1887–1960) settled upon the idea of using family budgets to map the contours of day-to-day life. He enlisted the services of two female investigators, each responsible for thirty families, who exhibited the necessary patience and perseverance to visit each family each day but Sunday to ask and record their daily expenses. The results of their work enabled him to begin filling the empirical hole about what constituted daily life of the Chinese people. Tao, who had trained with Sidney Webb at the London School of Economics and was a close collaborator with American social scientists as the director of the Institute of Social Research, first adopted Atwater's scale for calculating the equivalent adult male. The Atwater scale, devised by the American chemist Wilbur O. Atwater in 1886 to measure the relative energy requirements of persons of different age and sex, had by the 1920s become a standard tool for analyzing family-living data in the United States and in China.[70] Having converted all individuals to equivalent adult males, Tao assembled in a series of tables the average quantities bought and average expenditures used per family and per equivalent adult by kinds of food.

His classification of food was "made in accordance with the food habits of the Chinese and was adopted, because, it is convenient for calculating the specific elements of the Chinese food."[71] By this, he meant that he and his co-investigators found it more advantageous to ask the participants about their expenses in terms of cereals, vegetables, meat, and condiments. "The Chinese eats boiled rice, if he is a southerner, or corn or wheaten bread, if he is a northerner, with a little meat or its substitute, such as dried shrimps, vegetables and certain condiments to whet his appetite."[72]

What sorts of foods appeared regularly on the participants' tables? Tao noted with surprise the "limited variety of food articles in the table." Mouth-watering delicacies that were generally esteemed by Beijing people—egg-plants, radishes, pumpkins, cucumbers, crabs—were "conspicuous by their absence," although this may have been a consequence of timing, as his investigation was undertaken during the winter months. Instead of vegetables, one found a steady rotation of millet, corn flour, millet flour, wheat flour, cabbage, salted turnips, spinach, bean curd, onions, sesame oil, salt, soy paste, vinegar, and mutton. Meat consumption was low, and despite the reputation of the Chinese people as a "pork-eating race," Tao's data suggested a higher consumption of mutton than pork.[73] Fruits like persimmons and peas, "which grow plentifully in the vicinity of Beijing and as a rule, are displayed on the stalls in abundance on the streets," rarely appeared on the tables of his survey households—mostly likely on account of the "heavy octroi taxes and duties which have so raised their prices that they have practically become a luxury of the well-to-do."[74] The main distinctive features of food consumption of these Beijing families, Tao wrote, included the high proportion of food expenses dedicated to the purchase of cereals, the plentiful consumption of pickles and pungent and odoriferous edibles ("in lieu of meat and dainties"), the sparing use of fruits, and the near absence of milk and its by-products.

Rendering the patterns of food consumption of even a limited number of Beijing families into tables of average quantities and expenditures raised the constructive possibility of comparing the diets of different countries. Tao ventured to suggest that comparisons with Japan and India might yield interesting results. Since all three peoples were "essentially 'vegetarian' in the sense that they eat meat very sparingly" and use rice or wheat as their principal food, with other articles "such as meat, fish, vegetables, and condiments being consumed merely for the purpose of stimulating appetite," it quickly became apparent that diets of Beijing laborers compared favorably with those of Japanese prisoners and laborers (but not Japanese farmers) and Bengali families in comfort. This comparison when supplemented with a nutrient analysis of the various foods comprising the Chinese diet led Tao to conclude, "That great masses of the Chinese have been and at present are still under-nourished nobody could gainsay, yet it seems that, on the whole, the simple vegetarian diet would be sufficient to meet the bodily requirement of the Chinese." If the Chinese diet was found to be wanting, it was because "the Chinese diet of today is but that of the European peasant of yesterday." The root cause lay in China's material poverty that had left it "stranded on a barren shore and left there in a sad plight," as the "swift currents of modern scientific and industrial progress . . . buoyantly and triumphantly" rolled the West forward.[75]

The momentum generated by Chinese social surveys led many Chinese sociologists and intellectuals to identify "poverty" (*pin*) as one of the nation's most urgent problems. But in contrast to late Qing reformers who invoked *pin* as economic hardships specific to individuals or who correlated poverty to scenarios of possible national extinction, Chinese sociologists and intellectuals of the 1920s understood poverty as a distinctly *social* problem whose dimensions could be charted in terms of income and expenditures. It was, as Tao Menghe explained in 1920, "a social problem" that transcended individual circumstances and for which "an objective and universal standard" was needed. In other words, poverty became a normative concept for which one could define a minimum level of subsistence or the minimum cost of food, clothing, or shelter needed to sustain a life.[76] Preoccupation with urban poverty led Tao and his colleagues to initially downplay the significance of the Chinese diet. However imperfect it may be, the Chinese diet appeared both functional (i.e., sufficient to "meet the bodily requirement of the Chinese") as well as in keeping with China's spatial and temporal incongruence with the forces of modern scientific and industrial progress. It was, in other words, a backward diet reflective of China's backward state of development.

This sense that the Chinese diet, as revealed by social surveys, was basically sufficient did not last long. Chinese intellectual elites like Tao had initiated a wave of cost of living and livelihood studies for urban communities that reproduced American concerns and research methods, but alongside these efforts was a growing sense that the American model of social science and its implicit presumptions about the nature of Chinese society and people had its limitations. To quote the historian Tong Lam, "Although the imperatives of imperialism compelled Chinese social scientists to adopt the rhetoric of science and reason to reconceptualize China, they never felt comfortable with the image of China depicted by the Euro-American colonial gaze."[77] By the late 1920s, Chinese social scientists increasingly moved away from the problems of cities and their industrial workforces to investigate rural areas and the culture of the rural populace. The scale of this shift in focus was tremendous. Whereas rural studies constituted only about 6.5 percent of all surveys conducted in 1927, by 1935 nearly 38 percent of surveys focused on rural populations.[78]

What they found indicated greater cause for concern with respect to the Chinese diet itself. The very food categories Tao had used to determine his participants' daily expenditures—cereals, vegetables, meat, and condiments—became subject to intense scrutiny.[79] When coupled with the research coming out of medicine and biochemistry, the very foods social surveys indicated as regular and essential items of monthly expenditures increasingly appeared precarious and subject to hitherto unperceived deficiencies. The modern concept of the Chinese diet, quantifiable and comprehensible in terms of everyday purchasing decisions, still needed further biochemical refinement.

The process of indigenization that substantively redirected the Chinese social survey movement during the late 1920s and 1930s can also be seen with respect to the development of medical and biochemical research, which were also fields in which earlier research was largely conducted by Westerners. The chemist S. D. Wilson, who had completed his dissertation work at the University of Chicago before moving to China to work at PUMC, captured the general thrust of the initial Western-dominated period of nutrition research by focusing on identifying foods regularly sold at local markets and conducting chemical assays of such foods to determine their composition.[80] Early studies like Wilson's were primarily descriptive and largely in keeping with the ideas of practical economy Wilbur O. Atwater had advanced in 1887. Atwater, who had undertaken advanced graduate studies in agricultural and physiological chemistry in Germany and was keenly interested in the energy requirements of the human body at rest and in action, became an outspoken advocate for the importance of calorie knowledge when making food-related decisions. In 1896, he and his collaborator C. D. Woods published a compilation of approximately 2,600 analyses of American foodstuffs, which was later expanded to over 4,000 analyses in the 1899 reissue.[81] His tables of "fuel values" provided an essential reference for investigators working in China, who believed that the general level of poverty in China to be greater than elsewhere and that the Chinese lacked the necessary information to make better food selections. In the words of two of the earliest chemists working on Chinese foods, Hartley Embrey and Tsan Ch'ing Wang, "In a country like China—where the masses maintain themselves on a few coppers a day, where monotonous and often deficient diets are continued for long periods of time—the necessity of an increased public knowledge of the value of the local foods and of their proper use is even greater than in those countries where living is carried out on a higher level, where variety is possible on account of relatively full purses."[82]

As part of an emerging cohort of young Chinese intellectuals who had received advanced training in medicine and the laboratory sciences in the United States or Europe, had returned to China, and were training the next generation of research scientists, Wu Xian represented the changing face of science in 1920s China. His research crystallized a long-standing medical interest in the relationship between diet and health with the latest developments in laboratory sciences. The roots of his interest in the Chinese diet are unclear. His earlier professional achievements with protein denaturation did not obviously lead to his increased concern about the Chinese diet and its nutritional inadequacies, and yet from 1927 onward, his publication record included a growing number of synthetic as well as new treatises on food chemistry and nutrition.[83] The shift toward food chemistry and nutrition may have reflected changes in his personal life. Like many of his generation, Wu had been married at the age of eighteen to a girl of his grandmother's choice. His time abroad had changed his mental outlook, and when he returned to China and his wife in 1920, what he wanted was someone with whom he could share "the world he knew and enjoyed." His wife could not satisfy his desire for "a partnership in understanding and outlook," and they divorced. His second wife, Daisy Yen Wu, had also been an overseas Chinese student, who in 1923 was completing her master's in food chemistry and nutrition under the direction of Professor Henry C. Sherman at Columbia University. The two young scientists married in December 1924.

Wu's approach to the topic of diet and health broadly retraced themes similar to those raised by Western medical missionaries who had been ministering to the Chinese since the early nineteenth century. The historian Shang-Jen Li has suggested that, especially for the British, interest in Chinese dietary customs and the healthiness of Chinese food (or the lack thereof) served as a critical site of inquiry wherein Western medical practitioners navigated the physical vicissitudes of being in a foreign land as well registered the influences of place upon their national and racial identities.[84] Whether as an adaptive strategy for how to survive in "the tropics" or as part of a moral economy that sought to discipline individual colonial Europeans to "the biopolitics of racial rule," medical discussions of the Chinese diet by Western physicians relied on generalizable differences in the consumption of meat and alcohol.[85] Some, like John Dudgeon (1837–1901), a medical missionary of the London Missionary Society who also served as a medical officer to the Chinese Imperial Maritime Customs, praised the health benefits of Chinese food. The moderate consumption of meat and alcohol struck Dudgeon as both preferable and more healthful than the European diet, with its fondness for animal food.[86] Dr. Ernest C. Peake (1874–1950), also of the London Missionary Society, observed the low incidence of rheumatic fever in the country and attributed this to the Chinese "carbohydrate diet," which placed less strain on the kidneys and enabled "more perfect elimination of waste products from the blood." In contrast to the high rate of appendicitis among Westerners, the Chinese, Peake insisted, rarely suffered the affliction on account of their lower intake of "proteids" (proteins). It was the moderate nature of the Chinese diet—one more natural and simple than that of Europeans—that resulted in fewer diseases, "diseases [that were] more amenable to treatment," and "a greater freedom from acute and inflammatory affections of all kinds."[87]

Others, like Patrick Manson (1844–1922), who began his career in China and after his return to London established the London School of Tropical Medicine, espoused decidedly more negative views of the healthfulness of the Chinese diet. Seeing the food and diet as "agents" of national selection, Manson cautioned his fellow countrymen against adopting native foods in a quixotic attempt to acclimate to their new environs. The racial characteristics of the Chinese emerged from a process of natural selection that had worked itself over the course of many generations. The same could be said for the English. "Appetites bred through many generations become instincts, and an Englishman must have his beef." Evolutionary change did not permit sudden reversions of racial type. Manson explained, "You cannot altogether change your mode of living or the character of your aliment. Your stomach will no more obtain from the diet of a Hindoo all that is necessary for nutrition—though it may contain it—than it could in other circumstances from the blubber that delights while it nourishes an Esquimo."[88]

Be it positive or negative, this sense that diet shaped the racial qualities of a people resonated with Chinese medical researchers like Wu Xian working in the twentieth century. The key differences lay in scope and agency. For Chinese nutrition scientists, understanding the composition of the Chinese diet indicated the strengths and weaknesses of the nation itself. It also mapped out practical paths for intervention and change. The Chinese diet as a topic of scientific investigation indicated pathways by which local actors could reassert agency in the face of seemingly redoubtable challenges. If the Chinese diet proved anything less than adequate in light of modern nutritional knowledge, then the technical work of improving and transforming the diet represented essential tasks that proved to both the Chinese people and the world at large China's ability to rank itself among modern nations. In the words of one notable commentator about the critical value of nutrition, "Sound nutrition enables a body to receive all that it needs to grow. Those who are of sallow complexion, lacking of muscle, and infirm beyond one's years (*weilao xianshuai*) are suffering from insufficient nourishment (*yingyangbuzu*). For the individual, these [qualities] are [a sign of] misfortune; for a country, [a sign of] loss. That is why Europe and America have made it a duty to pay especial attention to the nation's nutrition and health."[89] Upon the Chinese diet, the fate of a nation rested.

The historian Michael Worboys has observed that nutrition science, in contrast to tropical medicine or tropical agriculture, afforded researchers a common approach for tackling diverse problems the world over.[90] Without requiring a separate medical epistemology, nutrition science, rooted as it was in physiology and chemistry, generated a vision of the universal man to underlie all nutritional investigations. Moreover, the thermodynamic theory of nutrition, which had emerged around the turn of the twentieth century, enabled the translation of specific types of food into a seemingly nonparticularistic language of uniform meaning and easily tabulated standard values. Nutrition scientists recognized that different local dietaries reflected different local ecologies, but so long as all food could be broken down into the same constituent parts, the overall value of any particular diet could be compared irrespective of its geographical origins.

With an eye toward the power and agency that comparison might afford, Chinese nutrition scientists who rose to prominence in the late 1920s and 1930s demanded more from the science than lists of food values for foods regularly sold at markets or appearing on people's tables. For them, the Chinese diet was a litmus test.

Wu Xian and his Chinese colleagues framed the question about the adequacy of the Chinese diet along two corresponding vectors of analysis: the nutrient profiles of local diets, and the physical and mental condition of the Chinese people. Formulated as questions, Wu challenged his students and fellow researchers by asking, Did the Chinese diet meet all known dietary requirements? And did the Chinese people display signs of malnutrition, as might be expected from living on diets lacking essential nutrients? Drawing together the work of William H. Adolph, a chemist who had studied under Edgar Fahs Smith before accepting a faculty position at the Shantung Christian University (later Cheeloo University), as well as recent surveys he had conducted in collaboration with his wife Daisy, Wu distilled the Chinese diet to the following essential characteristics: rice or wheat as the principal part of any meal, with other foods "used only to make these more palatable." Although all the available data sets came from North China—Adolph had surveyed 30 farming families (340 adults and 114 children) in Shandong, whereas Wu collected data from 35 families (146 adults and 47 children) in Beijing—Wu insisted that "the diets of the Chinese in different parts of the country cannot differ much from those shown" for North China and Beijing.

The Chinese diet in Wu's evaluation resembled in broad strokes the diet Tao Menghe had charted in his social survey of Beijing families. Adolph's North China and Wu's Beijing dietaries comprised many of the same food categories: cereals included wheat and wheat products, rice, millet, *gaoliang* (Chinese sorghum), and corn; "meat" included pork, mutton, chicken, fish, eggs, and milk; vegetables included melons, green vegetables, potatoes, turnips, and fruits; and "condiments" consisted of oils and "sugar & starch." But instead of calculating the average quantities and expenditures, Wu presented a further level of numerical abstraction by showing the "parts per 100" represented by each food item. For example, in North China dietaries, wheat and wheat products constituted 31.3 parts per 100; meat and chicken, 1.12 parts; and melons, 20.8 parts. Wu then tabulated the relative sums for each food category: cereals, 58.2 parts per 100; legumes and bean products, 7.3 parts; meat, 2.0 parts; vegetables and fruits, 28.2 parts, etc. The purpose of this form of enumeration was to justify his alarm regarding the low levels of meat consumption evident in local dietaries. Having transformed the Chinese diet into an aggregate set whose parts must add up to a singular whole, Wu shifted attention away from dietary sustenance and toward dietary optimality as the meaning and measure of adequacy. By highlighting the proportionality of any specific food category in relation to the whole, he raised the possibility that certain food categories should be treated as greater or lesser indicators of physical and national vigor. In this way, he introduced an argument for how to make the Chinese diet accountable.[91]

By treating the Chinese diet as a litmus test for the well-being of the nation, Wu recast the purpose of nutritional research in terms of optimality. "I wish to emphasize the fact that the goal of nutrition is the optimum and not the minimum. While the minimum of the essentials of life suffices to maintain and propagate the race after a fashion, it is only with the optimum which makes progress."[92] His biochemical colleagues agreed. Adolph, whose North Chinese dietary studies had been so integral to Wu's construction of the Chinese diet, observed, "The prosperity of the nation demands not mere maintenance, but an optimum metabolism expressed in terms of improved growth and vigor."

Conclusion

The conceptualization of the Chinese diet emerged as part of a broader epistemological shift in which Chinese intellectuals used claims of science and reason to construct new organizing principles for cultural production and political life. Faced as they were during the late Qing and early Republican years with the breakdown and abandonment of the old Confucian moral universe, Chinese intellectuals turned to science to reimagine their roles as both scholars and political subjects. Particularly during the iconoclastic New Culture Movement (ca. 1915–21) and the May Fourth Movement (1919), they vigorously embraced "Mr. Science" (Sai Xiansheng) and "Mr. Democracy" (De Xiansheng) as beacons of epistemological authority in a time of tremendous uncertainty and political disarray. Science, many believed, was a privileged way of knowing, because it (or more specifically, the scientific method) provided a correct path to knowledge that was impartial, objective, verifiable, and universally applicable. In looking back at indigenous approaches to nutritional knowledge, Chinese nutrition scientists bristled at their apparent lack of rigor and systematic explanation. However much the Chinese of yore might be acknowledged to have been food oriented, their concerns were misdirected and prone to eclecticism. What scientists like Wu Xian and Zheng Ji wanted was accountability, and a rich, diverse tradition of dietary combinations and prohibitions did little to satisfy their sense of political urgency and evolving cultural sensibilities.

Faith in science was coupled with boots on the ground, as young men and women fanned out throughout cities and the countryside to gather population statistics, ethnographic facts, economic data, and cultural artifacts; to conduct geological surveys and participate in archeological digs;

and to chemically analyze all the varieties of local foodstuffs in the expectation that such efforts would yield truth about the Chinese nation. These concerted efforts emerged from a backdrop of Western epistemic violence in which nineteenth-century Anglo-American ruminations about how and what the Chinese ate produced stronger ideological impressions of the imagined Chinese community than likely existed. Rendering the Chinese diet into quantifiable categories with universal applicability made it speak comparatively and across political boundaries. What nineteenth-century Anglo-American observers had hinted at and signaled to in varying degrees was effectively constituted through this growing body of research. The Chinese diet became not just the aggregate list of various foods grown and eaten by Chinese people but a way for Chinese intellectuals to communicate a sense of togetherness and simultaneity as members of an imagined community. Studies of living standards that indexed foods by classes and nutritive values, food analyses, dietary studies that rearticulated what people ate on a daily basis according to their chemical composition, experiments on the digestibility of foods, animal experiments on the nutritive value of different diets—all of this work made it possible to systematize and link together the wide variety of climates and food habits under the singular, overarching framework of "the Chinese diet."

With the discursive emergence of the Chinese diet, it became possible to capture the modern essence of how the foods Chinese people ate produced the people that were Chinese. This scientific enterprise strove to make legible nutritional comparisons across societies through the notion of a universal, biomedical body responsive to and reliant on a basic calculus of essential nutrients. But having a concept of the Chinese diet was not the same as demonstrating how the Chinese diet was adequate, and as Wu Xian himself posited, a notion of adequacy necessitated both empirical knowledge and an argument about the nation and prescriptions for daily life.

In Wu's estimation, the Chinese diet was inadequate for many reasons, the most important being the absence or minimal amounts of the right kinds of proteins. More consumption of eggs and greater encouragement of the use of milk and butter would dramatically improve the protein problem, but given prevailing economic conditions, this recommendation seemed unrealistic. A more straightforward step simply involved greater use of the soybean and its products. Such advice was eminently practical, difficult to fault, and nonetheless haunted by the spectral fear that the Chinese people were too small and too weak because they were not eating enough animal-derived proteins. How Chinese nutrition scientists mounted an argument for the inadequacy of the Chinese diet was inseparable from how they translated Chinese national development into a biochemical language of power and energy. The soybean's role within this emerging nutritional calculus of inadequacy was simple: if the Chinese diet was inadequate for the lack of proteins, then the soybean's high protein content represented a potential homegrown solution.

CHAPTER 3

Of Quality and Protein

Building a Scientific Argument of Chinese Nutritional Inadequacy

W HAT were Chinese foodstuffs made up of? How nutritional were they? What could be done to improve their nutritional values? For Luo Dengyi (1906–2000), who had recently graduated in 1928 from Beijing Normal University with a degree in agricultural biochemistry, these were questions that had accompanied him through the course of his studies. While clearly in dialogue with his academic interests, Luo nonetheless insisted that these questions were important, not because they represented specialist concerns but because they grappled with affairs that ordinary people needed to understand.[1] Writing in 1929 in the popular science journal *Natural World* (Ziranjie), Luo explained, "Food, clothing, and shelter are human necessities. Of these three, obtaining food is the most important and difficult to achieve. As has often been said, 'Ordinary prudence suffices to judge the adequacy of shelter and clothing, but neither instinct nor common sense is a reliable guide in the choice of foods.'"[2] Although Luo does not mention the biochemist Wu Xian by name, the oft-said phrase Luo used to preface his essay "On Chinese Foods" had originally been Wu's.

Wu's influence can be seen in the structure and progression of Luo's questions. What were Chinese foodstuffs made up of? How nutritional were they? What could be done to improve their nutritional values? These questions marked a trajectory in which Chinese foods functioned as terra incognita for China's newly trained young scientists. By testing, analyzing, and redefining local foods in terms of their chemical composition, Chinese nutrition scientists deemed science the true arbiter of the value of Chinese foods. Knowing the chemical makeup of everyday foods became the foundation upon which later interventions with the goal of improvement could be staged. But why did Luo implicitly characterize Chinese foods as somehow inadequate or deficient in the first place?[3]

Chinese nutrition scientists mounted a scientific argument for the nutritional inadequacy of the Chinese diet that privileged the importance of proteins in a modern progressive diet that supported national development. The social scientific and nutritional research of the late 1920s and 1930s had identified patterns of consumption that heavily prioritized grains and rice as the basis of the urban Chinese diet. The poorer the family, the greater the proportion of the monthly income spent on grains and flour.[4] In rural areas, the Chinese diet followed a similar pattern: a heavy proportion of grains and minimal to nonexistent amounts of meat. The sociologist Li Jinghan, for example, had found that the food and eating patterns of rural residents in Dingxian in the late 1920s were shaped, but not necessarily enhanced, by the three farming seasons (winter, planting, and harvesting).[5] What varied across seasons were not the kinds of foods eaten but rather the quantities, as if the farmers themselves had long since calibrated their food with their energy expenditure needs. During winter months, when agricultural labor was low, North Chinese farmers ate two meals (one in the morning, the other in the evening) consisting of a mix of sweet potato, millet, mixed grains, and vegetables. During the busier seasons, they ate three meals. Starting with the planting season, the quantities of food increased, but in strategic ways to stave off hunger. Millet constituted the majority of the daily diet, with mixed grains and dried sweet potato leaves added to round out the meals. Harvesting season witnessed a further increase, as millet came to dominate the daily diet.[6]

While sufficient in some thermodynamic sense to enable the farmers to work, these diets, by their lack of meat and dairy, suggested something demonstrably less than ideal. Wu Xian indicated as much when he wrote, "In a prosperous country like America, where food is plentiful and the average family has a good income, the danger of malnutrition is slight. But in China, where the majority of people are compelled to subsist on a diet limited in quantity and variety, it is highly important to know whether it is adequate in the light of our modern knowledge of nutrition."[7] Grains could provide sustenance and ensure subsistence. But progress and development required more. It required proteins—solid, dependable animal-derived proteins found in meat and dairy.

For Chinese nutrition scientists such as Luo Dengyi and Wu Xian, the inadequacy of the Chinese diet derived from its vegetarian cast: too many grains, not enough meat and dairy. In contrast to the bread-and-beef diet that signified power, wealth, and national advancement, Chinese people ate simply, poorly—"a diet limited in quantity and variety."[8] Little, if any, meat, no dairy, and few eggs had transformed the Chinese diet into maelstrom of difficult-to-digest grains and vegetables, all of which ranked low in their biological values, according to scientific thinking of the period. Although it was rare to hear a Chinese nutrition scientist advocate the outright adoption of a bread-and-beef diet, nevertheless their acceptance of the greater nutritional value associated with such a diet was clear. An adequate diet, they assured the Chinese reading public, ensured the progress of a nation, and for the Chinese nation to advance, its people needed proteins to grow.

Science provided the language and tools for understanding the inadequacy of the Chinese diet. Nutrition scientists endeavored to show how Chinese weakness of body and mind were attributable to the Chinese diet and its lack of animal-derived proteins. They used animal feeding experiments to highlight the nutritional perils of the largely vegetarian Chinese diet and communicated their message in specialist journals, family and women's magazines, and mainstream newspapers. The effort to scientifically demonstrate the inadequacy of the Chinese diet drew together a variety of intellectual professionals from professors of physiology and medical physicians to biochemists and public health reformers—engaging the public as nutritional activists and invoking the language of nutrition science to persuade the literate public that national vigor rested upon dietary reform.

But demonstrating the inadequacy of the Chinese diet was no simple matter, and although Chinese scientific consensus deemed the largely vegetarian Chinese diet to be an impediment for national development, what their research revealed about local dietaries, the vitamin profiles of common foods, protein and caloric intakes, and so forth yielded a more complex vision that had to be remolded to fit the argument that China's most pressing dietary problem derived from the deficit of animal-based proteins. This empirical complexity ultimately permitted space for negotiation and creativity as Chinese scientists became persuaded that the soybean, with its high concentration of protein, might furnish an answer to the problem of the Chinese diet.

The collapse of the dynastic order and the founding of the new republic in 1912 brought neither peace nor solidarity. The 1911 revolution, which had swept first through the ranks of the Qing dynasty's reorganized and modernized New Army but was ultimately led by intellectuals and urban elites, promised the creation of a strong and democratic nation. What unfolded in the subsequent decade tarnished the optimism and confidence of Chinese intellectuals that the Chinese people could rise above the politics of betrayal, terror, and factionalism that had become the order of the day. Without a functioning national government between 1916 and 1928, the country devolved into a period of warlordism and militarism. Domestic unrest and instability exacerbated the precarious state of Chinese sovereignty and reinforced the sense of national shame over China's inability to safeguard her own interests. In 1917, China entered World War I on the side of the Allies, and though no Chinese soldier fought in combat, some 96,000 were sent as laborers to the Western Front in Europe. Chinese participation in the Allied war effort yielded few political rewards; the Treaty of Versailles (1919) formalized arrangements in which Japan, not China, received possession of formerly German-occupied Shandong.[9]

The sense of failure to forge a strong and cohesive nation pervaded the intellectual landscape of the 1920s and 1930s.[10] Science, which Chinese intellectuals more generally esteemed for its putatively transhistorical and transcultural qualities, seemed to offer a proper method for reconstituting China as a modern nation within the global system of modern nation-states. Chinese nutrition research throughout the late 1920s and 1930s sought to establish the correspondence between collective survival and individual health, with the Chinese diet as a critical locus for scientific management of both the social and the individual body. Popular rhetoric based on analogies of race and the body postulated the reasons for China's decline as corollaries of what naturally occurs to the human body. Toxins in the body, bad habits, aging, senility—each of these could operate in parallel forms at the level of race to explain the decrepitude and frailty characterizing China's antiquated civilization.[11] Chinese adaptation of Western medical knowledge generated multiple connotations of health and disease and how bodily health might be instrumentalized to achieve social and political objectives. Not only as an issue of personal concern for the individual, bodily health was often construed in terms of Chinese national strength or racial fitness.[12] Popular acceptance and integration of modern sporting and physical culture forms in China from the early twentieth century further nurtured the idea among young patriotic Chinese that bodily health directly reflected national strength.[13]

Chinese nutrition scientists contributed to this pervasive sense of racial doom and gloom by producing empirical data to demonstrate the physical manifestations of a poor diet and pinpointing the lack of animal proteins in the Chinese diet as the source of Chinese weakness. Where others sermonized about the state of a nation's health in broad strokes, listing everything from the "illnesses of civilization" (*wenming bing*), like syphilis, tuberculosis, neurosis, and insomnia, to the "phlegmatic" nature of the Chinese, Chinese nutrition scientists mapped out the contours of national and racial crisis in the bodies of young children and students and in the very foods Chinese people ate.[14]

In the inaugural essay of a new series featuring the relationship between nutrition and the nation in the journal *Science* (Kexue), the biochemist Zheng Ji (1900–2010) painted a particularly grim picture of the Chinese people. Like many of this second generation of Chinese nutrition scientists, Zheng began his scientific training in China, before leaving for the United States to undertake graduate studies. He studied with the biologist Bing Zhi (1886–1965) at National Central University and then obtained a PhD in biochemistry from Indiana University in 1936.[15] Among the more prolific of nutrition scientists writing for both layman and specialist audiences, Zheng sketched the trajectory of poor physical health from childhood through adulthood.[16] Poor nutrition during childhood would result in incomplete development of the child's physical and intellectual powers—a body small and weak, a mind untapped and dull, and ultimately a child ever prone to disease. The effects of poor nutrition did not, however, end with childhood. Physically and mentally weak children grew into physically and mentally weak adults, and for a country whose long and storied past had imbued its people with tendencies that privileged arts and culture over physical culture and nutrition, the consequence was evident in the country's persistent state of enfeeblement. If the reader lacked a visual reference for just how pernicious China's nutritional woes were, Zheng Ji provided ample examples. "Most people in this country are humpbacked and have wallowed waists. Their facial color—particularly urbanites—is very poor."[17] He insisted that "very few of the country's primary and middle school youths possess[ed] fully developed, strong physiques."

Physical infelicities, even deformities, manifested themselves in dispositional ways that became pervasive national characteristics. Wu Xian attributed China's moral turpitude, as evidenced by ongoing political scandals and corruption, to its weakness of body and character.[18] Lacking physical fortitude, the Chinese were unprogressive, risk averse, and too easily satisfied with temporary ease and comfort.[19] He went further than most in suggesting that the Chinese had inherited such characteristics over the course of several generations.

The rhetorical power of these claims about national weakness depended on a vision of China's own past. As several writers reiterated, the ancient Chinese of yesteryear were more robust and vigorous than any Chinese found today. "Shen Nong lived to 101; Zhuangxu to 98; Emperor Ku to 108; Yao until 107; and Shun to 110. The average of these five men is 106 years. Compared with today, how rare is it to encounter a person a hundred years of age?"[20] Wu Xian also drew upon classical sources to demonstrate the greater physical stature of Chinese of yore. "It is mentioned in Mencius that Cao Jiao, who measured nine feet four, wondered why he could not be as great as Emperor Wen Wang and Emperor Tang, who measured ten feet and nine feet, respectively. Confucius also measured nine feet four."[21] Adjusting for differences in measurement, Wu maintained that "ancient celebrities" still measured six feet seven and though clearly not representative of the average height of the ancient Chinese, "the fact still remains that the height of the modern Chinese with the best physique do not even approach these figures."[22] For more contemporary evidence of Chinese dietary inadequacy, Wu continued, "The Chinese are small in stature compared, for instance, with the Americans and the English. They live shorter lives with higher mortality both among the adults and the infants. They possess low vital resistance, as evidenced by the prevalence of such diseases as trachoma and tuberculosis." To this, Wu added the further indictment of passivity and acquiescence. "[The Chinese] are over peaceful, non-persevering, non-aggressive, [and] non-enterprising, and are easily contented with the environment in which they find themselves."[23]

In linking individual nutrition to the health of the nation, Chinese nutrition scientists were invoking refrains about power and wealth with which the nineteenth-century literatus-scholar and translator Yan Fu (1854–1921) had himself grappled. As the historian Benjamin Schwartz has masterfully demonstrated, Yan Fu's complex engagement with specific strands of Western political thought (Herbert Spencer, John Stuart Mill, and Adam Smith) led him to champion two specific qualities, energy and the individual, as the prerequisites of wealth and power. The energy—intellectual, moral, and physical—that the West had exalted and that enabled it to achieve unparalleled industrial and military might had been, Yan Fu concluded, foundational to "[t]he Faustian nature of Western culture that had led to the Promethean conquest of external nature and the enormous growth of social-political power within human society."[24] Alerting the country to the perils of poor nutrition and bemoaning the lamentable quantities of proteins and vitamins consumed may seem a pale and unromantic corollary to Yan Fu's ruminations about energy and the individual, and yet at a practical level, the nutritional body and its attendant thermodynamic concerns channeled many of those same ideas. Nutrition scientists marshaled through their research a vision consonant with Yan Fu's conception of the individual whose energy, when consolidated with the energies of others in bureaucratic organizations, became enhanced and channeled toward constructive goals.[25] The nation as the cumulative social formation of individual energies depended upon sound, rationalized nutrition.

While lamentable for a country derided as an antiquated civilization (*wenming guguo*), the severity of China's physical and dispositional inadequacies could only be appreciated through comparison.[26] The Chinese were shorter than Americans and Europeans. Infant mortality rates, as best as they could be determined, exceeded those in advanced nations, and some suggested that the Chinese suffered from heightened susceptibility to disease on account of their diet.[27] In Zheng Ji's summation, "Our mortality rate is higher than that of the Europeans, Americans, and Japanese; our lifespan significantly shorter. These sorts of phenomena directly contribute to the disadvantage of the individual and indirectly to the disadvantage of our national race." The consequences of inaction were disastrous, and Zheng, who had a tendency for the maudlin, characterized the threat of poor health to be greater, "a thousand times worse than our enemies' guns and bombs."[28] National and racial survival was at stake.

To some extent, the growing body of anthropometrics supported these assertions.[29] Arising out of public and private initiatives, studies of Chinese heights and weights proliferated throughout the 1920s and 1930s.[30] The Nationalist government sponsored studies measuring the heights and weights of primary school students as part of its development of a national student health program. Researchers at private institutions like the Peking Union Medical College and the Henry Lester Institute for Medical Research in Shanghai undertook measurement studies as part of larger projects to understand the nutritional implications of the Chinese diet, as well as the quantitative dimensions of Chinese basal metabolism. What they found appeared to support popular stereotypes about regional as well as racial physical variation. Northern Chinese were on average taller and heavier than inhabitants of Central and Southern China.[31] British and American children, especially after puberty, were typically taller and heavier.[32]

But while roughly consonant, studies of Chinese anthropometrics also challenged the belief that physical and physiological differences were "truly racial" and not "mainly the accumulated effects of a particular type of nutrition and environment."[33] P. G. Mar of the Henry Lester Institute for Medical Research (Shanghai) obtained the physical measurements of 267 Cantonese schoolboys in Shanghai and then compared their mean heights and weights and nutritional quotients to boys from the British Isle of Ely, sons of Shanghai refugees and factory workers, and Cantonese boys raised outside of China proper (e.g., Hong Kong and Hawaii). While one might naturally expect that Mar's Cantonese schoolboys were taller than those "living in Shanghai under poor nutritional conditions, viz., the refugees and factory workers," they also turned out to be "slightly superior in stature as compared with the British and Chinese standards, and more so when compared with Cantonese from Kwantung and abroad."[34]

Mar stopped short of drawing any definitive conclusions—hoping instead to stimulate "the interest of those who are in a position to collect similar data, on Chinese subjects both here and abroad"—but his hesitancy to attribute his findings to either racial or environmental factors did not dissuade other scientists from forming their own conclusions. The physiologist Wu Xiang (1910–1995), who had been on the faculty of National Central University Medical School in Nanjing, emphatically asserted the importance of environmental and social factors by writing, "Physiological differences [in terms of measurement] can seem similar to the morphological differences emphasized in anthropology. To be sure, physiological difference among races can be explained by genetics, but for the majority of physiological characteristics (*shengli tezheng*), we must look to life habits (*shenghuo xiguan*) and social environment (*shehui huanjing*) to understand their true significance."[35] Diet as one of the foundational yet malleable elements of daily life represented one of the most important factors shaping the expression of the national physique. To address Chinese physical and dispositional inadequacies then, one needed to attend to the Chinese diet and confront directly its primary weakness: the lack of proteins to support proper growth and development.

PROTEINS AND GROWTH

The 1920s and 1930s were exciting and heady decades for nutrition science research in China, much of it focused upon topics pertaining to the quality of one or another aspect of the Chinese diet. In part, Chinese scientific interest in the issue of quality, especially with respect to proteins, reflected recent advances in the global science of nutrition. Western scientific thinking in the late nineteenth century had held that health depended on sufficient energy intake (i.e., the calorie content of the diet); that the three major components of the diet (carbohydrates, fats, and proteins) could replace each other in proportion to their calorific content, although some amount of protein was essential to provide nitrogen; and that different proteins had equivalent nutritive values. More sophisticated animal feeding experiments revealed that these three suppositions did not hold, and as yet unidentified dietary components that could not be measured in nitrogen or calories played a vital role in maintaining the condition of normal health.

In 1912 Casimir Funk, a 28-year old Polish chemist, attempted to isolate the factor in rice polishings at London's Lister Institute, and in the process, advanced a new hypothesis that there were at least four organic compounds that must be present in the human diet to prevent beriberi, scurvy, pellagra, and rickets. Each compound, Funk suggested, contained an amine group— hence his denomination of these vital factors as *vitamines*. For the next 30 to 35 years, research devoted to establishing the identity of these new organic nutrients dominated publication lists. Although it soon became clear that not all of these organic nutrients were "amines"—thus the shortening of the term to *vitamins*—the discovery of vitamins rearticulated the parameters of nutrition science research and foregrounded the importance of quality. The idea that one could become sick from ingesting a foreign agent fit with older sensibilities as well as the germ theory of disease, which had consumed the intellectual energies of the international scientific community from the 1880s onward. What "the newer knowledge of nutrition," a coinage of the American biochemist Elmer V. McCollum (1879–1967), demonstrated was that one could become ill and even die as a consequence of the *absence* of certain essential elements.[36] A deficit of a single vital nutrient (micronutrient) could be just as debilitating as carrying a microbe, and for many in the medical community, this constituted an intellectual leap of faith in an opposing direction. That disorders could spring not only from the presence of foreign, noxious agents but also from the absence of something benign contradicted all nineteenth-century medical teaching. In the words of Albert Szent-Györgyi, the Hungarian physiologist who is credited with discovering vitamin C, "A vitamin is a substance you get sick from if you don't eat it."[37]

In light of the major advancements in nutrition science involving vitamins, one might naturally expect a similar locus of generative fascination among Chinese scientists. Investigations of the vitamin profiles of local Chinese foods did emerge as an early topic for research, and while never abandoned, the primary focus of Chinese scientific energy targeted proteins, rather than vitamins, as more critical for evaluating the quality of the Chinese diet.[38] Proteins were a subject of intense intellectual interest, because, as Luo Dengyi explained, "Since Mulder first proposed in 1835 that proteins constituted an essential constituent of organic life and coined the word 'protein' on account of its Greek roots meaning 'of first importance,' nearly a century of research has shown that proteins play a fundamental role in cell reproduction and are essential to one's existence."[39] Mulder's intimations became Justus von Liebig's mantel. Von Liebig (1803–1873), the father of modern nutrition science, crowned protein in the 1840s and 1850s as one of the three foundational elements of human nutrition and celebrated it as a muscle-building substance absolutely necessary for human strength.[40] By the late nineteenth century, investigators of the physiology of nutrition who had worked in the language of quantitative chemistry had expanded von Liebig's original claims and built a broad consensus about the relations between diet, protein, and physical vigor.

Vitamin research, through its implicit invocations of questions of dietary quality, helped spur investigations into the chemical characteristics of proteins and what made some proteins apparently of higher nutritional value than others. Although chemists in the 1830s and 1840s had identified amino acids as the much simpler crystalline products obtained when subjecting proteins to boiling with either strong sulfuric acid or a strong alkali, they could not explain the precise nutritional value of amino acids within one's diet. Evidence from digestibility studies showed that there was a complete breakdown of proteins into amino acids before absorption, yet feeding studies indicated that amino acids could not replace protein. The isolation of tryptophan in 1901 by Sir Frederick Gowland Hopkins at Cambridge University, the subsequent identification of the twelve essential amino acids (i.e., ones that the body cannot synthesize itself and must be supplied in the diet), and an effort to develop standardized methods for assigning reproducible numerical values to different individual proteins consolidated scientific consensus around the idea that the nutritional adequacy of a diet depended upon its proteins and ability to promote growth. By this measure, animal-derived proteins, in contrast to plant-derived proteins, garnered scientific vindication as the more superior proteins for consumption.

In 1928, Wu Xian, working alongside his wife Daisy Yen Wu, a former student of the biochemist Henry C. Sherman, initiated a series of rat experiments on the Chinese diet. Their object of inquiry involved the attempt "to construct a purely vegetarian diet, which when tested with rats is as good as a well balanced mixed diet."[41] Since the diet of the majority of the Chinese people were largely vegetarian, Wu explained, conducting feeding experiments of vegetarian diets on an omnivorous animal like the rat could provide "more conclusive evidence" of the inferiority of vegetarian to mixed diets.[42] Wu and Wu designed a series of diets consisting of a cereal, a legume, and a leafy vegetable that was then fed to four rats, two of each sex, for a period of four weeks. His suspicion that the Chinese diet, with its high proportion of grains, minimal quantities of meat, and lack of dairy, failed to meet modern nutritional requirements had been expressed in 1926 when he gave his lecture, "Chinese Diet in the Light of Modern Knowledge of Nutrition." But to counter the strong cultural and religious sympathy that existed among Chinese laymen and professionals who did not consider vegetarian diets to be inherently inferior, or even the Chinese diet in particular to be demonstrably deficient, Wu and Wu needed to marshal the powers of science.[43]

The importance of the Wus' feeding experiments lay not in their novelty in China or elsewhere. More than a decade prior, the American physiologist James R. Slonaker (1866–1954) and the biochemist Elmer V. McCollum had separately investigated the growth and infant mortality of rats fed vegetarian diets of varying degrees of strictness.[44] The conclusions drawn from these earlier studies varied in degree. Slonaker, who only fed vegetable foods to his rats, concluded that strictly vegetarian diets were unsuitable for the nutrition of an omnivorous animal. McCollum and his different collaborators hesitated to condemn vegetarian diets as ill equipped to satisfactorily nourish "an animal of omnivorous type," but they also expressed serious reservations about how one might achieve "the optimum of well-being with vegetarian diets." Wu doubted his results would deviate much from earlier findings, but in recasting the rat feeding experiments as a scientifically rigorous analysis of the nutritional merits of the Chinese diet, Wu linked what might otherwise be esoteric, laboratory-based discussions of the value of vegetarian diets to the fashioning of a modern China.

What about the Chinese diet so concerned the likes of Wu Xian and his scientific colleagues? Put simply, rats fed a Chinese diet that lacked animal-derived proteins failed to grow as robustly as rats fed a control diet consisting of whole milk powder and whole wheat.[45] "Protein," Wu explained, "is an important constituent of cells. Plants absorb from the air and soil simple inorganic compounds that they turn into proteins. Animals, however, must either rely on plants or eat other animals to obtain the proteins they need. Thus, if food is lacking sufficient or appropriate proteins, the ability of cells to properly grow and the functioning of the body's various organs are both compromised."[46] Wu, alongside his international colleagues, identified the physiological value of protein in its ability to assist and spur human growth—one of the four principle nutritive functions of food.[47] A diet that supplied the necessary substances for growth and repair of the organism, as well as the energy for the production of animal heat and muscular work, achieved the goals of basic nutrition. Foods, contemporary nutritional wisdom maintained, could be further categorized into "energy-bearing" foods (rich in calories) and "protective" foods (rich in minerals, vitamins, and proteins).[48] An adequate diet comprised both types of food, but an optimal diet clearly required more of the latter.

Nutritional investigations of the Chinese diet had revealed an alarming imbalance in these two types of foods. The Chinese diet, with its heavy reliance upon the five grains, provided sufficient coverage in terms of "energy-bearing" foods. Recent studies by Ruth Guy and K. S. Yeh at the First Health Station of the Beiping Municipality; Zheng Ji, Tao Hong, and Zhu Zhanggeng of the Nanjing Biological Research Center (Nanjing Shengwu Yanjiusuo); and Ge Chunlin of the Chemistry Department, Shandong University all provided extensive evidence justifying the conclusion that in terms of numerical value, local Chinese diets could and did afford sufficient caloric coverage that matched or exceeded caloric standards set by mainstream textbooks of chemistry or those propagated by the League of Nations.[49] But in terms of "protective foods," the Chinese diet appeared demonstrably inadequate.

"Protective foods," according to the League of Nations Health Committee, denoted "a foodstuff which is especially rich in those nutrient principles, 'good' protein, vitamins, or minerals, in which the principal foods of any geographic area are deficient."[50] For the United States, milk and leafy vegetables formed the most important protective foods. But as the League of Nations Health Committee observed, what served the role of a protective food in the American context did not necessarily apply elsewhere. "In other regions where the protein content of the diet is either too low or of poor quality (e.g., Asiatic diets consisting chiefly of polished rice or soja bean [soybean], with a small quota of green vegetables), meat would provide a highly valuable protective food."[51]

This gesture of geographical sensitivity was both sincere and yet inconsequential when followed by an explication of the existence of a hierarchy of protective foods. Regardless of the region in question, milk, milk products (including butter), and eggs consistently outranked other protective foods like green-leaf vegetables and fruits. Dairy milk especially was increasingly touted by nutrition scientists as nature's perfect food and was even designated the most important alimentary factor in the rise of modern civilization.[52] McCollum—who has been credited with the discovery of vitamin A, a key agent in enabling growth in animals and humans that he had isolated from the fat of whole milk—insisted that "the consumption of milk and its products forms the greatest factor for the protection of mankind."[53] The normalization of milk-drinking as an integral, if not essential, part of dietary balance and health cast a heavy shadow on diets lacking such an important protective food. The social and cultural consequences of these dietary differences were stark.

Given the heavy preponderance of grains, the absence of milk, and minimal presence of eggs and meat, the Chinese diet appeared imbalanced and regressive in comparison with American and European diets. What the Chinese diet lacked were "good" proteins from protective foods. Chinese nutrition scientists determined that some 95 percent of average Chinese protein intake derived from vegetable sources, with the remaining percentage coming from animal sources. That a diet should obtain protein from a variety of sources was understood and accepted, but nutrition science also increasingly emphasized the importance of protein of "animal origin," which many considered essential to healthy growth.[54]

Social scientific research further corroborated the nutritional concern expressed over Chinese dietary proteins. Tao Menghe, Li Jinghan, and others had described consumption patterns heavily tilted toward grains and flours. In the 1930s, the agronomist J. Lossing Buck (1890–1975) surveyed 3,200 families in 150 different localities in more than three provinces. He and his colleagues consistently found diets in which cereal seeds constituted the bulk of the diet. In Pingding, Shanxi, 97.4 percent of total calories consumed by adult males came from cereal grains (namely, corn), with the remaining calories coming from legume seeds and vegetables. In Ping Tsih (present-day

Pingxiang), Jiangxi, 89.7 percent of calories came from cereal grains (rice), 1.2 percent from legume seeds, 3.0 percent from vegetables oils, 3.2 percent from animal products, and 2.6 percent from vegetables. The case in Huaming, Shandong, differed in that 62.4 percent of total calories consumed by adult males came from cereal seeds. But while the proportion of the diet occupied by grains was significantly less than what was found in Shanxi and Jiangxi, the difference was made up by legume seeds and not animal products. The pattern was clear: the Chinese diet was primarily vegetarian and lacking animal-derived protein. Quoting William H. Adolph, "Taking the country as a whole, . . . with its 400,000,000 of population, and keeping in mind particularly the large agricultural areas of the interior, we have here a very close approximation to a real vegetarian diet on a large scale!"[55]

The physiological value of proteins, while universally recognized, did not translate into obvious prescriptions for how much protein ought to be consumed daily, although the scientific impulse tended toward the high end. Individual scientists like the German physiologist Carl von Voit (1831–1908) and the American chemist Wilbur O. Atwater (1844–1907) established dietary norms in the late nineteenth century, which later became scientific standards, especially with regards to protein. For both men, as well as their colleagues working in the field of labor physiology, the purpose of standards lay in their technical ability to address sociopolitical issues concerning labor and food supply. As the historian Dietrich Milles has suggested, "nutritional knowledge was an early attempt to analyze and combat the consequences of industrialization with scientific instruments."[56] Speaking before an audience composed of people with responsibility for providing food in different kinds of institutions, von Voit recommended a daily per person intake of 118 grams of protein, with at least one-half of the amount coming from animal sources. Interestingly, the human subject von Voit had in mind was not the average man but rather "a physical worker, that is, a necessarily well-muscled person."[57]

By establishing his baseline as a man who could maintain physical work for ten hours per day at a trade such as carpentry or bricklaying, von Voit inextricably linked protein to both physical activity and strength.[58] In his nutritional surveys of American working-class households, Atwater largely accepted von Voit's standards and even modified them upwards to take into account the higher "plane of living" of the people of the United States and their greater quantities of food consumption.[59] The justification for high protein consumption intertwined ideas of physiological need with national and racial fitness and the expression of political might. As Francis G. Benedict (1870–1957), a student of Atwater and director of the Carnegie Nutrition Laboratory, observed in 1906, "Dietary studies made in England, France, Italy, and Russia show that a moderately liberal quantity of protein is demanded by communities occupying leading positions in the world."[60]

The modest amount of scientific pushback against high protein consumption that existed came from the physiologist Russell H. Chittenden (1856–1943), the first director of Yale University's Sheffield School of Science. Although Chittenden's primary research involved the action of different digestive enzymes on food proteins, his acquaintance with Horace Fletcher, a wealthy middle-aged American who attributed his good health to thorough mastication of each mouthful of food (100 chews before swallowing), led the former to investigate in a more systematic fashion reduced intake of protein and its effects upon physical vigor. Chittenden rejected the protein standards set out by von Voit and Atwater as too high, and instead suggested reduced standards along the order of 60 grams.

Chittenden's studies caused a considerable stir in the scientific community, especially as his research could not be easily dismissed.[61] Nonscientist faddists like Horace Fletcher and Dr. John Harvey Kellogg, as well as religious groups like the Seventh-Day Adventists, had also extolled the virtues of low-protein diets, but their claims ran toward the sensational and depended, in the estimation of mainstream scientists and physicians, too much on personal experience and not enough on science. Chittenden's scientific colleagues could not find fault with the quality of his research, and yet accepting his conclusions proved too difficult. Benedict, for example, expressed admiration for Chittenden's research but reiterated the conviction that the proportion of protein in a diet appeared to be one of the determining factors in the productive capacity of a nation: "The negro and the poor white of the South, the Italian laborer of southern Italy, all partake of diets relatively low in protein. That their sociological condition and commercial enterprise are on a par with their diet, no one doubts. . . . Furthermore, it seems clearly established that when people accustomed to a low protein diet are fed on a higher plane, as is the case when the southern Italians come to America, their productive power increases markedly."[62]

Wu Xian shared Benedict's conviction that dietary protein indexed the productive capacity of a nation and its people. In his evaluation of Chittenden's low-protein experiments, Wu highlighted the short period of experimentation as the critical factor diminishing the suggested health benefits of a low-protein diet: "The only weakness of Chittenden's study is the short duration of experimentation, which makes it difficult to take [his results] as the norm. What is suitable [to eat] for a short period of time is not necessarily appropriate for an entire lifetime. In other words, eating a low-protein diet for nine months may not manifest any harm, but over a period of several years, harm may occur to one's general health or lead to obstacles in growth."[63]

Wu's skepticism likely arose from his tendency to apply a diachronic view to Chinese nutrition. His earlier examples of the physical height and vigor of ancient Chinese, in contrast to the smallness and pettiness of his fellow compatriots, rested on the assumption that the Chinese diet was the outgrowth of long-term structural forces and the historical outcome of deep fissures in the country's economic bedrock. Writing in 1932 for the journal *Independent Thought* (Duli pinglun), Wu postulated that in the early history of mankind, humans depended upon hunting for obtaining nourishment. The discovery of fire and cooking transformed life by making even the hardest of grains edible. "In China," Wu wrote, "agriculture developed early, and by the third century, the people's diet already emphasized the five grains. A leisurely survey of the classics shows several references to hunting during this period as well. The land was plentiful and population light, such that the people did not suffer from economic pressures, and food could be obtained at will."[64]

As idyllic as ancient times might sound with its ample land, generous eats, and a sparse population, the development of a sedentary, agriculture-based society was not without its advantages. Hunting culture receded, and in its place arose an agricultural civilization with a booming population. Wu neither celebrated nor disparaged this growth but rather emphasized that with the decline in hunting during the Qin (221–206 BCE) and the Han (206 BCE–220 CE) dynasties, the Chinese diet assumed a more vegetarian nature. The factors facilitating the growth of a major civilization were the same factors leading to a depreciation of the standard of living and greater competition for limited resources. Agriculture had become the foundation of the country (*nong wei bang ben*), and as eating grains constituted a lesser financial burden than eating meat, the people's diet gradually became thoroughly vegetarian. Wu explained, "Eating meat was expensive, whereas eating grains was not. In addition, with the introduction of Buddhism to Chinese society [during the Six Dynasties period, 220–589 CE], its devotees (literally "superstitious followers," *mixin zhi tu*) believed that killing animals was immoral. Although the number of people adhering to the Buddhist practice of abstaining from meat and fish was not great, the idea that vegetarianism was a moral good permeated people's consciousness and definitely influenced the Chinese people's diet."[65]

With respect to the Chinese diet, the protein problem, as Chinese nutrition scientists understood it, was both more subtle and pernicious, because despite the obvious absence of meat and dairy, the Chinese diet seemed to include sufficient quantities of protein. If one only considered gross metrics, for example, the total daily caloric intake or average protein intake, the Chinese diet appeared satisfactory. Wu himself proffered a handy "rule of thumb" for calculating the appropriate amount of dietary proteins: proteins should constitute 10 to 15 percent of one's total caloric intake. For a person who consumes 3,000 calories daily, his diet needs to include between 75 and 112 grams of protein.[66] William H. Adolph's work on North China dietaries estimated an average protein intake of 80 grams per capita per day.[67] Wu Xian and Daisy Wu calculated an average protein intake of 91.7 grams for their Beijing participants.[68] Zhu Zhenjun examined the diets of Shanghai families in the winter of 1931 and found an average daily intake of 86.6 grams of protein (in summer months, an average of 85.8 grams).[69] The average body weight of the adult Chinese male was 55 kilograms. With the standard protein requirement determined as one gram per kilo of weight, one might reasonably reach the conclusion that the Chinese diet afforded sufficient protein coverage. One would, however, be mistaken.

If growth was the precondition for a people's productive power, then laboratory-controlled experimentation that yielded poor growth analogically explained the physical and dispositional problems pervasive in Chinese society. In Wu's vegetarian feeding experiments, he and his wife consistently found subnormal growth among the laboratory rats. They had devised a number of cereal-legume-vegetable combinations simulating the Chinese diet as the basal ration: the cereals used were wheat, rice, corn, sorghum, and millet; the legume of choice was soybean, since it was commonly used in China; and for vegetables, they selected spinach, cabbage, and *xiao baicai*, which Wu translated as "small cabbage."[70] With spinach as the primary vegetable, the rats developed signs of rickets (i.e., a chalky appearance, a curved shape to the teeth) and growth at about half the normal rate.[71] Cabbage produced similar results, which led Wu to discontinue the trials in favor of another vegetable. The only exception involved *xiao baicai*, which he and his collaborator had introduced to the rats that had previously been consuming cabbage. The transformation was shocking. "To our surprise, all the rats, which were growing at approximately half the normal rate, suddenly began to make great gains in weight." Signs of rickets disappeared. Wu initiated four series of experiments with *xiao baicai* as the primary vegetable, and the results confirmed "the conclusion already reached." Rats grew at comparable, even better, growth rates than stock rats. They evinced no signs of abnormality, and their fertility appeared normal. The only hitch with this surprising series of results emerged with the second-generation rats, which were "undersized." The unexpectedly promising results associated with *xiao baicai* led Wu and Wu to experiment with other local vegetables like *youcai* (*Brassica chinensis* L.), *gaicai* (*Brassica* sp.), *ganlan cai* (*B. oleracia* L.), and *jiecai* (*B. juncea* Coss.), although none of these achieved the same growth curves as *xiaobai cai*.

An inadequate diet in light of modern scientific knowledge, as Wu and others were quick to point out, yielded deficiencies in one or more of the four essential factors: calories, proteins, vitamins, and minerals. Though the Chinese diet was heavily tilted toward one food group (grains), Chinese nutrition research nonetheless failed to unearth obvious deficiencies in any of the four dietary factors. This raised the possibility that by some unanticipated measure, the Chinese diet might actually have been adequate. But Chinese nutrition scientists insisted that this could not be. "An adequate diet may be defined as one which assures uninterrupted growth to the full adult size, high fertility, low infant mortality, perfection of teeth and skeleton, resistance to infection, and maximum span of life possible for the species. A diet which is adequate for growth may not be adequate for reproduction or conducive to long life, but one which fails to support normal growth certainly cannot be regarded as an adequate diet."[72] Such a definition ensured that individual examples and suggestions to the contrary could be reintegrated into the fold of a larger narrative of national deficiency.

To recognize the inadequacy of the Chinese diet, one needed to see the diachronic implications laden in synchronic snapshots. "Experiments with animals have shown that, when the diet is not markedly deficient in any one of the dietary factors, the animals do not develop any well defined disease. Their appearance remains such that they could have been regarded by [any-one] to be normal."[73] But lest one jump to the conclusion of the apparent health or healthfulness of the Chinese diet, Wu cautioned against rash celebration. Appearances can be deceiving. "Their fertility may not be decreased, but infant mortality is high. Growth is slow, body weight is below normal, and the size diminished from generation to generation."[74] In other words, a population raised on a nutritionally inadequate diet may continue to increase in total size, but its constituent members increasingly manifested signs of regression and even devolution. He emphasized that "conditions like this must exist among human beings. . . . And it is this lowered vitality and increased mortality among the human beings caused by improperly constituted diets, rather than deficiency diseases with marked symptoms, which are the real menace to public health."[75] Wu concluded his findings by stressing, "We may thus conclude that we know of no vegetarian diet at present which would afford optimum nutrition for an omnivorous animal, the albino rat. Since the metabolism of the rat has been shown to be very similar to that of the human being who for many thousands of years has been also omnivorous, it seems justifiable to conclude that optimum nutrition of human being [sic] cannot be obtained with purely vegetarian diets."[76]

By predicating the inadequacy of the Chinese diet upon its being vegetarian, Chinese nutrition scientists endeavored to alert the Chinese people of the menace in their midst. The very foods they ate unthinkingly and by custom endangered the nation's ability to achieve wealth and power. At best, the Chinese diet was a diet of subsistence and maintenance, but what was needed was one of health or optimum metabolism and growth.[77]

CONCLUSION

By drawing upon modern science to demonstrate the social and scientific problem that was the Chinese diet, Chinese scientists claimed for themselves the moral and political authority that derived from science's epistemological authority as a privileged way of knowing—one, it was believed, that provided the correct path to true knowledge, which was impartial, objective, verifiable, and universally applicable. The Chinese diet in biochemical terms could be assessed and critiqued. It could be compared with other national diets, and it could serve as a gauge by which to evaluate China's standing within an emerging capitalist world order that fetishized qualities like efficiency and productivity. But once translated into calories, carbohydrates, proteins, and fats, the Chinese diet also emerged as a technical problem that the Chinese themselves were best equipped to solve.

The inadequacy of the Chinese diet was a technical problem, requiring a technical solution, and in this sense, soybean research yielded possible solutions, because the soybean was fungible and adaptive to the nutritional demands of a modern diet scaled for optimality. Although clearly plant derived, soybean proteins could nonetheless serve a critical role in improving local dietaries and aiding growth. Wu Xian, for one, encouraged the increased consumption of leguminous plants and tofu for the general populace on account of their availability and positive nutritional profiles, although he demurred about the long-term prospects of such consumption. In terms of nutritional research, Zheng Ji highlighted both the urgency and practical benefits of further research on plant proteins. In a country like China, whose poor economic conditions necessitated dietary reliance on plants and legumes, Zheng insisted that it behooved Chinese researchers to advance scientific understanding of the nutritional value of plant proteins, especially those found in soybeans and grains.[78] How to pair or combine foods for maximal nutritional coverage, identifying nutritional equivalences between plant and animal proteins, and investigating vegetable oils and their nutritive function in local diets indicated pathways by which a more rational and scientific approach to the Chinese diet could yield positive effects and uplift the population.

Thus, one way in which Chinese nutrition scientists deployed nutrition science so as to articulate forms of political action involved redefining the debate about poorer-quality proteins in terms of energy-bearing carbohydrates and legume (especially soy) proteins. As research progressed through the 1930s, Chinese nutrition scientists increasingly shifted their attention to the crucial importance of total daily caloric intake in securing minimum health and to promoting soy proteins as viable alternatives to the absence or deficiency of animal-derived proteins. They played an especially prominent role in rethinking the value and importance of child growth and the use of soybean milk as a healthy, hygienic substitute for cow's milk for infants and children.

CHAPTER 4

Which Milk?

Soybean Milk for Growth and Development

I N the early twentieth century, milk became important to how Chinese intellectuals and scientists thought about China and its place within a wider world. Although dairy products and processes had been continually introduced and reintroduced during earlier historical periods, milk represented otherness, in light of its connection to the nomadic and seminomadic peoples living in Central Asia and along the northern borders of the empire.[1] Milk was mainly considered a medicine or tonic for the elderly, and sometimes the young, and when discussed in culinary treatises, milk was typically integrated into the cooking process—fermented, curdled, or cooked—as opposed to consumed raw or fresh.[2] Even after the birth of a nascent dairy industry in several Chinese treaty-port cities, such as Shanghai, Harbin, and Beijing, from the mid-nineteenth century onward, milk remained largely peripheral to the Chinese worldview. But as European and American conceptions of milk shifted over the course of the nineteenth century, and more and more Westerners came to drink and consider milk an indispensable food, so too were the Chinese increasingly confronted with ideas of milk's essential goodness, its place in a scientific world order of modern nutrition, and its role in making healthy, strong bodies. Earlier notions of otherness were not so much eclipsed as reoriented as milk became a symbol of Western wealth and power.

The idea of milk's importance to the modern Chinese pursuit of wealth and power generated its own discursive and material experimentations with milk alternatives. Almost as soon as the Chinese found themselves faced with presentations that identified milk as the foundation of a modern diet that fueled the success of modern nations, they began exploring other possibilities that better suited China and the Chinese people. Spurred by the propagation of a nutritional paradigm that identified dairy as an essential food category in the human diet and milk in particular as a critical protective food whose consumption ensured both individual and national fitness, Chinese entrepreneurs and scientists in the 1910s and 1920s began experimenting with ways in which to refashion a common food, *doujiang*, which could be consumed alone but more often served as an essential ingredient in the making of tofu. Through the efforts of men such as the anarchist Li Shizeng and the pediatric physician Ernest Tso, *doujiang* was reinvented and discursively constructed as a healthy, more hygienic, technologically sophisticated alternative for cow's milk.[3] Similar in color and rich in nutrients, soybean milk could be made to signify China's own indigenous contribution to the global pursuit of greater nutritional health.

As milk drinking became increasingly construed as integral to a normative diet, not drinking milk became a problem whose tidy resolution marked a first step in creating and nourishing a modern China. By the 1930s, milk drinking became linked to concerns about child growth and development. Drawing upon developmentalist thinking in which the child became the repository of developmental aspirations and whose ascent to adulthood functioned as the physiological manifestation of China's own developmental path, Chinese nutrition scientists and other nutritional activists positioned the figure of the child as the primary recipient of their reforms. The struggle to identify practical fixes for rectifying the Chinese diet became a struggle to save the health and vigor of the Chinese child, whose poor nutritional health was evidenced by the smallness of his stature. Nutrition and medical scientists targeted customary practices associated with infant and child feeding for reform and reevaluated the sorts of foods deemed appropriate for growth and development.

For many, the soybean, as a protein-packed, locally sourced food that could be adapted to serve the needs of growing children, offered a glimmer of hope for China's nutritional quandary. Economical, amenable to scientific engineering, and more easily digestible, the soybean, especially in the form of soybean milk, articulated a Chinese path of development whose merits aligned with the nutritional needs of a modern nation. Much of the advocacy in favor of soybean milk was premised upon the idea that it was a distinctly Chinese food whose functional role in the Chinese diet was akin to that of dairy. Whether or not this was in fact true mattered less than the implicit challenge to the bioculturalist assumptions of universality embedded in the celebration of milk.

The Milky Way

Scientific interest in milk and its chemical properties arose in the nineteenth century when scientists in Germany, France, and England, using newly developed techniques of analytical chemistry in the laboratory, began investigating the chemical composition of foods, body fluids, and tissues. In 1827 the English physician William Prout (1785–1850) identified three elemental units of human sustenance—"the *saccharine*, the *oily*, and the *albuminous*"—that constituted the building blocks of flesh, bones, and human energy. Later chemists modified the terminology of this classification of ultimate foodstuffs: *carbohydrates*, coined in 1844 by Carl Schmidt and covering sugars and starches; *fats*; and *protein*, that is, substances that, like the white of an egg, coagulate on heating.[4] Milk, human and bovine, was one of the foods that contained all three elements. Prout extolled milk as both a universal and providential form of nourishment. "Of all the evidences of design in the whole order of nature," he argued, "milk affords one of the most unequivocal." He continued, "It is the only aliment designed and prepared by nature expressly as food; and it is the *only material* throughout the range of organization that is so prepared. In milk, therefore, we should expect to find a model of what an alimentary substance ought to be—a kind of prototype, as it were, of nutritious materials in general."[5]

Prout's celebration of the powers of milk traveled across the Atlantic and deeply impressed Robert Milham Hartley (1796–1881), a religiously inspired temperance and social reformer in New York City and first director of the New York Association for Improving the Condition of the Poor. Hartley was keen on improving the supply of milk for infants of the poor. The growth of American cities had led to a decline in breastfeeding, and mothers, especially among the well-to-do, turned to cow's milk as an alternative to wet-nursing. But the most commonly available milk came in the form of cheap "swill milk" produced by cows fed on the by-products of urban breweries. Hartley decried the use of "swill milk" as a dangerous product and expended considerable effort demonstrating the moral and physical dangers of consuming such milk. His campaign to rid New York City of its swill milk system and replace it with "pure" country milk brought into the city by rail was coupled with the fervent conviction that milk was an intrinsically desirable, God-given food for humanity that was also "the most perfect of all alimentary aliments."[6] Hartley's bête noire was the swill milk system, not milk per se. Indeed, his objective was "to reunite the city public with its biblical fresh milk drinking legacy."[7]

Hartley's voluble celebration of milk as the perfect food for everyone befitted his role as a milk reformer but largely overstated milk's place within American diets in the first decade of the twentieth century. Initially, at least, milk reformers were mobilizing to increase the consumption of milk among a select population, namely infants, and later the infirm. Although widely used as a kitchen ingredient, consumption of milk as a beverage, especially in American cities, remained low. It was not until after World War I, at least in the United States and Britain, that milk came to be seen as a good food for everyone; in part, this shift reflected how the discovery of vitamins and other micronutrients radically altered the way Western scientists understood diet and nutrition. In seeking to understand the function of vitamins, scientists like Elmer V. McCollum and F. G. Hopkins found that milk, when added to inadequate feedings of purified substances, seemed to impart quite miraculous growth effects upon laboratory animals. American farmers had witnessed similar effects when they added milk supplements to their livestock feed. Prout's earlier demonstration of milk's unique standing—it offered the dietary trinity of carbohydrate, protein, and fat—was vindicated to different effect with the discovery of milk's vitamin-bearing properties. In McCollum's words, "the composition of milk is such that when used in combination with other food-stuffs of either animal or vegetable origin, it corrects their dietary deficiencies."[8]

Milk's elevated nutritional status also raised its profile among American practitioners of the emerging field of pediatrics, who argued that milk could prevent childhood deficiency diseases. Medicalization of infant care had begun prior to the turn of the century, as American physicians became increasingly involved in determining the root causes of infant mortality. Many medical writers and research-oriented physicians attributed high infant mortality rates to improper feeding and food, and although breast milk was generally believed to be the best infant food, most physicians doubted the existence of "the ideal breast milk" and instead encouraged women to use alternatives.[9] Cow's milk was touted as the best and most available alternative. As one prominent American pediatrician asserted, "The fact cannot be challenged that for children under two, other than those breast fed, cow's milk is an absolute necessity if disease and death are to be kept within bounds and if the coming generation is to survive and is to sustain national standards."[10]

Praised as nature's perfect food, dairy milk was even designated the most important alimentary factor in the rise of modern civilization. McCollum, who had identified the substance in the fat of whole milk that acted as the key agent in enabling growth in animals and humans (vitamin A), insisted that milk and related products were essential, if not the best, protective foods, whose presence or absence within local diets predicted social, cultural, and scientific achievement.[11] Writing in 1918, McCollum suggested that the world's people could be divided into those whose diets included milk and those that did not. On the one side, "represented by the Chinese, Japanese, and the people of the Tropics, generally," were people who "employed the leaves of plants as almost their sole protective food. They likewise eat eggs and these serve to correct their diet." On the other were the peoples of North America and Europe who have "likewise made use of the leaves of plants, but in lesser degree, and have, in addition, derived a considerable part of their food supply from milk and its products." The social and cultural consequences of these dietary differences were dramatic. "Those people who have employed the leaf of the plant as their sole protective food are characterized by small stature, relatively short span of life, high infant mortality, and by contended adherence to the employment of the simple mechanical inventions of their forefathers. The peoples who have made liberal use of milk as a food, have, in contrast, attained greater size, greater longevity, and have been much more successful in the rearing of their young. They have been more aggressive than the non-milk using people, and have achieved much greater advancement in literature, science, and art."[12]

McCollum's celebration of milk and his rhetoric that causally linked together Western political and economic success, body size, and dairy culture might have been dismissed as one man's fancy were it not for its general acceptance in the scientific community.[13] Based on the lectures McCollum gave at the Harvard School of Public Health in 1918, *The Newer Knowledge of Nutrition*, which celebrated the "gospel of milk," sold fourteen thousand copies in its first three years and went into five editions by 1939.[14] Popular and widely read, *The Newer Knowledge of Nutrition* sacralized the milk-intensive

Yankee/Northern European diet for a general audience inside and outside of the United States and, as the sociologist E. Melanie Dupuis has shown, canonized a politics of purity in which one particular diet was promoted as perfect and healthy, while all others (i.e., racial, ethnic, and regional ways of eating) were denigrated as indigestible and evidence of degeneracy.[15]

As a ranking member of the League of Nation nutrition committee, McCollum occupied a position that conveyed his influence in a variety of ways. His unequivocal affirmation of milk as an essential component of a good diet was evident in the League's 1936 *Final Report*, which defined "correct nutrition" on the basis of "good" proteins (i.e., those of animal origin) and protective foods. Milk was among the highest-ranked protective foods on account of its "good" proteins, minerals, and vitamins (A, B, C, and D).[16] In cross-national investigations of nutritional adequacy conducted by League of Nations experts, "superior health" was often attributed to the consumption of milk, as represented by, for example, the African Maasai and Indian Sikhs.[17]

Such transformations to the importance of milk in a healthy, modern diet did not escape Chinese attention. Milk advertisements began to appear in Chinese journals and magazines such as the *Ladies' Journal* (Funü zazhi) and *Shenbao* in the 1910s. By the 1930s, popular representations of milk as both modern and scientific abounded.[18] Between 1927 and 1937, an average of one milk advertisement could be found on the pages of each daily edition of *Shenbao*.[19] Milk's association with geopolitical wealth and power and its repositioning as a kind of nutritional wonder food that could prevent disease and promote growth appealed to Chinese reformers who sought to restore China by destroying traditional forms and patterns and rebuilding it according to Western models. Family reformers such as the Shanghai dairy entrepreneur You Huaigao (1889–?), elaborated a vision of the modern nuclear family that reimagined its role in the production of the Chinese nation. You's conception of the *xiao jiating* (literally, small household) emphasized the family's economic productivities and intertwined the consumption of material goods with the pursuit of intellectual and spiritual cultivation. He argued that the nation could be strengthened through the family's rational exercise of consumption, and among the various commercial goods he encouraged his readers to adopt was milk, whose nourishing properties would ensure the proper development of healthy, strong Chinese babies.[20]

You's suggestion that a healthy nation depended on healthy children resonated with contemporary readers, because it spoke directly to contemporary social and political fears about Chinese weakness. Growing concern about the kinds and qualities of proteins in the Chinese diet—and how such proteins (or the lack thereof) debilitated Chinese bodies—became increasingly intertwined with the idea that children have different nutritional needs from adults and hence require a different diet.[21] This emphasis on children and their nutritional needs unfolded amid an unprecedented explosion of discourse and political activity for and about children, childhood, and child development. New academic disciplines (child psychology and educational psychology) emerged and worked to instill new ideas about the science of age development into school curriculums.[22] New organizations dedicated to child welfare and promoting child health and education cropped up in urban areas. The National Child Welfare Association of China (Zhonghua Ciyou Xiehui), for example, which was established in 1928, operated a series of programs, which included welfare homes, nurseries, and child sanitariums in Shanghai and Nanjing; the publication of a monthly magazine, *Modern Parents*, and a series of books on proper methods of child disciplining and parent training; and radio broadcasts of lectures on child welfare.[23] Scientific and practical knowledge about the nature of children and childhood development circulated to an eager and engaged reading public.

Fascination with the figure of the child also permeated cultural criticism and literary discourse, especially between the advent of the New Culture Movement in 1917 and the outbreak of full-scale war with Japan in 1937. Whether in the form of new literary and musical works for Chinese children or the development of mass-market magazines like *Children's World* and *Little Friend*, discursive interest in the child fueled the burgeoning Shanghai culture industry. That the figure of the child should come to generate such intellectual activity depended on a particular sort of mirage, which the historian Andrew F. Jones has called "an immaculate conception of history," in which the child is figured as an agent of national redemption.[24] For its part, the Nationalist government sought to capitalize on popular enthusiasm by inaugurating a National Children's Day in 1932.[25]

For Chinese nutrition science, the child occupied a position of singular importance, because of its physiological enactment of the process of transformation. Children, in contrast to adults, occupied a stage of continuous growth (*fayu*) and development (*fazhan*). "All of a child's vital functions depend on the transformation and oxidation of nutrients (i.e., proteins, carbohydrates, fats, vitamins, and minerals). In order to insure complete growth, normal development, and the proper use of these vital functions (*shenghuo jineng*), there must be enough fuel (*ranliao*) to make up for that which is expended and advance tissue reproduction."[26] As many commentators noted, children did not just live (*shenghuo*), they grew (*shengzhang*).[27] "When a child is growing, his skeleton, muscles, and even his various organs are changing from small to big, short to tall. At no point can the child do without the nutrition obtained from food that ensures robust and flourishing vitality."[28] Good nutrition enabled a child's body to fulfill certain essential tasks: build tissue; generate energy (*jingli*): replace used-up, worn-out components; and regulate vital functions.[29] It ensured that growth unfolded unimpeded and to its greatest potential.

Poor nutrition, which directly affected growth, scarred a child and imperiled her future abilities to navigate and succeed in a social Darwinian world:[30] "If a child does not get enough food, then he lacks the essential raw materials (*yuanliao*) [for growth]. . . . Growth becomes sluggish. A child's growth and development becomes delayed; his nutritional health compromised; and not only does his physical well-being suffer, his various organs will lose their natural capabilities and become susceptible to disease."[31] This concern for how nutrition shapes a child's growth can be seen in closer detail in the differentiation between the physiological functions associated with protein digestion in children and adults. "A child can assimilate (*tonghua*) large amounts of amino acids, because his body is growing. An adult assimilates amino acids for the purpose of metabolism (*xinchen daixie*); a child for the purpose of development (*fada shenti*)."[32] The different physiological functions achieved by proteins in adults and children meant that the latter needed more. According to one popular nutrition piece, "During childhood, growth is especially fast, and children need proteins to make new cells. Thus a child's daily protein needs per kilo of body weight are higher than an adult's."[33]

Speaking of the proteins in the Chinese diet, Wu Xian stressed that what might prove serviceable for an adult would, for a child, "inhibit her ability to grow fully or optimally."[34] Chinese scientific nutritional reasoning pivoted on the idea that for an adult, since protein needs were determinate, anything more was largely wasted (*wangfei*) and expelled in the form of urine. That which the stomach did not digest and the kidneys did not convert to urine became fat. Physiologically, such wastage did not occur in children, who benefited from more proteins obtained from foods like cow's milk, *douzhi* (fermented mung bean drink), meat, and eggs.[35] As one prominent educator explained, "Many Chinese people think that child nutrition and adult nutrition are the same, but [what they don't understand] is that an adult has completed his growth and has developed an appropriate capability for storage and self-protection, such that instances of poor nutrition do not lead to maladies. A child is not the same. Abnormal nutrition renders it more difficult for a child to maintain his healthy disposition, because his body quickly exhausts the available nutrients and requires more to replenish and rebuild what's been used up."[36] In other words, while adults needed nutrition for maintenance purposes, children needed nutrition for growth and development.[37]

What did a well-nourished child look like? A well-nourished child was rosy in complexion and vivacious in character. His body grew normally—his weight always in balance with and appropriate to his age. In contrast, a malnourished child possessed a sallow complexion, a stuffed-up nose, and flaccid skin. Listless and easily startled, the child (and his weight) never matched expected norms. He was unable to endure hard work and was physically weak. Chinese layman and specialist writers who promoted the importance of scientific nutrition, and especially child nutrition, repeated this litany with understated relish.[38] Chen Bangjian (1889–1976), a student of the famed polymath Ding Fubao (1874–1952) and prolific scholar of the history of medicine, distilled the lessons of good nutrition to a series of bullet points: children needed protein to grow, and protein of certain types (e.g., eggs, cow's milk, beef, soybeans, and corn) was especially advantageous.[39] As the future guardians of the Chinese nation, children represented both seeds of happiness and vectors of destruction.

The discourse of child development as a kind of microscopic figuration of national development dominated the growing body of popular science literature on child nutrition. The child, or so the popular refrain upheld, was the seed of the future. "The child is the primary factor of mankind, and mankind's happiness rests upon the child's body."[40] As a microcosm of a larger collective (i.e., the Chinese people, or *minzu*), children represented both mutability and potentiality. Their presence signified a commonly shared past as well as the potential for development and improvement. "School-age children are our nation's most important [form of] property (*caichan*)."[41] Such property required nurture and investment to ensure appropriate growth, because the linkage between children and nation lay in children's future responsibility as the nation's adults. "In a situation in which China represents the 'sick man' of Asia, if we want to revitalize the Chinese nation (*fuxing zhonghua minzu*) and revive national power (*guoshi*), it is even more imperative that we earnestly work [on the problem of child nutrition], because national rejuvenation (*fuxing minzu*) depends on a health citizenry, and without healthy children, how can there be a healthy nation?"[42]

Child development predetermined national development by recasting the physiological processes of growth and development as naturally occurring steps in the production of the nation's workers. Good nutrition began during childhood, and as children were a nation's future adults, the industrialization and economical development of the country depended upon strong and able workers who were not persistently plagued with illness and disease. At the physiological level, poor nutrition depleted the body's reserves of potential energy (*chuxuli*). Without sources for replenishment, the body became increasingly weak and feeble.[43] Because growth was seen as a continuous process connecting child bodies to their adult forms, what happened in childhood necessarily impacted one's future course. In the words of one nutrition educator, "Nutrition strongly influences a person's choice of work, most commonly in the sense that malnutrition can lead to an occupational disease. Children, as the future's adults, must contribute their bodies to society by taking on work and standing on their own two feet."[44] The problems resulting from poor child nutrition appeared in two forms: high mortality even before children reached working age, and high susceptibility to occupational diseases. In the latter case, Chinese writers endeavored to illuminate for their readers the close association between certain forms of work and specific diseases wrought by poor nutrition: factory work and tuberculosis; lead industry and lead poisoning; sugar industry and loss of teeth and stomach problems; ceramics and digestive problems; distilleries and paralysis, loss of memory, and a weak heart.[45] The reasoning, however specious, indicated that proper nutrition could prevent or forestall such debilitating conditions from occurring.

A VEGETAL SOLUTION

How nutrition scientists answered the question of what proper nutrition for children entailed depended on how the researchers framed the long-term objectives of growth and development. For physicians and chemists of missionary background—men such as John Hammond and William H. Adolph—investigations of Chinese standards of health and their relation to diet tended to elicit gentle surprise and admiration of the unintended yet surprisingly durable ways in which Chinese obtained health. Although handicapped by a variety of environmental factors, including overpopulation, limited food resources, and poor hygiene, the Chinese, they believed, nonetheless managed to exhibit signs of health in keeping with their economic environment.

In 1925, John Hammond, a pediatrician working in the Peking Union Medical College's Department of Medicine, published a report with his collaborator, Hsia Sheng, on the physical measurements and diets of ninety-six Chinese boys living in the School for Poor Children in Beijing, many of whom were orphans or waifs from famine areas of Zhili and Hunan.[46] In their attempts to determine the normal growth standards of the Chinese child and the specific role played by "the food factor" in the development of such standards, Hammond and Sheng compared their measurements with growth curves taken from children of various summer schools in Beijing and corresponding curves for American boys.[47] They identified regular disparities in growth curves for Chinese boys living in the School for Poor Children when compared with their American counterparts as well as the wealthier children at Beijing summer schools, that is, consistently lower weights and smaller statures.

When they evaluated the diets actually consumed, they found similarly stark differences.[48] Largely composed of corn meal and wheat *mantous* (steamed buns)—the specific quantity eaten depending on the age of the boy and ranging from four to twelve at each meal—a smattering of vegetables (i.e., Chinese turnip, eggplant, and white pumpkin) in the morning and the evening, and bowls of millet or wheat gruel, the Chinese diet yielded a total daily caloric intake that was half the amount of American children, with moderately low protein and fat consumption and high intake levels of carbohydrates. They consumed no milk, butter, or eggs. Even fruit lacked a place within the diets of these poor boys.

And yet, for Hammond and Sheng, these differences did not indicate a poorer state of health so much as a path of evolutionary development that harmonized the human body to the prevailing social conditions. "We have here, apparently, a large population which must be rationed in the most economical manner. . . . We believe that it is possible that the Chinese have developed a diet, in an evolutionary manner, which embodies great economy, and which gives a maximum result for a minimum intake."[49] The results of such evolutionary adaptations were physical bodies free of fat and the excesses of modern development. They were smaller than their American counterparts, but not necessarily less healthy. Indeed, one of the more unexpected discoveries broached in their study involved the "surprisingly fine condition" of the Chinese boys' mouths, mucous membranes, tonsils, glands, and teeth. Despite the generally dismal, dirty appearance of the boys' teeth, Hammond and Sheng found few cavities and, shockingly, "perfectly white enamel underneath" the "peculiar yellow coat" on their teeth.[50] "[The Chinese] seem to have 'cleared for action,' to have trimmed themselves down to a physique suitable to the economic environment."[51] Such findings indicated the possibility that what constituted the Chinese "normal" and the American "normal" occupied different planes.

Hammond and Sheng's conclusion resonated with observations Adolph had also made about the nutritional value of the Chinese diet. The longevity of Chinese civilization had led to a kind of unintentional and blind form of experimentation. The Chinese did not knowingly discover the principles behind food economics and nutrition science, and yet through centuries of trial and error, they had managed to adopt practices that achieved outcomes in adherence with these various principles. Adolph noted approvingly how the Chinese seemed to implicitly understand the attendant "transformer loss" of raising meat. It was thus only natural for the Chinese to conclude that cereal grains were most economically employed directly as human food.[52] The Chinese preference for pork was explained in light of what modern science had proven, namely, that an acre of ground in the form of pasturage produced two pounds of pork for every pound of beef or mutton. According to Adolph, "The laws of economics have dictated far more of the actions of the Oriental than we realize."[53]

These unintentional "discoveries" resulting from blind experimentation—"that guiding angel of the Orient"—had enabled China to achieve a state of stable equilibrium. Despite having a diet low in dairy and meat, the Chinese had developed alternatives to meet the basic nutritional need for protein and vitamins. Shen Nong, the Chinese farmer-dietician, "thousands of years ago, chose to develop and retain in his agricultural repertoire just that one variety [of the soybean] which contained the highest percentage of protein, and also the highest percentage of fat"—and thereby made up for the lack of meat in China through legumes. Nutrition science had determined that wheat protein and rice protein were incomplete proteins and therefore suggested combining different flours to achieve a more effective nutritional balance. For the Chinese living within vicinity of Beijing, combining corn meal and soybean meal was a long-standing practice and generally regarded as producing a more nourishing food than wheat alone.[54] Vitamins too, though not consciously theorized and understood by the Chinese, were nonetheless addressed by dietary habit through the regular incorporation of green vegetables, spinach, and cabbage. In a jocular tone, Adolph retorted, "And we of the Occident, having just discovered vitamins, are now busy haranguing our housewives and urging greens in the diet—and often with ill success."[55]

As impressive as it was that China had achieved a "finely balanced solution to her food supply problem," it was ultimately not enough. What struck Hammond and Adolph as positive forms of nutritional subsistence bode ill for progressive-minded Chinese intellectuals intent upon transformation and uplift. A modern nation, as opposed to an aging civilization, however finely tuned, required "growth and vigor."[56] The goal of nutrition, Wu Xian and other Chinese nutrition scientists insisted, was "the optimum and not the minimum." In Wu Xian's words, "While the minimum of the essentials of life suffices to maintain and propagate the race after a fashion, it is only the optimum which makes progress."[57] Like a child whose optimal growth and development depended upon sound nutrition, so too the Chinese nation required more than blind forms of evolutionary adaptations wrought from centuries of trial and error. In this respect, Chinese scientists offered a more proactive approach for addressing China's nutritional needs.

Social and scientific concern over the nexus of relations linking nutrition, growth, and children converged in the debate over infant feeding.[58] Chinese medical physicians, researchers, and public health educators underscored the social imperative of "the problem of caring for infants" (yuying wenti) for the development of the nation, and their efforts to encourage new or more scientifically informed practices of care constituted an important subset of a broader debate concerning the role of women in the emergence of a new China. Reformers drew from a wide variety of sources, including republican motherhood campaigns in colonial America, Japanese "good wife, wise mother" (liangqi xianmu) language, as well as fascist German and Italian pro-motherhood arguments.

The Nationalist government after 1927 seized upon popular discourse for its own purposes and promoted the idea of a "Republican" mother (guomin zhi mu), who was "an informed citizen who transmitted her well-grounded opinions to her children, educating her sons and daughters to lead patriotic and virtuous lives."[59] The Nationalist ideal of healthy, educated mothers producing citizens of sound mind and body was featured prominently throughout popular media, even as it never succeeded in obtaining complete consensus—calls for women to eschew, or at least delay, reproduction in favor of joining the workforce remained a vital component of this public debate. Nevertheless, public and private conversations on the importance of maternal and infant health helped advance an idealized form of modern reproduction for Republican mothers that drew on the appeal of contemporary eugenics and science.[60]

The soybean provided a possible solution to the "problem of caring for infants." The idea that cow's milk nurtured both strong nations and strong children had been popularized in China by the 1930s, but most Chinese had little, if any, access to the drink. The availability of fresh cow's milk was limited by geographic and economic factors. Large-scale dairying in several Chinese cities like Harbin, Beijing, and Shanghai emerged after foreigners began settling in treaty ports from the mid-nineteenth century onward. Shanghai, where dairying developed most extensively, accounted for almost half of total Chinese milk production in the 1930s.[61] The nascent dairy industry, nurtured and developed by a group of enterprising, foreign-educated Chinese businessmen in Shanghai, nonetheless experienced significant difficulties associated with sanitation, transportation, and the high cost to the consumer.[62] However limited the actual scale of operations may have been, the idea that cow's milk represented Western modernity and science enjoyed disproportionate influence. Drinking cow's milk was universally recognized as a Western practice alien to the Chinese but whose adoption could signal China's conscientious striving for success in the evolutionary struggle to survive.[63]

But as B. S. Platt, an associate researcher in the Division of Clinical Research of the Henry Lester Institute of Medical Research (Shanghai) stated, "The facilities afforded in China at the present time for introducing such substitutes for human milk are so limited that no useful purpose can be served by extended discussion."[64] Indeed, when researchers fanned out from their laboratories to investigate local feeding practices, they identified zero instances in which fresh cow's milk was used for infant feeding and only six instances out of 422 case histories where imported milk powder was employed.[65] In Platt's evaluation, any attempt to improve the dietary health of a community must evolve from existing practices, and in China, dairying required "too much land to be a practical measure." Furthermore, "the

Chinese cannot, in general, afford to buy imported preparations of [cow's] milk."[66]

Without a national dairy industry and lacking economical ways to obtain imported milk products, nutrition reformers focused on soybean milk as a locally available and affordable alternative to cow's milk that could nonetheless achieve comparable physiological results. Ernest Tso (Zhu Shenzhi), who was the first researcher in China to study the application of soybean milk for the purposes of infant feeding, framed the significance of his research in terms of long-term growth prospects and the extent to which nondairy diets satisfied the nutritional prerequisites of Chinese children.[67] Tso invoked the authority of Elmer V. McCollum and repeated McCollum's assessment that "the diet of China, Japan, and other countries in which the same general habits prevail [i.e., a lack of cow's milk] is not suited for the proper nutrition of young children."[68] In McCollum's original words, "The final goal is to strive to discover whether any dietary regimen in use by man best promotes his vitality to the maximum. There is good reason to believe that the Oriental diet of the type under discussion, is at best but a second-rate one, and that it is not capable of meeting the needs of a growing child except in special cases where the most fortunate selection of articles is made. It does not, in general, support vigorous health and stimulate effort to an advanced age."[69]

By citing McCollum, Tso seemed to suggest that the absence of cow's milk in the Chinese diet posed serious problems to child growth and development. He insisted that the not-uncommon situations in which "a mother's milk fails" or "the family cannot afford either the employment of a wet-nurse or artificial feeding with cow's milk" raised serious concerns about what kind of nutrition Chinese infants were getting, if at all.[70] With neither breast milk nor cow's milk, Chinese infants faced severe and potentially life-altering challenges that delimited the extent to which they could mature into robust, vigorous adults. Thus, from both an economic and a physiological standpoint, Tso argued, investigating the growth effects of a soybean milk diet on young infants warranted attention.

Scientific interest in soybean milk as infant food did not arise out of an attempt by the Chinese scientific community to also demonstrate the nutritional inadequacy of mother's milk.[71] The extent to which Chinese mothers during the 1920s shifted away from breastfeeding to artificial feeding methods is difficult to determine. Greater female participation in the burgeoning urban and industrial workforce may have decreased breastfeeding rates, although further research remains to be done to substantiate this point. At

the very least, Chinese medical emphasis on the importance of breastfeeding may have functioned as a defense mechanism to stem the actual or perceived tide of women forgoing breastfeeding for alternative methods. It may
also have reflected the medical community's concern for the impracticality
of cow's milk as an infant food in China, given the limited extent of dairying and the prohibitive costs associated with buying fresh and canned milk.[72]

Throughout the 1920s and 1930s, popular and specialist journals printed
column after column urging mothers to breastfeed their babies.[73] Medical
experts emphasized the nutritional importance of breast milk to infant
growth and development. Many physicians argued that breast milk was the
best prophylactic against diarrheal diseases and the best nourishment for
the superior growth and development—mentally and physically—of the
infant child, and for building resistance to infection.[74] As one "Young & Old"
explained, "Mother's milk is suitable for infant digestion. It is neither too
thick nor does it cause diarrhea. There's no other food as exquisite and
healthy in the world that can beat mother's milk."[75] Popular press pieces in
support of breast milk emphasized the economic extravagance, as well as the
questionable cleanliness, of tinned cow's milk. They characterized breast
milk as the natural product of motherly affection—a form of nourishment
that benefited both the infant and the mother.[76] Some even drew on the rhetoric of the National Goods Movement (Guohuo Yundong) and attempted
to translate breast milk into "national goods" (guohuo), consumption of which
aided China's economic independence.[77]

For situations in which a woman has been chronically ill or unable to produce breast milk, the popular press provided instructions on how to introduce and provide artificial milk (rengong yingyangfa).[78] The more common
practice prior to the twentieth century was to employ a wet nurse. To this end,
classical medical authors expended considerable effort in detailing the
importance of obtaining a wet nurse with the right sorts of physical qualities and character attributes. The emphasis on artificial milks, be they from
an animal or plant, was a part of the larger project of modern motherhood
that re-rendered "natural" acts as transparent acts (i.e., descriptions and
images of how gestation and birth actually occur), guarded the nuclear family
against interlopers (e.g., wet nurses), and overlaid female reproduction with
responsibilities to the nation-state.

To guide women in their selection of which artificial milk to choose,
advice, which arrived in translation from foreign experts such as Japanese
physician Dr. Hirota Tsukasa (1859–1928) and American public health activist

Dr. S. Josephine Baker (1873–1945), characterized fresh cow's milk as the best nutriment to serve as an alternative to breast milk, because of the former's nutritional advantages.[79] "Cow's milk has exceptional nutritional value, because it contains lots of proteins and fats."[80] It could be served in the morning or for a snack, and so long as the original animal source had been determined to be free of disease, cow's milk provided all the nourishment growing infants needed.[81] In a similar fashion to Japan, popular prescriptions tended to organize one's options into a hierarchy of milks, with cow's milk (i.e., tinned milk) dominating the list as the best alternative in cases in which the mother could not breastfeed her infant.[82] Tso's research on soybean milk should be seen as an example of economic pragmatism through the language of nutrition science.[83]

Chinese investigation into the nutritional benefits of the soybean aimed to recast a local foodstuff as a scientific food. Clinical researchers associated with the Peking Union Medical College (PUMC), Yenching University, and later the Henry Lester Institute of Medical Research in Shanghai, examined not only the chemical composition of soymilk and other soy-derived products but also their place in local diets and their effects on growth and development. Much of the experimental work utilized laboratory animals (rats and guinea pigs) as test subjects, but even as early as 1927, Tso had already begun investigating the physiological effects of a soybean milk diet on an infant six weeks of age. He carried out his examination and observation for eight months on Baby Yao, who had been born in the PUMC Hospital on August 27, 1926. Because the growth record of the child during the testing period compared favorably with "the average development of breastfed infants," Tso concluded that a diet mainly of soybean milk, "properly supplemented, . . . can be more or less comparable to cow's milk in nutritive properties."[84]

Tso's research marked the beginning of a series of medical attempts in China to apprehend practical solutions to the problem of infant feeding. Researchers investigated the concentration of vitamins B_1 and B_2, the bone-building potency of soybean diets, protein digestibility, and nutritional differences associated with soybean milk made from roasted soybeans instead of the usual wet-grinding method.[85] They experimented with different soybean milk formulas to determine greater nutritional optimality. Soybean milk for infant feeding was a practical alternative, although not necessarily a perfect one. In at least one experimental feeding trial, the results of the soybean milk preparation, which included fresh egg yolk, produced tragic results that ultimately led to the deaths of the two infants involved.[86] Most medical soybean research from the late 1920s through the late 1930s, however, did not result in such tragedy. Instead, the primary focus lay in performing chemical assays comparing the nutritive properties of soybean milk and cow's milk and running experiments on animal subjects.

Tso's research on the positive growth effects of a soybean milk diet for infants quickly reached urban audiences. Within a year, Chinese reprints and summaries of his work had appeared in public health and medical journals. In 1933, the bimonthly *Kwang Chi Medical Journal* (Guangji yikan), edited by Ruan Qiyu (1891–1946), reported that the city government of Nanjing had implemented a trial program to distribute soybean milk to infants to combat malnutrition. Initiated on National Day (October 10, 1933), the program had been designed to provide poor families with a nutritious and affordable infant food that had been properly and scientifically produced. "Many of the city's infants suffer from poor nutrition. Infant nutriments like cow's milk and milk powder are too expensive," the organizers lamented. In 1935, the pediatrician Su Zufei cited Tso's research in her recommendation that soybean milk could solve the pervasive threat of undernutrition that haunted Chinese children. "Our standard of living is so low that [if faced with the following situations, that is,] low supplies of cow's milk, insufficient breast milk, or recently weaned children, there's always a fear of undernutrition." Legumes, Su continued, were full of nutrients, and this fact was well understood by the general public. So long as soybean milk was scientifically produced to yield "4.4% of protein, 1.8% of fat, and 9.5% of water-carbon," its benefits for infant nutrition were proven.[87] At a price point significantly cheaper than cow's milk (a tenth as much!), soybean milk was affordable for middle-class and poor households. As further support for the value of soybean milk to infant nutrition, Su highlighted the decision by the Beiping Health Demonstration Station to use soybean milk in its infant feeding programs.[88]

That such nutritional benefits could be derived at lower expenditures was touted as one of soybean milk's advantages as an alternative to cow's milk. But its advantages were not limited to cost. A young female dietician writing for *Women's Youth* (Funü qingnian) in 1934 also highlighted the fact that soybean milk did not curdle or congeal in the stomach, as cow's milk was thought to do. In other words, soybean milk was more easily digestible—an argument that had also been advanced by an earlier generation of Chinese proponents for modern vegetarianism.[89] In this case, soybean milk's greater digestibility was especially important, as an infant's stomach was vulnerable during its first year of life, so the easier it was to digest, the greater the influence it would have on proper growth and development.[90]

Not only was soybean milk more digestible, it was, some argued, more hygienic because it was specially bottled and delivered to one's home.[91] Although an observant commentator could minimize this apparent advantage by pointing out that cow's milk was also bottled and delivered, medical proponents of soybean milk for infants highlighted two additional distinguishing features: first, because soybean milk came from a plant, one need not fear contamination or illness resulting from a sick cow's milk production, and second, one could easily produce soybean milk at home, thereby circumventing concerns about poor packaging or mishandling.[92] By providing an affordable but also accessible alternative for cow's milk in infant feeding, soybean milk promised the nutritional advantages of cow's milk in a more digestible form. Its goodness derived as much from its nutritional profile as from its low cost and sanitary properties—all of which is to say that soybean milk was deemed a modern good food for growing the Chinese body. In the words of Wen Zhongjie, writing for *Science Collectanea* (Kexue congkan), "One can little hardly believe that soybean milk has all that we need nutritionally and is so affordable. If we Chinese can use it regularly, then the less well-off can still obtain good foods and infants without mother's milk can still obtain proper nutrients (*zhengdang zhi yangliao*); they need not worry about [not] building a strong body or a robust race (*jianshen qiangzhong*)."[93]

CONCLUSION

By the early twentieth century, the Western scientific community had come to extoll the virtues of milk as an integral component of human nutrition, nature's perfect food, and later an essential protective food whose presence in local dietaries could serve as the alimentary benchmark for determining the rise of modern civilization. Nations could be ranked according to what they ate, and without milk, the likelihood of such a nation rising to the ranks of the progressive few was small. Without milk, as chemists like Elmer V. McCollum explained, such nations suffered from poor physiques, shortened lives, high infant mortality, and stunted literature, science, and art. To be without milk was to be excluded from human progress and modern civilization.

This message of dietary destiny and the importance of the "power cuisines" of nineteenth-century imperialist nations informed the mindset and activities of nutrition scientists and physicians like Ernest Tso, who internalized the modernist demand for milk but attempted to subvert its universalizing reach by querying which milk.[94] That the cow should be the primary or sole benefactor of such nutritional and civilizational goodness seemed to contravene the wealth and diversity of China's own experiences. That the world over might esteem cow's milk and its products did not, in and of itself, necessitate that the Chinese too should do the same. If anything, modern science and the language of biochemistry testified to the power of alternatives like soybean milk to achieve the same ends. With the proper engineering, the goodness of cow's milk could also be found in soybean milk.

By the late 1920s, the importance of soybean milk as a Chinese alternative to cow's milk grew in significance alongside growing concern for Chinese infant and child health. Ernest Tso framed the quest to improve infant and child health as an economic and social problem for which soybean milk was uniquely advantaged to solve. As a local customary food and by-product of the tofu-making process, soybean milk was both more available and more affordable than cow's milk. With medical research undertaken to confirm its nutritive properties and positive influence on child growth and development, medical proponents of soybean milk also characterized the drink as more digestible for infant stomachs and hygienic for its association with modern bottling and distribution. That soybean milk could also be made at home suggested a degree of control and security not otherwise available with fresh or tinned cow's milk. The importance of milk and its alternatives for Chinese intellectuals and scientists from the 1910s through the 1930s delineated a broader concern for how China ought to develop and its place within a global community of modern nations. For them, "got milk" may have been the prerequisite for modern progress, but "which milk" represented the more pivotal concern.

CHAPTER 5

Doujiang as Milk

Hybrid Modernity in Soybean Milk Advertisements

I N autumn 1934, inspectors from the Food, Dairies, and Markets Division
of the Public Health Department of the Shanghai Municipal Council (SMC)
began touring Chinese soybean milk manufacturers in Shanghai. They visited local facilities and inspected the grounds and equipment. They collected
advertisements, and they took samples for the purpose of conducting bacte-
riological and nutritional analyses. Their subsequent reports revealed a fluid
landscape in which customary practices blended into new experimental ventures that brought the material trappings of modern industry. "Nearly all
bean curd shops," the inspectors observed, "make this liquid [i.e., soybean
milk, or "bean curd milk"] as a side line, and have been doing so for many
years."[1] Food stalls were also known to sell soybean milk. But for reasons
unclear to the inspectors themselves, a crop of "proper" manufacturers of
soybean milk, that is, those set up with the express purpose of making and
selling only soybean milk, had taken root in Shanghai's commercial landscape. Although significantly fewer in number than tofu shops and food
stalls, inspectors identified at least fifteen manufacturers whose operations were located in or near the borders of the International Settlement.[2]

What struck SMC inspectors as a sudden burst of commercial soybean
milk production was more like the crest of a wave that had broken upon settlement soil and thereby attracted Western attention. Chinese observers would
not have been so surprised. Throughout the 1920s and 1930s, a veritable

groundswell of interest had arisen around soybean milk and its economic and nutritional advantages. Scientific concern for the Chinese diet and the growth and advancement constraints it imposed on the Chinese people, especially the young, had sparked a lively debate about ways in which to reform the Chinese diet. Scientists, educators, and public health advocates argued about everything from the merits of cooking techniques (and their impact on nutritional values) and increasing meat consumption to the right or best sorts of plant proteins and practical ways to improve infant and child nutrition. A vital thread linking these topics was the conviction that certain foods could achieve multiple goals in multiple registers. Soybean milk represented one such food. With proper attention and scientific management, the development of commercial soybean milk articulated a path forward—a path resplendent in nutritional virtue and economic strength.

As a result of rhetorical strategies that commercial vendors and soybean milk proponents pursued to make soybean milk attractive to a discerning Chinese public, soybean milk came to represent a form of modernity that could be imbibed. Starting in the early twentieth century, Chinese nutrition scientists and physicians began experimenting with ways in which to refashion a common food, *doujiang*, into a modern good food that we know as soybean milk (*douru* or *dounai*). Their efforts were spurred by the development of industrial food production and the propagation of a nutritional paradigm that identified dairy as an essential food category in the human diet and milk, in particular, as a critical protective food whose consumption ensured both individual and national fitness. Nutrition scientists in and outside of China increasingly construed milk drinking as integral to a normative diet. Not drinking milk became a problem whose tidy resolution marked a first step toward creating and nourishing a modern China.

Despite the best attempts of Chinese nutrition scientists, this refashioning of *doujiang* involved combining elements from China and the West to produce a polyphonic, hybrid modernity. Commercial purveyors of soybean milk marketed it as a scientific, hygienic foodstuff that bridged traditional and modern values. Using the language of classical Chinese medicine and allusions to Daoist pursuits of longevity to describe their product, they also highlighted the modern conveniences of standardized and sanitized glass packaging and bottle caps. Through their packaging and advertisements, commercial soybean milk companies promoted—in indirect, and sometimes contradictory forms—cutting-edge vernacular knowledge about scientific nutrition that mixed old and new. In the case of *doujiang*, macro- and micronutrients became key players alongside older dietetic ideas about digestion and seasonality.

The hybridity exhibited in soybean milk advertisements did not, however, disguise the differential power relations between the various elements employed. All things traditional and modern were not equal, and over time, the language of Chinese medicine and Daoist longevity diminished in prominence, while claims of science and scientific nationalism became more robust. The gradual eclipse was never complete, but by the early 1940s, advertisements increasingly foregrounded children as the proper subjects for the consumption of modern soybean milk and science as the definitive measure for both the social and commercial value of the product.

Advertising for the Modern Consumer

Ephemeral yet dialectical advertising images speak to both the immediacy of a past time as well as a longing for the future. Chinese advertising from the Republican period enables contemporary historians to consider "society" or "the social," as theorized at the time, as the essential ingredient to modernity.[3] The advertising image, like other dialectical images, is not referential, because advertisements do not simply represent existing social forms. Instead, they enact conditions in which possibilities for how we imagine and understand modern society endure. Advertising serves as the material content by which a new social theory of personhood, society, and modern conduct were put into play for the Chinese consuming public.

An immanent critique of commercial advertisements for soybean milk uncovers a similar logic in which a form of neotraditionalism is cast as modernism.[4] But rather than expressing an imagined world of elite everyday life in which homosocial relationships between gentlemen (*junzi*) are registered in terms of hobbies and connoisseurship—as was the case for New York–brand cigarettes—soybean milk advertisements invoked the language of Daoist body cultivation and redeployed it alongside and in combination with scientific nutritional ideas. Individual striving for a finer and subtler energetic configuration of the body, the pursuit of longevity, and Chinese medical ideas for fortifying the body and preventing disease became, in the hands of the advertisers, natural companions to a biochemical interpretation of food and eating. Moreover, such claims of fortitude and life-nourishing advantages were materially supported by the cutting-edge packaging and distribution system set up to ensure that the eager consumer had a fresh and steady supply each morning.

The Beneficial Soybean Milk Company (Youyi Douru Gongsi), which operated out of a factory on Tatung Road (present-day Xinqian Road) in Zhabei, placed half-page ads for its natural (*tianran*), life-nourishing (*yang-sheng*) soybean milk. Sold throughout Chinese neighborhoods in the International Settlement, Beneficial Soybean milk presented itself as the lodestar for longevity and a kind of medical panacea for fortifying the body against disease.[5] Casting forth a kindly tale of hope and generation with a proactive moral, the advertisement begins its narration, "All people hope for a long life, but we have never heard of one who didn't first study the arts of 'nourishing life' and yet lived to an old age. The path of 'nourishing life' is not initiated when sick." To begin caring for the body at its moment of distress was both foolhardy and ill-timed. Foresight and studious cultivation of nourishing life were much more effective strategies for caring for one's body and extending life. Resonant with one of the household maxims by the Ming neo-Confucianist Zhu Bolu (1627–1698), studying self-preservation was like "repair[ing] the house before it rains" and not waiting until "one is thirsty to build a well." Indeed, Confucius himself, as the advertisement reminds us, recognized the value of mindful, preventive practice when he said, "A man who does not think far ahead must soon confront more immediate worries."[6]

To cultivate one's *jing qi shen*, foresight and active preparation in the service of disease prevention and longevity were essential. On this matter, the advertisement did not equivocate. Qi is the foundational energy of the universe, the life force of the human body, the basis of all physical vitality, and the very stuff of the Dao. But to achieve longevity, one who nourishes life must transform the gross material experienced every day to higher-level, more subtle energy networks. *Jing*, which is the most tangible and strongest of the various kinds and levels of qi in the body, is central to any discussion of ideas of health and illness. In its dominant form, *jing* is sexual potency—semen in men and menstrual blood in women—and its loss was seen as a source of qi loss that could cause physical weakness, lead to disease, and precipitate early death. But even without massive *jing* depletion caused by unforeseen circumstances, a body's vital essence naturally diminishes over a lifetime. Its rise and decline essentially defines human life. Moderation and economy became the watchwords for regulating and slowing this natural process of decline, keeping the *jing* within the body, and reversing the downward movement of qi.

Because one's qi is in constant exchange with the outside world—breath, food, drink, physical contact, sexuality, emotions, and so on—taking care to align one's qi, to keep it proper and flowing smoothly, serves as the basis by which to deter or forestall wayward, heteropathic, misaligned, off-track, and harmful qi. Learning how to keep one's qi harmonious and right is difficult, but the rewards include greater qi refinement and circulation to subtler and more cosmic levels. Qi that has transformed into the finest internal energies and that flows with the vibrational frequency as the gods themselves is *shen* (spirit). People who have increasingly transformed their qi into spirit are more like spirits, gods, and the immortals. Drinking Beneficial Soybean milk would not immediately bestow such rewards, but as the advertisement nonetheless insisted, intensive study of everyday foods and their medical efficacies was the best way to achieve longevity. To this end, Beneficial Soybean milk, which had been assiduously investigated and shown to possess a variety of efficacies, could serve as part of a regular regimen for nourishing life.

Although Beneficial Soybean did not include references to the seasonality associated with drinking soybean milk, other purveyors did. Nourishing Life Soybean Milk Company (Shengsheng Douru Gongsi) labeled its drink an "autumn supplementing product" (*qiuji bupin*). Federal Soybean Milk Company (Fada'er Dounai Gongsi) encouraged wintertime drinking of its "winter supplementing product" (*dongji bupin*). Minor differences aside, these modern soybean milk companies positioned their goods as vital food products whose benefits correlated with the seasons.

Although the advertisement does not mention Chen Yingning (1880–1969), who was one of Republican China's most influential theoreticians and a practitioner of the Daoist self-cultivation practice known as "inner alchemy" (*neidan*), its characterization of the proper dietary relationship one ought have is strongly reminiscent of modern Daoist appropriation and synthesis of scientific nutrition. For Chen and other modern Daoist practitioners, an improper diet disturbed the qi equilibrium of the body. Placing stress on the appropriate ingestion of necessary nutrients (*yingyang*), Chen drew on scientific theories of nutrition. Carbohydrates (*tanshui huahewu*), proteins (*danbaizhi*), and fats (*zhi fang*) constituted the three essential nutritional components for a modern practitioner's diet. To maximize the qi-nourishing power of different foods, a practitioner should be attentive to a number of factors, including freshness, proper preparation, the practitioner's own physical constitution, and its interaction with the nutritional makeup and properties of the food ingested. Modern Daoist dietary regimes blended scientific nutrition with ideas and categories from Daoist dietetics, traditional herbalism, and Chinese medicine. As the historian Liu Xun has persuasively argued, Chen "integrated his knowledge of modern theories of nutrition with his erudition in Daoist dietetics. Modern theories of food and nutrition were adopted as means of understanding and interpreting the traditional categories of food properties for a modern audience."[7]

Soybean milk, while not a specific food advanced by Chen Yingning in his recommended dietary regimens, nonetheless capitalized on the modern Daoist synthesis of scientific nutrition and the art of cultivating life. In this sense, Beneficial Soybean milk represented a wonderful amalgam of tradition and modernity. Having set forth a general framework for seeking longevity and health, the advertisement for it proceeded to highlight the biochemical value of soybeans: "Soybeans are rich in nutrients, sweet in taste, mild in nature, and full of proteins, as much as 35%, surpassing all other plant foods."[8] The Good Fortune and Health Soybean Milk Company, which largely replicated the text used in the Beneficial Soybean Milk advertisement, indicated that its product contained as much as 35 percent protein. The makers of Glycine Soybean Compound (Gainaisheng) claimed its product possessed vitamins A, B, C, D, and G, as well as carbohydrates, fats, protein, phosphorus, iron, and sodium.

This focus on the protein-richness of soybeans had become a regular refrain in media invocations of soybeans in the 1930s. As discussed in chapter 4, medical experts like Ernest Tso (Zhu Shenzhi) and Hou Xiangchuan celebrated the soybean for its potential to spur growth in China's young. But their interest was directed fixedly toward the biochemical properties of soybeans and rooted in their interests and training in Western medicine. In contrast, popular advertisements like those issued by the Beneficial Soybean Milk Company embedded biochemical properties in a broader matrix of apparently complementary knowledge systems. That soybeans possessed 35 percent more protein than other plant foods was simply further demonstration, by other means, of the inherent value of the plant for nurturing life. As the advertiser indicated with appropriate humility, this discovery of the soybean's biochemical advantages constituted a natural extension originating from discipline and cultivation of life. "My humble self has devoted considerable attention to selecting the best soybeans whose essence is combined with wheat essence to make soybean milk that would satisfy the requirements of a 'nurturing life' (yangsheng) expert."[9]

Lest the reader continue to hesitate about the value of soybean milk, the advertisement emphasized that drinking Beneficial Soybean milk would "supplement the brain and calm the liver, benefit the marrow and moisten the lungs, stimulate essence and enrich yin, nourish blood and drain fire, normalize qi and moisten the throat, disperse phlegm and promote elimination, quicken the pulse and moisten skin."[10] The list, expansive and generous, provided the reader with an assortment of therapeutic actions from which to choose—too many to be in keeping with genuine medical expertise, and yet technical enough for the reader to recognize its purported medical efficacy.[11] The claims made by the Beneficial Soybean Milk Company were not unduly extravagant, although the combination of actions may indicate a degree of creativity on the part of the advertiser. Another commercial purveyor, the Nourishing Life Soybean Milk Company (Shengsheng Douru Gongsi), emphasized soybean's lack of "floating heat" (wu fu huo). A piece published in 1930 in Commonsense Drugs (Yiyao changshi bao), a weekly journal that covered Chinese medicine and drugs, characterized soybean milk as cooling in nature and endowed with the propensity to "drain fire" (xiehuo).[12] In cases in which a person suffered from urinary incontinence or cloudy urine, soybean milk possessed contrasting efficacies comparable to other popular formularies involving ginkgo seeds (baiguo yanfu), which could help prevent urinary incontinence, or the "six-one dispersal" infusion (liu yi san chong fu), which promoted urination and drains heat.[13] Soybean milk was also recommended for cases involving yin depletion.[14]

This deliberate mixing of old and new, Daoist with Chinese and Western medicines constituted an important feature of soybean milk advertisements in the 1930s, and it reflected patterns other scholars have identified as constituent to Chinese media culture. The visual and textual strategies adopted by soybean milk companies were the same as those seen in medical advertisements.[15] The foreignness conveyed by glass bottles, bicycle delivery, and industrial-style hygiene via pasteurization were offset by more Chinese images and references to supplementing the brain and draining fire. The Good Fortune and Health Soybean Milk advertisement featured an image of what must be Shouxing, the god of longevity (figure 5.1). Dressed in long robes and carrying a long cane with a carved bird at one end and a gourd hanging from the top, Shouxing represents not only the aspiration for long life but also the very vision of fulsome jingqi (seminal essence). His forehead literally swells with jingqi. By directly appealing to those among the reading

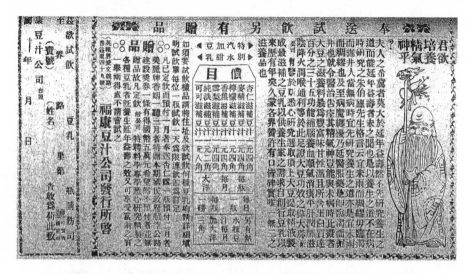

FIGURE 5.1. Shouxing in an advertisement for soybean milk. Folder U1-16-1745, Shanghai Municipal Archives.

audience keen to cultivate their *jingqi*, Good Fortune and Health Soybean Milk cast its product as the ultimate tonic. Produced from the essential essence (*jingye*) of soybeans, soybean milk would nourish and meet the exacting requirements of a Daoist acolyte of "nourishing life" for years to come. What the historian Barbara Mittler has described as "multiplicities in time, space, language, and imagery" as conveyed through the incorporation of foreign objects and images operated in similar fashion for soybean milk advertisements, with their alternating invocations of Daoist longevity, medical balance, and nutritional health.[16]

Advertisers nested the nutritive properties of soybean milk—rich in protein and fats, with various vitamins and minerals to boot—within this broader matrix of life-enhancing and medical benefits. Their espousal of Daoist and Chinese medical efficacies did not prevent them from also incorporating visual and material motifs of more foreign extraction. In certain instances, the foreign elements dominated the advertisement. Federal Soybean created a trademark featuring a nuclear family gathered around a table enjoying the delights of soybean milk (figure 5.2). With the father seated—his elbow casually resting on the table while the other hand holds a glass of soybean milk—the mother pours another glass for a child whose back faces

標 商

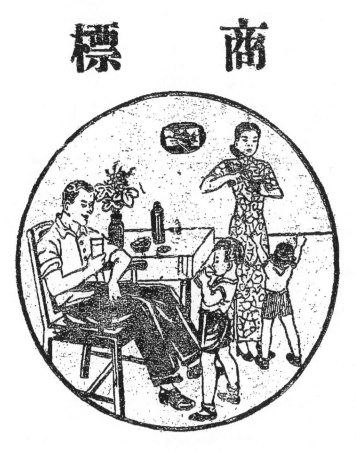

FIGURE 5.2.
Trademark for
Federal Bean Milk
Company. Folder
U1-16-1745, Shanghai
Municipal Archives.

the reader. The other, older child, drinking a glass of soybean milk, stands opposite the father, and on the table one finds a second thermos of soybean milk. Everything from the furniture to the family composition to the clothing suggests an idyllic, hygienic modern lifestyle.

Federal Soybean Milk enacted a scene of modern domesticity that prioritized youthful growth and nourishment, in contrast to the previous invocations of long life. The slogans—"Make the nation powerful and prosperous!" (*wei guo qiangsheng*); "Nourish and strengthen the body!" (*zibu qiangshen*)—called forth a world in which strength and vigor are essential qualities, and the imperative of fortifying young bodies pervades daily life. The overt focus on the specific form of the container (i.e., a thermos) also distinguished Federal Soybean milk as a modern industrial commodity, unlike the local *doujiang* one might purchase from the nearby tofu shop or food stall. The advertisement explained, "We have spared no expense in using the finest quality ingredients. We invited a chemical expert [*huaxue zhuanmen jishi*] to supervise the production of each type of soybean milk. To aid the drinking experience, we have arranged for a custom-designed hot-water bottle made of smelted metal that can be sent out each day. The customer can drink the soybean milk at any time without having to first cook it."

What further separated these manufacturers from the bean curd shops and the food stalls that traditionally sold *doujiang* could be found in the details. Joined by an explicit intention to sell only soybean milk, these companies packaged and delivered their goods for the convenience of their customers. *Doujiang* is most commonly derived as a by-product when making tofu or bean curd. This process involves wet-grinding soybeans to produce a slurry that is then strained. The resulting liquid can be sold separately as *doujiang* or coagulated with gypsum or other coagulants that cause the proteins to precipitate and form a whitish mass that, once strained and pressed, becomes tofu.[17] Leaving off the coagulant step gives one *doufu jiang*, or *doujiang*, but this liquid cannot be immediately consumed without causing indigestion—hence Federal Soybean Milk's reference to cooking soybean milk. It was quite common for *doujiang* and its modern counterpart soybean milk to be sold with the understanding that once home, the consumer would cook the liquid before consumption.

The convenience marketed lay in the packaging. Some companies bottled their milk in beer bottles, mostly green in color and corked at the top. Others used milk bottles with cork stoppers, or "tomato-sauce bottles." Bottles were typically unlabeled, but in a few instances, the manufacturer had conscientiously marked each with text "solely in the Chinese language" detailing the "name of the factory, trade name, and telephone with address," as well as a pithy tagline like "Nourishing food for winter" (*dongji bupin*).[18] Delivery might occur by foot or bicycle "by coolies, each with two baskets on bamboo," who fanned out into Shanghai's various districts early in the morning, roughly from 5 until 8 a.m., to deliver fresh soybean milk by monthly subscription. One could also purchase fresh, hot *doujiang* outside, which would be consumed in situ. But Federal Soybean Milk's innovation, which it foregrounded in the image of a thermos flask, was to transpose the public experience of *doujiang* to one's private, domestic space, within which soybean milk could be enjoyed at one's leisure (figure 5.3).

This decidedly modern spin on a local practice might lead one to assume that such claims about soybean milk's efficacies in draining fire or supplementing the brain, normalizing qi, moistening the lungs, dispersing phlegm, and so on would have no place in Federal Soybean Milk's advertisement. But in fact, Federal Soybean Milk, like its competitors, Beneficial Soybean Milk or Nourishing Life Soybean Milk, stressed the power of its product to moisten the lungs and remove phlegm (*runfei huatan*) and supplement the brain (*bunao*)—all with a fresh and pleasing taste (*xianmei shikou*). Indeed, even with the specially designed thermos and an appeal to bourgeois domesticity, Federal Soybean Milk defined its product as the only, truly nourishing, body-strengthening "nourishing life product" (*yangsheng pin*).

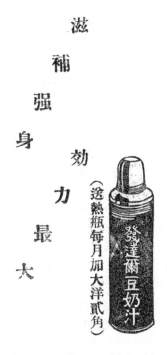

滋
補
強
身 効
力
最
大

（送熱瓶每月加大洋貳角）

發達爾豆奶汁

FIGURE 5.3. Close-up of Federal Bean Milk's thermos with inspiring slogans. Folder U1-16-1745, Shanghai Municipal Archives.

The neotraditionalism evidenced by soybean milk advertisements came in several forms—the emphasis on seasonality, associations with the *yangsheng* tradition and longevity, the purported Chinese medical efficacies—and yet its most distinguishing mark lay in the embrace of multiplicities of time, space, language, and imagery. These seemingly traditional elements were neither radically different nor temporally dislodged from the seemingly more modern characteristics associated with an industrial commodity: economy, bourgeois domesticity, and scientific nutrition. Mixed together and bridging old and new, East and West, soybean milk advertisements represented the power of reinvention and creativity. Consider the palate to which these soybean milk companies appealed. All soybean milk companies produced and sold soybean milk in its original flavor, but several offered soybean milk in flavors such as salty, sweetened, almond, "snow pear" (*xueli*), lemon, banana, orange, and chocolate.[19] Glass bottles, thermoses, and bicycles—all signifiers of Chinese modernity—elevated these soybean milk companies above the common fray of bean curd shops and food stalls. These modern purveyors promised convenience and age-old wisdom, bottled and brewed to achieve cleanliness and sanitation.

THE COW OF CHINA

Manufacturers like Beneficial, Nourishing Life, and Federal knitted together a variety of associations in presenting their soybean milk products as modern. But the extent to which they cast soybean milk as an alternative for cow's milk depended on their identification of the appropriate target: the elderly or the young. For companies like Beneficial Soybean Milk and Nourishing Life Soybean Milk, the primary audience for their milk appears to have been adults, especially those who might be looking for supplements to bolster their aging bodies. Their advertisements did delineate how their products would benefit different groups of people—the elderly (*nianlao zhe*), adults (*zhuangnian*), youths (*qingnian*), and infants (*yinghai*)—but the emphasis was skewed toward the older population. Mothers of frail constitution or whose breast milk was insufficient could feed soybean milk to their infants as a milk replacement. Youths who drank soybean milk would benefit from its brain-nourishing and spirit-raising effects (*bunao zhenjing*).[20] Adults, especially those involved in physical labor or serving the nation (*fuwu shehui*), would benefit from the high protein content. And the elderly—especially those who had not undertaken sufficient preparation in the arts of "nourishing life," whose qi and blood (*qixue*) were weak and degenerate, who suffered from asthma, phlegm-stasis, aching bones, and so forth—would gain the most, when they found that drinking soybean milk pacified the liver, cleared the lungs, made qi smooth, vacated phlegm, strengthened bones and muscles, and rendered skin moist and soft.[21] This list suggests that children were not necessarily the primary targets for these drinks. Even Federal Soybean Milk, with its depiction of family life and the visual inclusion of young children drinking soybean milk in its logo, continued to emphasize the more adult-oriented benefits of soybean milk as a health-bolstering tonic.

By the late 1930s, however, soybean milk advertisements increasingly prioritized children as the primary beneficiaries. This shift in focus occurred within a heightened climate of fear and uncertainty as the prospect of war with Japan shifted from speculation to outright certainty when the refugee crisis that erupted after the Japanese attack on Shanghai in the summer of

1937 created conditions that nurtured a new kind of social activism that made soybean milk a critical component of its nutritional programs for Chinese children (see chapter 6). Soybean milk, nutritional activists argued, offered an indigenous solution that could be mobilized efficaciously and quickly to meet the nutritional needs of refugee children.

The increasing prominence given to children as the principal beneficiaries of soybean milk can also be seen as a popular reflection of a nutritional paradigm that asserts the universality of dairy's importance to all human diets. Nutrition science's celebration of dairy, and cow's milk in particular, knew no geographic constraints, and Chinese scientists joined their international colleagues in promoting the nutritional value of cow's milk for child growth and development.[22] The nutrition scientist Shen Tong (1911–1992), like many of his contemporaries, considered cow's milk the "perfect food" for its provision of the most "complete proteins," that is, all the amino acids one needed for proper growth.[23] Wu Xian argued that however much calcium one might derive from a vegetarian diet, for the growing young, a milk diet was vastly superior for supporting growth and development.[24] Their nutritional colleague Hou Xiangchuan described milk as a superior food that "contains the best type of proteins and is rich in calcium, vitamins A, B, and G, and small amounts of other nutrients."[25] The only thing that milk lacked was iron, but even this lack, as the League of Nations 1936 nutrition report testified, could be recast as a positive trait. "Milk, although itself poor in iron, renders more effective the iron contained in the diet."[26] These qualities, particularly its high concentration of protein, represented the fundamental ingredients that made up Western wealth and power, such that to drink cow's milk served to transmute the mundane experience of eating into a highly politicized act of national well-being.[27] What China lacked in cows could, nonetheless, be made up with science. In the refashioning of *doujiang* as soybean milk, science played the role of fairy godmother.

In 1939, Dr. Harry Chan (Chen Daming) invented a soybean milk formula that he marketed under the name of "Glycine Soybean Compound" (Gainaisheng Yingyangfen). Born in 1893 to Chan Tong Ork, a prominent overseas Chinese merchant based in Victoria, Canada, Dr. Chan was raised and schooled in Canada before returning to China after 1926. A licensed physician who had worked in hospitals in Montreal, Canton, and Shanghai, Dr. Chan developed a multipronged advertising campaign to promote Glycine as the most nutritionally sound, general substitute for cow's milk available on the market. His goal was to popularize soybean milk consumption in order to improve the health of the masses.[28] According to a 1944 biographical entry, which Chan himself likely authored, he and several colleagues undertook a series of experiments in which they devised a new formula for soybean milk that was both tasty and nutritious. With a new formula in hand by 1939, Chan initiated "numerous clinical trials with gratifying results."[29] Armed with scientific evidence and a penchant for self-promotion, Dr. Chan trade-marked "Glycine"—after the soybean's scientific name—and marketed it throughout Shanghai.

To pique public interest and spur sales, Chan responded to inquiries to the "letters to the editor" section and placed several articles in Shanghai news-papers extolling the virtues of soybean milk. The company sent form letters to local physicians recommending its product and produced a multipage pam-phlet detailing at length Glycine's nutritional profile and the various benefits derived from drinking it. Its logo consisted of a cherubic baby, sitting astride, presumably, a tin of Glycine. In Chan's words, "Soybean is a concentrated food and is called the 'Cow of China.'"[30]

This phrase, "cow of China," came directly from Julean Arnold (1875–1946), an American businessman. Born in Sacramento, California, Arnold had been sent to China in 1902 as a student interpreter at the American Legation in Beijing. He worked for the US Consular Service until 1914, when he took up the position of US commercial attaché for China, a position he served in until 1940. A most vocal proponent for the development of a Chinese soybean milk industry, Arnold had developed an interest in Chinese soybeans before he left his government position. His advocacy intensified, however, after 1940, when he began using his extensive network of contacts to generate popular support for soybeans.[31] Arnold was an attentive and dutiful disciple of the task of promoting American trade interests and yet however much he was keen to advance American commerce, he seems to have been sincerely fond of China and the Chinese people. His emphasis was on a kind of business practicality interwoven with idealism. He became, especially in the 1940s, an outspoken proponent for developing the Chinese market so that it served both American and Chinese interests. To this end, Arnold was eager to assist Chinese busi-nessmen and intellectuals in seizing the possibilities before them. When Japan invaded in 1937, Arnold stepped forward and provided both financial and public support for using soybean milk as a form of nutritional relief.[32]

His dedication to the project of economic uplift for the Chinese people manifested itself most vividly in his promotion of the humble soybean, and especially soybean milk. In a land without a developed dairy industry, the "modernization and popularization of the little soybean as the cow of four hundred million of Chinese" was of critical importance. Nutritionally rich and yet affordable, soybean milk symbolized, in commodity form, the country's broader transformation into a modern civilization. In Arnold's words, "The soybean is a Chinese product, owes its origins to China and has had a long history of development in that country. However, it is only within recent years that such a thing as a standardized soybean milk has been made possible. . . . It requires a scientific manner of handling to insure against the introduction of a large amount of water than consistent [sic] with the requirements as food. It also demands [an] appreciation of the importance of dietetics to handle intelligently the addition of ingredients essential to making the solution a substitute for cow's milk."[33]

For both Arnold and Chan, science was the key. Science provided the technical know-how to standardize everyday recipes. Science could rectify any nutritional inadequacies and counteract potential contamination. Moreover, if properly supervised and managed, science ensured that the latest technological developments could be applied to small-scale and local production in a bid to transform such industries into something more expansive and modern. In this sense, Arnold and Chan were retracing a path blazed more than a decade earlier by Li Shizeng and his Parisian soybean foods factory (see chapter 1).

With Glycine, we see science cast front and center as the critical factor separating it from its competitors. Glycine, as its sales pamphlet proclaimed in English, "is the latest food product from scientific laboratories, the result of years of research conducted by nutritional specialists, and pronounced by the medical profession as a practically perfect food—for infants, children, and adults."[34] In Chinese, the emphasis was similarly placed on the involvement of nutritional specialists (yingyang zhuanjia), who had invented a food that satisfied one's vitamin and mineral needs. In addition, because Glycine adhered to a scientific method (kexue fangfa) in its manufacture and packaging, the consumer could rest assured that the product at hand had been sterilized (xiaodu) and was of the highest quality. Scientific engineering was a badge to be worn proudly, and in the case of Glycine, scientific research and validation functioned as the putative foundation upon which the product could present itself as a "complete food," a "vitamin food," a "protective food," and an "ideal food."

A "complete food," the Glycine advertisement explained, was a food that contained all the nutritional elements required for growth and maintenance of body tissues. Proteins, carbohydrates, fats, vitamins, minerals—Glycine had it all! But most importantly, its biochemical makeup enabled one to confidently conclude that Glycine was "more nourishing than cow's milk"—more digestible, less likely to engender allergic reactions, and 100 percent pure, without any risk of diseases like "hoof and mouth disease, dysentery, typhoid, undulant fever, streptococcal infection, etc."[35] If these salubrious effects were not enough, the advertisement added a further enticement: Glycine was less expensive than cow's milk.

Although Glycine also referenced its beneficial qualities for adults (for example, strengthening the body [qiangshen] and helping to maintain a youthful appearance [yangse]), its primary claim of nutritional efficacy was directed toward children. Moreover, in prioritizing children, Glycine recast those older preoccupations about replenishing qi and soybean milk's tonifying effects as part of a linear progression of development. In bold-faced type running vertically as its own subheading, a Glycine advertisement proclaimed, "Children who drink [Glycine] as a substitute for milk powder will grow faster (shengzhang xunsu) and be of a lively/vivacious yet sweet disposition (huopo tianzhen)." Efficacious and rapid growth ensured continuity of health between childhood and adulthood. After all, the advertisement hinted, were not healthy, vigorous adults once healthy, vigorous children?

Glycine's vision of scientific nourishment can also be seen in its instructions for how to feed it to children, especially infants. These instructions invoke a refrain of scientific regularity and order. From one week of age, one should only feed an infant every four hours or so. For example, the advertisement explains, one should prepare Glycine (in a 6:1 ratio of hot water to Glycine powder that has been quickly heated through after mixing) at 6:00 in morning, 10:00 in the morning, 2:00 in the afternoon, 6:00 in the evening, and 11:00 at night. As the child grows, one should add another half teaspoon of Glycine to each preparation. There are other nutritional supplements, the advertisement assures, one can add to a child's diet to gain extra nutritional advantage: cod liver oil, orange juice, and vegetable soup. However one chooses to proceed, the key to determining Glycine's nutritional efficacy involves the child's weight. Weekly weighings will help one determine if a child is gaining a normal amount of weight (about five liang per week). If a child does not achieve this goal, one should simply increase the amount of Glycine used in each preparation. This is, according to the advertisement, "the most scientific and convenient method for feeding [a child]."[36]

Science went hand in hand with wealth and power. To visually communicate this idea, Glycine devised an advertisement composed of serialized images and captions (figure 5.4). Moving from the top left-hand corner down, the images and captions enact a set of causal relationships whose conditionality is reaffirmed by the top-down presentation. If one uses old practices, like wet nurses, then a child will not grow properly. Wet nurses are conduits for poison that harm a child. Their room and board is expensive and therefore not cost-effective. In contrast, new-style parents use Glycine so that their children will be lively, cute, and successful. Highly nutritious—even more so than cow's milk—Glycine is also economical. Smart heads of households know this. While the message, and its derogation of wet nurses, is unsurprising, the selection of images accompanying this message is.[37] Old

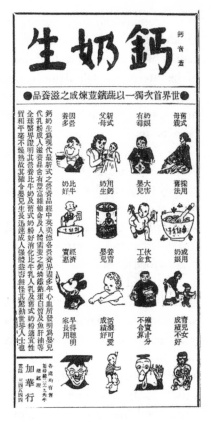

FIGURE 5.4. Glycine advertisement. *Shenbao*, January 14, 1941.

practices are represented through skeletal bodies: the poisonous, emaciated form of the wet nurse whose malevolent influence produces an equally emaciated child. A rice bowl whose contents have attracted a bevy of flies is juxtaposed against the sterility and safety of the Glycine tin. Mickey Mouse designates economic value, while a duck raising his hand (?!) signifies the unfortunate consequences of being fleeced. Even Popeye makes an appearance as the putative champion of greater nutritional value who enjoys drinking a cup of Glycine.

Glycine was not alone in casting itself as the amalgam of modern scientific endeavor. Another soybean milk purveyor, Green Spot Vito-Milk, listed the names of several scientific bodies in and around Shanghai as confirmation of its nutritional merits and of the scientific standards employed in the manufacture of its product. "[Vito-Milk] is manufactured in accordance with the directions and supervisions of the Society for the Advancement of Children Nutrition, the various medical bodies of whole Shanghai [sic], specialists of nutrition of medical research institutes, the Health Department of the International Settlement, and the Health Department of the French Concession." If the list should strike one as suspiciously long, the advertisement assured the public that they had "proper analytical certificates, health permits, and licenses, etc." as proof.[38]

Green Spot's hyperbolic expression of scientific credentials irked J. H. Jordan, the Commissioner of Public Health for the SMC, not because they were entirely fabricated but rather because these claims refashioned the significance of existing institutional measures to regulate food production under SMC jurisdictional authority. As Jordan explained, "It is clearly the duty of a Health Officer when inspecting new enterprises, designed to produce specialized food for the population, to make sure that as far as possible they shall be conducted in a proper fashion."[39] Health inspections of facilities and grounds, as well as the chemical testing of product samples, were part of the institutional routines deemed compulsory for the maintenance of modern public health. Green Spot's reference to scientific bodies like "the Health Department of the International Settlement" reframed perfunctory administrative visitations as hallmarks of scientific evidence for a curious public. This, in Jordan's opinion, was going too far. "To use my inspection visits," Jordan exclaimed," as a means of advertisement is in my view entirely unethical, and something should be done to stop this sort of thing."[40] Jordan's displeasure did not halt Chinese entrepreneurial manipulation of institutional credentials. Indeed, despite the back-and-forth expressions of disappointment and consternation, as well as internal reports chronicling the claims made by "popular science" types like Dr. Chan, soybean milk purveyors like Green Spot continued to blur the lines between fact and fiction, science and tradition.[41]

Conclusion

Throughout the 1930s and 1940s, Chinese soybean milk purveyors appealed to the Chinese public through a mixture of visual and textual tropes that refashioned *doujiang* as soybean milk. But where the earlier advertisements lent equal, if not greater, weight to corporeal efficacies associated with Chinese medicine and Daoist pursuits of longevity, by the 1940s, the scales had shifted. Gone were the visual markers of long life and the extended ruminations of soybean milk's medical efficacy for the pulse or other organ systems. And in their place was found greater emphasis upon the conjugal family (*xiao jiating*), children as the primary recipients, and the language of science and scientism writ large.

Visual advertising evidence does not *illustrate* an already present world; it presents "a world in which precisely the ideology of progress and discovery of society emerge into thinking and into the physical environment."[42] It functions as a dreamscape that enables visualizations of the passions shaping modern social behavior to appear. To drink soybean milk, as the advertisements suggested, was to participate in a larger social order, whose constitution presupposed a shared logic and understanding of ideas about self and society, progress, and a future when China would belong to the family of advanced nations. The visual celebration of science and children evoked a world in which the Chinese could be born anew—raised above the mire of pestilence and profanity that seemed the more conventional order of the day—with a single modification to one's everyday life, a glass of soybean milk.

In the Glycine logo (figure 5.5) composed of bodies in calisthenic assemblages, we can read the logic of progressive time into each character. Moving from the top to the bottom, each character that makes up the Glycine name (gai-nai-sheng) is composed of differently aged bodies in anxious or excited reiterations. The first character, *gai*, which

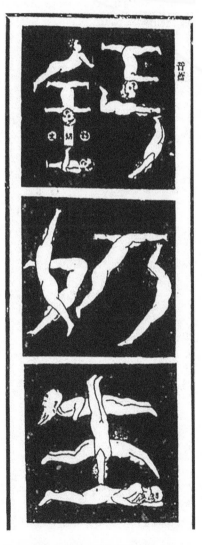

FIGURE 5.5. Close-up of the Glycine logo showing the growing body in calligraphic configurations. *Shenbao*, January 8, 1941.

is the scientific character for the chemical element calcium, consists of child bodies in playful contortion. The second character, *nai*, which designates the breasts and "milk" (be it breast milk or some other typically animal "milk" used in feeding infants), consists of youthful bodies, and the last character, *sheng* (life) comprises elderly bodies whose most distinguishing feature is the long beard. Through these three characters, we can trace the contours of a life cycle from childhood to old age, where the limberness and precocity of youth persists. But we can also map a trajectory that begins with science and the chemical fruits of modern life and culminates in a life emboldened with eternal vitality and vigor. Modern soybean milk, we are allowed to imagine, is a form of liquid life, born in the laboratory yet resplendent in the essential vitalities to sustain aging bodies. Soybean milk as a bodily restorative or a tonic for nourishing has not been replaced so much as repositioned in the temporality of modernity.

CHAPTER 6

The Rise of Scientific Soybean Milk

Nutritional Activism in Times of Crisis

IN the spring of 1938, the English-language periodical *China Quarterly* published a series of photographs depicting the citywide relief work undertaken to deal with the influx of refugees who had poured into Shanghai's foreign settlements since early August 1937.[1] In a bold maneuver to deflect the Japanese from their military campaign in North China, Chiang Kai-shek launched the bulk of his best German-trained divisions against Japanese naval fleets in the Shanghai area. Rumors of the Nationalist attack and the resulting Japanese retaliation sent people living in the rural communities adjacent to Shanghai and in the Chinese-controlled parts of the city desperately scrambling for safety. By the time the Chinese forces began to retreat westward on November 11, 1937, the world's fifth-largest city, which formerly had an estimated population of 3.5 million, was struggling to cope with the human consequences of direct military action. An estimated one million people fled from their homes during the crisis.[2]

The resulting refugee crisis engulfed the city, and the urban landscape of the foreign settlements became a patchwork of makeshift refugee camps with varying degrees of official sanction.[3] Disorder was not, however, the ruling visual imperative of the *China Quarterly* photographs. Instead, we see children, bundled and round with winter layers, standing in line beside a matshed building (a makeshift, box-like structure with mats on the roof); a line of elderly women with their hands folded inside their jacket sleeves, seated before a young woman at a podium; a child lying on a small padded mat out on the sidewalk; young women with the Red Cross emblazoned on the fronts of their long white dresses; and even a delousing station staffed by two men all in white except for the cross stitched upon their shirts.

In showing the kinds of scenes they do, these photographs present the case that the overall organization and administration of relief was guided by a modern, rational sensibility. Refugees stand in queues, medical and relief aid personnel are uniformed in white, and productivity appears to be the guiding discipline in ordering the daily lives of refugees, who are marshaled into school, taught to weave baskets or embroider, and in general kept busy so that time may not be wasted and the old adage that God helps those who help themselves may ring true.

This sensibility is particularly evident in the three photographs depicting children and soybean milk. In terms of objective and sensibility, the initiative undertaken by local elites, Chinese and foreign, to remedy what many perceived to be the hidden cost of war—child malnutrition—was decidedly modern and, perhaps more importantly, self-consciously scientific. The Refugee Children's Nutritional Aid Committee (Shanghai Nanmin Ertong Yingyang Weiyuanhui; henceforth, the Refugee Children's Committee) was unique among the various private and governmental emergency relief initiatives, because it alone did not attempt to provision or provide for the refugees' basic necessities: food, shelter, or clothing. Instead, it spearheaded a program to produce and distribute fortified soybean milk and other nutritional supplements to refugee children. Convinced that the typical refugee diet furnished at the camps was inadequate for the needs of young children, the Refugee Children's Committee members brought together members of Shanghai's professional elite, particularly from the biomedical sciences, and drew upon such expertise to craft a relief program that placed a biomedical conception of nutrition at the heart of its efforts. Their goal was not basic sustenance but rather better nourishment.[4] And to this end, they expended a great deal of effort to come up with a scientifically tested formula for soybean milk and bean residue cakes (douzha bing), which were distributed to an estimated 10,000 to 15,000 refugee children a month between November 1937 and March 1938 (figure 6.1).[5]

What began in 1937 as emergency relief for refugee children transformed into a national initiative for spreading the gospel of soybean and nutritional health. War had served as the initial instigator for the nutritional activist work in Shanghai's numerous refugee camps, but as fighting spread, the

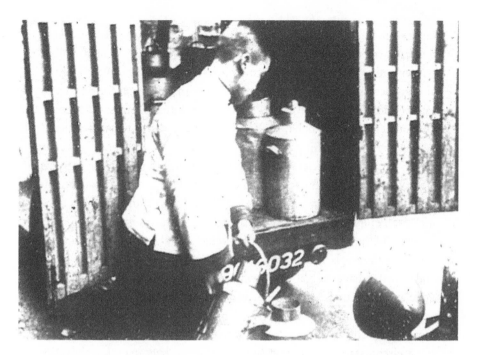

FIGURE 6.1. "A delivery of soya bean milk for a refugee camp." Original caption from *China Quarterly* (Winter 1937–38).

activists involved in the Refugee Children's Committee, and its successor organization, the China Nutritional Aid Council (Zhonghua Yingyang Cujinhui), came to see long-term value in extending the work of nutritional activism into the Chinese hinterland (for more on the China Nutritional Aid Council, see chapter 7). Today, many take for granted nutrition science's integral role in shaping food and diet, but in China during the early twentieth century, the advent of a scientific approach to nutrition as a way to improve the vitality of populations as well as intervene in crisis situations was neither self-evident nor universally accepted by the general public. Efforts to introduce nutritional concepts, for example, calories, vitamins, proteins, and so on, to the broader Chinese public had been piecemeal and unsystematic since the late nineteenth century, but with the Refugee Children's Committee, and later the China Nutritional Aid Council, a more organized and deliberate attempt to educate and transform people's dietary habits arose as a kind of alimentary defense in the face of national crisis.[6]

The soybean was especially important to their work, as it offered an obvious and locally available protein source. Working with local elites, businessmen, and missionaries in and outside occupied areas, Chinese nutrition scientists deployed the soybean as a weapon to combat malnutrition and instill a modern scientific consciousness. Their work was not always successful, but it represented a line of thinking and form of social intervention that we more commonly associate with modernist doctrines of development than the older, but still publicly espoused, tenet of imperial governance of "nourishing the people" (*yangmin*).

The Refugee Children's Committee's soybean milk distribution programs were an important example of a living empirical ideal: a rational, scientifically driven program for both saving the Chinese nation and building up the most vulnerable (in the bodily sense) during a time of great distress. Its selection of the soybean as the primary vehicle for achieving modern nutritional health reveals how nutrition science converged with national interests and helped reshape the history of soybean food patterns in Republican China. Popular understandings of soybean milk were already shifting toward a more child-centered and scientific one (see chapter 5), but with the nation in a state of war, the Refugee Children's Committee was able to capitalize on exceptional circumstances to domesticate this vision of soybean milk as the rational solution for the Chinese diet.

REFUGEE EMERGENCY

Tension between China and Japan had been mounting since the Japanese seizure of Manchuria in 1931. Further encroachments into northeastern China rocked the popular consciousness and provoked major social disruption. Rehe, just north of the Great Wall, fell to the Japanese in early 1933, and by 1935, Japan had assumed control of the northern province of Chahar, west of Rehe. This expansion of Japanese military presence came on the heels of three decades of increasing Japanese involvement in Chinese social and economic life. From the turn of the century, Japanese had been pouring into China in large numbers, and in contrast to their Western counterparts, they did not limit themselves to treaty port enclaves or missionary stations in the interior. By 1930, there were more Japanese in China than all British, American, and other Westerners combined.[7] By effectively exploiting and expanding the unequal treaty system, Japan succeeded in creating a vast informal empire in China. With the Marco Polo Incident on July 7, 1937, in which a missing Japanese soldier became the pretense for an exchange of fire between

Japanese and Chinese troops, Japan initiated steps to transform its informal empire into a formal one.[8]

In the days leading up to the Japanese attack on Shanghai on August 13, 1937, rumors of the impending crisis flooded the city. The *North-China Herald* estimated that roughly 50,000 refugees had entered the Settlement from Zhabei from July 26 through August 5. Citing growing concern for the "large-scale departure of Japanese residents from China and the presence of sandbags in certain isolated sections of Chapei [Zhabei]," refugees piled their belongings "high in lorries and rickshaws, on handcarts and even carried by coolies, [and] poured into the International Settlement from Chapei [Zhabei] and Chiangwan [Jiangwan]."[9] One family suffered a "double misfortune" when two handcarts, laden with family property consisting of $3,000 worth of cash, jewelry, and clothing, "disappeared in the stream of lorries and other forms of transportation which poured into the Settlement and the French Concession."[10]

The majority of the displaced sought refuge with friends and family in locations deemed safer and temporarily free from fighting and bombardment, which in practice meant heading toward Shanghai's foreign concessions. For those unable to secure such refuge, accommodation assumed a myriad of irregular and even unconventional forms. Refugee camps of every shape and size, and with varying degrees of official sanction, dotted the urban landscape. One of the largest camps was situated in a temple, adjoining "foreign style dwelling houses" on Xinza Road in the Western District, and housed approximately 8,000 refugees.[11] Medical officers from the Shanghai Municipal Council (SMC) Public Health Department characterized the premises as "dirty," with "insufficient water supply." They noted "only a very small stove" and "no possibilities of providing water for washing purposes."[12] Buildings in states of disrepair and neglect were just as likely to become refugee shelters as schools, universities, temples, and churches.[13]

Native-place associations, as well as provincial guilds and benevolent societies, played a crucial and early role in the establishment of refugee camps. They organized materials and resources to house and feed refugees, coordinated evacuations from the city to home villages, and functioned as the main financial supporters of the committees later created to address the problem of refugee assistance.[14] Native-place associations also worked as public advocates and mediators for the refugees residing in camps under the direct jurisdiction of international agencies like the Shanghai International

Red Cross and concession authorities.[15] The relationship, however, was a complex one. In one instance, the Cantonese Residents Association both telephoned and sent a written request to Judge C. Franklin, chairman of the SMC, demanding immediate attention to the provision of "hospital facilities in the Settlement to take care of sick and dying refugees."[16] Having unsuccessfully attempted to move three dying refugees into nearby hospitals, all of which refused them admittance, the Association was fuming at the injustice. "All the hospitals are full at present. We could not send our sick refugees to any one of these hospitals, and we have no extra space for accommodating them. Some of these cases are very bad infectious ones, which is a menace to the general health of the whole camp."[17] The SMC Acting Commissioner of Public Health adamantly disagreed with the Cantonese Residents Association's assessment, insisting that measures were in place, space was available at area hospitals, and in addition, "a hospital to deal solely with sick refugees has been established in the premises of the Hangchow Restaurant, 1454 Avenue Edward VII."[18] He did not, however, reject all of their claims and insisted that the names of the offending hospitals be reported.

Statistics on the total number of camps and their occupancy is difficult to ascertain, as archival sources reveal disparate methods for counting and reporting. The SMC Public Health Department recognized 161 camps with an estimated occupancy of approximately 97,000 refugees for December 1937, while newspapers of the time cited figures closer to 137,000 refugees in an unspecified number of camps at the end of November 1937.[19] Based on the work of historians Feng Yi and Christian Henriot, the total number of camps in the International Settlement seems to have peaked on December 6, 1937, with 158 camps housing 95,336 refugees. In the French Concession, the number of camps fluctuated between 40 and 47 between August and December 1937, for some 23,000 to 27,000 refugees.[20] The majority of refugees came from the ranks of the urban petty bourgeois (*xiao shimin*), and its composition was weighted heavily toward women and children.[21]

For the Shanghai Municipal Council and the Shanghai International Red Cross, the administration and maintenance of refugee camps ought to have been a regulated affair, with regular inspections, official assessments, and punitive sanctions to enforce order and discipline. Care, and in particular the efficacy of care, depended upon a well-ordered system composed of specific committees with delegated tasks. Based on information gathered during regular visits by two or three persons from the International Red Cross (IRC) to camps throughout the International Settlement and the French Concession,

N. B. Doodha, the chairman of the visiting committee of the IRC, observed, "The degree of organization runs from a low standard where the refugees are counted and given some sort of nourishment, to where there is high efficiency in management and a good diet is provided." To ensure proper care and to "improve the lot of Chinese refugees," however, "some sort of more or less standardized system which could be practiced throughout" would have to be created. He maintained that the ideal camp held upwards of four or five thousand inmates—"It is felt that the smaller camps are generally inefficiently operated, and that they show a comparatively higher cost per capita than the larger camps"—and had an internal organization and management that adhered to a clear and systematic division of labor and responsibility.[22]

Transparency and the production of data were key elements to Doodha's conceptualization of camp organization and the delivery of care. Refugees, insofar as they provide the human referents for the slew of numbers and figures a well-run camp continuously gathers and collates each day, are comprehensible only so far as their needs and general affairs are quantifiable. He recommended immediate registration of each person upon their entry to a refugee camp and the assignation of serial numbers, one per refugee, for identification purposes. Camps units—the generalized, abstract term for a hut, a room, or a floor, depending on the specific construction of the camp— functioned as part of the denomination process, while also serving as an organizational device for the implementation of camp discipline and routine. Camp records, which included statistics reflecting the number of refugees in the camp each day; numerical breakdowns in terms of men, women, and children; the total number of sick, and so on, ought to be readily accessible and available for public examination by being posted on public bulletin boards near the entrance of the camp office.

In practice, these expectations for institutional order, though implemented at the administrative level, were often confounded by the local realities on the ground. With most camps under the direct supervision of various native-place associations, guilds, and benevolent societies, the Public Health Department and the Medical Committee of the Chinese Medical Association encountered a variety of red-tape complications, misunderstandings, and conflicting interests in their attempts to oversee the health and welfare of refugees.[23] The attendant complexities and challenges are evident in the SMC Public Health Department's attempt to control the spread of infectious diseases. The scale of the emergency relief effort had necessitated the voluntary cooperation of all manner of medically trained personnel throughout the city.

The SMC Public Health Department deployed medical officers and inspectors to ascertain the state of camp life, helped secure material support for inoculations and vaccinations, and administered a system of sanitary control to help prevent or contain the spread of infectious disease.

The SMC Public Health Department depended upon the cooperation of not only the on-the-ground medical personnel (Chinese and Western-style physicians, nurses, and student volunteers) but also the camp's management. In the case of the New World camp, which had been financially supported and administered by the Cantonese Refugees' Relief Committee (Guangdong Youhu Tongxiang Jiuji Nanmin Weiyuanhui), medical officers from the SMC Public Health Department reported on August 18, 1937, that medical care at the camp was provided by one Chinese male nurse and one female Chinese doctor.[24] Both individuals offered "to help spot cases of communicable diseases in order to isolate them in time."[25] But less than a month later, on September 3, 1937, Robert C. Robertson, who headed the SMC Public Health Department's committee on refugee problems, complained to the Secretary of the SMC, "My medical officers inspecting this Camp urgently report to me that there is great difficulty in impressing upon the Cantonese volunteer doctors, the importance of preventing epidemics, and that they are not cooperative in the Health Department's recommendation." Robertson further stated, "One case of Cholera has been found to date in this badly organized, overcrowded, and much too big camp."[26] Although details are scant, the New World camp was reorganized and improved along the lines demanded by the SMC Public Health Department. Organized evacuations of the refugees by the Cantonese Refugee Association helped to reduce the total camp population, and by September 23, 1937, the *Shanghai Times* reported of the New World camp, "What was once a rather objectionable spot is now a habitable center housing 4,000 inmates."[27]

As an administrative organ delegated with the primary task of protecting the public's health to the extent that it had "the right, even the duty, to impose hygiene and sanitation regulations on private citizens for the public health," the SMC Public Health Department possessed rather limited resources to enforce compliance within the various refugee camps. Camps that failed to take the necessary measures to, for example, prevent fire risks from unrestricted cooking, remove "unlicensed hawkers . . . selling foodstuffs which, in many cases, are unfit for human consumption," and maintain latrines and drains "in a sanitary condition"[28] received constant scrutiny from the Public Health Department as well as other related departments (e.g.,

Public Works, the Fire Brigade, and the Municipal Police). The Public Health Department could and did ration provisions, particularly in the form of drugs, allotted to the specific camp, and it could and did withhold financial support if it deemed an errant camp unreliable for the funds.[29] The department was willing to use public censure through the presses and, in the most severe cases, even threatened to "ship them [the refugees] back to their own country."[30] But even with these measures at hand, enforcing compliance was by no means a straightforward task.

Despite these difficulties, the SMC Public Health Department was far from unsuccessful in overseeing the infrastructure for the care and maintenance of refugee health. Refugees underwent mass inoculations, delousing, and quarantine measures when necessary.[31] The Shanghai United Epidemiology Committee organized and administered delousing and bathing services for refugees.[32] From November 1, 1937, through January 31, 1938, mobile delousing units visited four hospitals, 69 camps (once), 29 camps (twice), and three camps (three times); 47,663 refugees and 1,957 garments and beddings were treated. During that same period, the mobile bathing unit visited twelve camps and treated 4,069 persons.[33] Through the winter of 1937, the Shanghai International Red Cross supported "nineteen camps clinics (catering to a refugee population of 24,000) and nine mobile clinics (reaching 65 camps with a refugee population of 58,000)."[34]

The Chinese Medical Association, working in conjunction with the Shanghai International Red Cross, set up six camp clinics and eight mobile clinics that visited an average of six to seven camps daily between 8:30 a.m. and 4:30 p.m. to provide curative and preventive medical aid. Camps with populations over 1,000 were outfitted with a clinic, while camps with fewer than 1,000 refugees were served by mobile clinics.[35] The Chinese Medical Association created a Central Medical Supplies Depot under the supervision of Drs. Bernard E. Read and T. C. Chi that functioned as a depository from which refugee clinics and hospitals could obtain drugs. "A simple [pharmacopoeia] was worked out for the use of refugee clinics, all approved clinics [and hospitals] being permitted to apply for drugs and supplies listed in this [pharmacopoeia] up to their respective quota."[36] The Chinese Medical Association also organized a Public Health Nursing Service with a staff of ten public health nurses, whose responsibilities included assisting the work of doctors and clinics and giving lectures and demonstrations in health education, as well as a Sanitation Service comprising five sanitary inspectors assisted by a labor corps of selected refugees. "Each sanitary inspector [was] assigned to one of five districts and under their direction the refugees them-selves [were] organized to carry out daily routine cleansing. Selected refugees [were] organized to form labor corps to undertake technical work such as construction of privies, installation of water and sewage, road building, etc."[37]

The overall effect of this concerted municipal program for addressing the medical and health needs of refugees was the expansion of the sphere of day-to-day interactions refugees had with Western medicine. Although Shang-hai possessed an outstanding proportion of the country's registered Western-style medical doctors (22%), the vast majority of Chinese lived and worked outside the penetration of the biomedical gaze.[38] The concentration of Western-style doctors in Shanghai did not translate into a greater propor-tion of the urban population served by Western medicine, and whether on account of preference or cost, most Chinese continued to seek medical relief and health advice from indigenous sources, such as practitioners of Chinese medicine.[39] With the social upheaval and general displacement of the popu-lace resulting from the outbreak of fighting, this disjunction separating Western medicine from the Chinese population was upset. Mass inoculation, compulsory vaccinations, delousing, bathing, and feeding schedules were all concrete ways in which Western medicine, backed by state power (in this case, the foreign concession of the Shanghai Municipal Council), inter-vened directly in the lives of Chinese refugees. It is within this context of organized third-party medical interventions that the nutritional activism of the Refugee Children's Committee took root.

NUTRITIONAL CRISIS

The Refugee Children's Committee, formed in November 1937, was one such program attempting to bring order and relief to the city. Composed mainly of Shanghai's professional elite, the committee was international in both membership and orientation. Pediatricians, nutritional specialists, public health officials, and social workers of both Chinese and foreign nationalities cooperated to devise a workable plan for producing and distributing soybean milk and related nutritional supplements to refugee children in camps located throughout the city.[40] The committee's initial operations were funded by a $6,000 donation by the German community. The Shanghai International Red Cross and China Child Welfare later provided regular monthly stipends to ensure the continuation of its work until disbandment in 1939.[41]

To attend to the nutritional health of refugee children, the Refugee Children's Committee mapped onto the city's existing infrastructure a complex network of production, distribution, and experimentation channels. It divided the city into six districts, each with its own distribution center serving the refugee camps within its domain. In addition to the six distribution centers, it also operated a main office from the premises of 65 Moulmein Road, which was home to the Hospital for Refugee Children. It contracted with local bakeries, such as the Shanghai Wing On Bakery, to produce the bean residue cakes. The grindstone used in making soybean milk was "donated by a generous Chinese friend." The delivery carts came from a local milk dairy whose plant had been bombed, and even a truck from a local garage was procured.[42]

Although the documentary record for the committee's operations during the first six months of its tenure has not survived, it is clear from the extant monthly reports that the program maintained a permanent staff of managers, assistant managers, inspectors, delivery coolies (by bicycles), bean milk makers, cleaners/sterilizers of milk containers, and female distribution workers. The organization of work seems to have been gendered: the scientific testing was performed almost exclusively by male physicians; the actual distribution of the milk within the camps was performed by young professional females who had been trained in social work, home economics, or nutrition. The total number of employees fluctuated according to the conditions of the time, a reduction in the size of the refugee population and the closing of camps by municipal authorities being the main reasons for a reduction in the number of employees.[43]

How the Refugee Children's Committee settled upon fortified soybean milk as the optimal nutritional supplement to distribute is a story that mixes the melodramatic with the pragmatic. It is a story that grounds the scientific endeavor of preventing child malnutrition in a social concern over mother's milk. Nellie Lee, a young Chinese woman born in New York City, educated at Mt. Holyoke College, and responsible for the Refugee Children's Committee's field operations, rooted the committee's origins in the lamentations of women with barren breasts and the cries of young infants. Lee was the administrative secretary in charge of local operations. She described the flurry of phone calls and the desperate pleas to cow dairies in town for milk donations—all in the hopes of pacifying the hungry cries of refugee babies. In the absence of breast milk, cow's milk was the first alternative sought. But the distance from cow's milk to soybean milk was a short one, and when Lee encountered difficulties securing enough cow's milk supplies, she naturally turned to soybean milk.[44]

In contrast to Lee's emotional description of the crisis, the popular press account attributed the committee's organization to Dr. Ting'an Li, Public Health Commissioner of Greater Shanghai, and his administrative acuity.[45] Dr. Li was prescient enough to recognize the looming threat of nutritional deprivation and its effects on the child refugees. "Adults can withstand nutritional deprivation for a certain period of time, for there are reserves to draw on, but growing children need vital materials to build up their bodies, otherwise they will become easy prey to diseases, or their physical development may be so impaired as to affect the health of their lifetime."[46]

These two seemingly contrasting accounts of the committee's origins and interest in soybean milk can muddle the historical clarity of the situation. And yet, the discrepancy highlights two important factors for understanding the committee's work and its situation within contemporary Chinese society. Nellie Lee's account highlights the human and maternal aspects of the refugee crisis: thousands upon thousands of mothers—traumatized by the bombings, fearful of what is yet to come, struggling to manage on limited, perhaps even nonexistent, resources to feed their babies, their bodies increasingly malnourished and stressed. Juxtaposed against this scene of strain and struggle is calm and rationality. A male Chinese physician, who also serves as one of the leading public health officials, oversees the campaign. His administrative acumen and professional expertise, coupled with a strong sense of civic duty, leads him to begin marshaling human and organizational resources to prevent a human disaster of epic scale. Children, the bearers of the future and the leaders of tomorrow, are physiologically ill-equipped to deal with long periods of nutritional deprivation. Dr. Li thus mounts a campaign to prevent malnutrition and nutritional deficiency diseases. He, and presumably his colleagues, draws upon medical science to instill order and rationality on a scene fraught with disorder and chaos. Whereas Nellie Lee focuses on the emotions of the moment, the newspaper account homes in on order and rationality. Soybean milk, for Nellie Lee, is the salve to stop a child's sorrow over the lack of mother's milk. Soybean milk, for Dr. Li and his medical counterparts, is the nutritional fix-it to avert a physiological catastrophe, that is, the stunting of China's next generation of citizens. Though seemingly divergent in tone and objective, both accounts situate the soybean as the foundation for relief, and it is this convergence

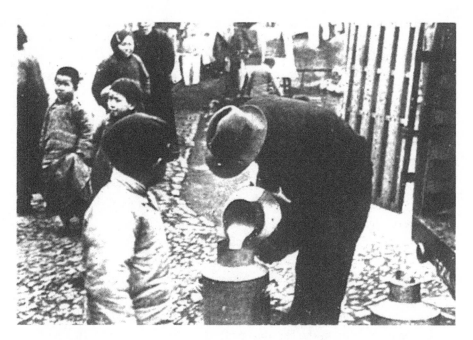

FIGURE 6.2. "Milk from the soya bean, the 'Cow of China,' affords nourishment for refugee children at the low rate of 1.8 cts. Mex. per pound." Original caption from *China Quarterly* (Winter 1937–38).

between the medical and maternal spheres that came to typify relief work with the soybean.

The soybean represented both modern scientific advancement and home-grown ingenuity during a period of national distress (figure 6.2). In its official explanation explaining the selection of the soybean as the primary ingredient for its nutritional supplement, the Refugee Children's Committee drew upon medical research to justify its choice.

Several years ago in Peiping [Beijing] experiments were made with soya bean milk and found that it is comparable to cow's milk in vitamin A and richer in vitamin B. It is deficient in minerals, particularly calcium and that is added to the milk. It has been experimented [*sic*] that a six weeks old infant was successfully fed to 9 months on soya bean milk, supplemented with cane sugar, cod liver oil, orange juice, rice porridge, spinach puree, and sodium chloride. The mental, muscular development and nutritional status in general appear to be as good as other normal infants reared on mammalian milk diets. It was found that a formula could be evolved which, with the addition of calcium and sugar, produced a bean milk which closely approximated the food value of cow's milk.[47]

That the soybean was already a feature of regional Chinese diets, the Refugee Children's Committee argued, provided further validation. "The soya bean has long been popular in the diet of the Chinese. It can be prepared in many forms and it has been said that one can have a complete feast in which every dish is a soya bean dish but each one so different from the last as to make one feel no sense of duplication."[48]

There are two reasons for questioning the Refugee Children's Committee's narrative about selecting the soybean. In the first case, its invocation of nutrition science, and the experimental work on soybean milk conducted just a decade previously, serves to normalize the comparative relation between cow's milk and soybean milk in infant diets. Though not specified by the organization, the broader medical community's fascination with soybean milk as a cow's milk alternative was quite recent and, in China, reflected a growing medical concern over the state of child development in the country (see chapter 4). What this sanitized, logical explanation excludes is how important—and emotionally charged—the issue of milk and the feeding of the young was throughout the Republican period, but especially at this moment of all-out war with Japan. Furthermore, the insistence that soybean milk was a staple component of the Chinese diet reflected less an accurate description of contemporary eating patterns than a growing cultural consensus about the soybean's indigenous status and pervasive presence.

RATIONALIZING RELIEF

The growing certainty of war with Japan in the years preceding 1937 magnified the social and moral impetus for improving the Chinese diet. Chinese commentators writing for the literate elite bemoaned the severity of China's "nutrition problem" (yingyang wenti).[49] War was a state of emergency (feichang shiqi), and with the Chinese nation under imminent attack, addressing the nutrition problem through the establishment of nutritional standards represented a basic, essential form of preparation. The stakes were high; national and racial survival depended on the procurement and maintenance of a proper diet.

The refugee crisis in Shanghai in 1937 brought this point home, but it also enabled an intellectual shift toward greater scientific penetration of non-laboratory settings. The outbreak of war afforded a unique opportunity for nutrition scientists and researchers to combine academic research with social action by exploring the logistics and complexities of applying medical knowledge born in the laboratory outside in the "real world." This melding of scientific and social praxis in the name of national salvation is amply visible in the activities of Hou Xiangchuan, an associate researcher in the Division of Physiological Sciences at the Henry Lester Institute of Medical Research and active member of both the Refugee Children's Committee and its successor organization, the China Nutritional Aid Council. The most direct application of his biomedical expertise is evidenced in his preoccupation with constructing a scientifically nutritious and economically sensitive refugee diet. A single meal whose composition had been carefully calibrated to satisfy essential nutritional requirements could function as a prophylactic against the outbreak and spread of nutritional deficiency diseases. Hou, who served as chairman of the Shanghai International Relief Committee's subcommittee on refugee health and wrote extensively about refugee diets, related a complicated tale of precarious living for most refugees: "During August 1937 when the Sino-Japanese hostilities broke out in Shanghai the number of refugees gathered in empty houses and matshed camps rapidly exceeded two hundred thousand. Practically all of them had to be fed by charity. Most were given only polished rice gruel and a little salted turnip, others were given steamed bread and salted vegetables."[50]

Initially, "many of [the refugees] however were able to purchase at least for a time additional foods like vegetables, fish or meat with the little cash which they carried with them upon evacuation."[51] But as hostilities deepened and personal cash dwindled, the food provided by the camps, which Hou characterized as "not up to the minimum dietary requirement," failed to protect the refugees from nutritional disorders. Hou wrote, "For fear of further outbreaks of nutritional disease, camp authorities were urged to provide a better diet for refugees. A diet consisting of several common and inexpensive foods similar to the Chinese dietary standard . . . was recommended to the organizations sponsoring the camps through the good offices of the Municipal Public Health Department [in the International Settlement]."[52]

Crafting dietaries represented one form of scientific intervention in social relief. But because these dietaries adhered to criteria distinct from economic supply and demand, as well as customary tastes, the necessity of demonstrating the nutritional efficacy of these diets also arose. The scale of the refugee crisis in Shanghai had necessitated the proliferation of initiatives by all kinds of competing national, international, and local institutions and associations, whose various prerogatives often led to lively political battles over influence and resources.[53] Scientific reporting helped differentiate certain kinds of relief work as more efficacious and could be used to demonstrate local fitness in international terms. As part of the Shanghai International Red Cross's organizational activities, which had the support of the foreign consular corps and the Nationalist government, Hou would have been sensitive to the need for demonstrating the efficacy of his dietaries in politically legible terms that had what the historian and political theorist Timothy Mitchell has called the "character of calculability."[54]

Hou and his colleagues conducted epidemiological surveys to determine the incidence rates of various diseases and investigations into the health of refugees. Chemical and biological assays of various Chinese foods had been undertaken since the early 1920s, but nutritional surveys, which evaluated both food and the resultant state of nutrition in the individual, did not appear in the medical literature until the mid-1930s. The refugee situation in Shanghai was certainly not the desired environment for scientific research, and yet few denied the substantive opportunities war afforded medical specialists seeking to explicate the relationship between food and health within specific populations. Hou, like many of his research colleagues, obtained valuable access to refugees as participant subjects for his various nutritional studies.

Hou's highly specialized training and clinical experience in creating viable nutritional standards for refugee diets shaped his work with the Refugee Children's Committee and the Nutritional Council. Moreover, his research methodology established a pattern for how these organizations presented the significance of their work to international funding agencies and the broader Chinese reading public. The key to nutritional activism lay in the mutually reinforcing construction of science as both the method for delivering social relief and also the justification for the content of such relief. Scientific expertise formulated the proper dietary instructions to which the committee adhered. Scientific expertise demonstrated the efficacy of such instructions through systematic clinical observation and measurements. Thus, for the Refugee Children's Committee, testing, experimentation, and clinical trials were mainstays of the relief program itself.

One of the first issues Hou tackled for the committee involved the adjustment and refinement of a soybean milk recipe that satisfied requirements on nutritive, economic, and practical levels. In a lecture before the Shanghai YMCA, Hou characterized the soybean milk nutritional supplement as "up to nutritional standards [yingyang biaozhun]" because it was devised from research methods (yanjiu zhifa) and regulated ingredients (guiding chengfen).[55] Hou reported, "The preparation of soybean milk was carried out according to the usual age-old Chinese procedure, namely that the soybeans were first weighed and then washed thoroughly in several changes of clean water."[56] After soaking the beans for ten hours, the entire batch was put through a stone mill and ground into a thick creamy paste. The paste was transferred to a clean muslin bag from which the liquid milk was filtered. Water amounting to eight times the amount of soybean was regularly added during the process of filtration, after which the milk was boiled for approximately twenty minutes and then poured into distribution cans.[57] Hou adapted his recipe from an earlier one devised by Dr. Ernest Tso of the Peking Union Medical College. The main difference distinguishing the two recipes was calcium lactate, which Hou added to ensure the requisite calcium intake.[58] To help diminish the "beany taste" often associated with soybean milk, Hou added molasses and native brown sugar. With these adjustments in place, Hou argued that the Refugee Children's Committee had achieved a nutriment that was both nutritiously rich and tasty.[59]

Hou's suggestion of traditional craftsmanship highlights a curious ambiguity about the soybean milk production process. Although he characterized the preparation of the soybean milk as "the usual age-old Chinese procedure," the fact that a Western-trained physician, as opposed to the common tofu vendor, produced the milk seemed to lift the entire enterprise into the realm of scientific technique. Once the recipe had been determined, Hou proceeded to introduce the laboratory analysis of the quality of soybean milk into the Refugee Children's Committee's set of production protocols. Each batch of milk made for refugee children had to meet the same set of nutritional criteria in terms of its protein, vitamin, and calcium content. Regular milk testing was supplemented with scientific investigations of the milk's effects on refugee children. Hou and his assistants visited camps and conducted physical examinations on the refugee children. His adherence to the dictates of science reframed the work of Refugee Children's Committee as necessarily scientific, objective, and right.[60]

The extent to which nutritional activism departed from other kinds of food relief is attested by the prominence given to scientific studies demonstrating the efficacy of calculated dietary interventions. Although these studies appeared primarily in medical journals, their influence was not limited to a specialized readership, as précis of the studies often reappeared in popular journals like *Science* (Kexue), *Science World* (Kexue shijie), and *Women's Journal* (Funü zazhi). From November 1937 through the spring of 1940, at least four different medical studies were published in connection with the Refugee Children's Committee's work. Most of these were in the form of height and weight surveys of refugee children. Hou and his assistants visited 20 camps and measured 1,028 children and found that the children receiving soybean milk experienced an appreciable increase in weight when compared to children who had refused the milk.[61] Hou explained, "The present studies were not planned and started as an experiment but arose from an urgent need to supply a nourishing cheap food to refugee children whose diets were inadequate for normal health and to infants whose mothers could not supply sufficient milk. This afforded an unusual opportunity for observing on a large scale by taking body measurements the possible nutritional value of soybean milk as a supplementary food."[62] Hou's findings functioned as demonstrable proof that relief work fashioned in accordance with scientific principles produced positive results in the fight against child malnutrition.

Relief operations across the city began winding down by late summer 1938 as Shanghai fractured along competing wartime jurisdictions: Japanese occupation of the formerly Chinese-controlled areas and the tenuous continuation of foreign rule in the foreign concessions, at least until December 1941, when Japan assumed complete authority over all parts of the city. The Refugee Children's Committee too shifted its orientation, as plans were launched to expand its nutritional program into the southwest interior (see chapter 7). Its influence, however, preceded the operational logistics and administrative reappraisals. Its dual focus on soybean milk and the nutritional health of children, its commitment to rational, scientific practice for the formulation and management of relief, and its insistence that nutrition science could solve the intransient problems of the day became a blueprint for subsequent experiments in soy-based nutritional feeding programs.

The idea of feeding the population in times of crisis was hardly new when the Refugee Children's Committee began introducing its brand of nutritional activism to local communities in Shanghai. "Nourishing the people" (yang-min) has long been recognized as a foundational tenet of imperial governance. The idea of the ever-normal granary, in which officials bought grain when the price was low and sold it when the price was high, thereby keeping grain prices low and stable, has been attributed to Mencius.[63] The administration of official disaster relief (huangzheng), which took form as both preventive and ameliorative measures, ranging from building granaries and maintaining river control to issuing tax dispensations and sponsoring famine relief, represented a vision of sage rulership that shaped expectations of imperial and bureaucratic responsibility.

Although the practice and implementation of these principles varied by time and place, it is clear that during the high Qing period, the state had organized a system of large-scale relief works to a degree of efficiency unseen in earlier times. Characterized as the "golden age of famine administration" by the historian Pierre-Etienne Will, the eighteenth century marked the high point in the state's capacity, in terms of both money and grain, to marshal its resources and successfully tackle the twin problems of agricultural reconstruction and famine prevention.[64] By establishing and maintaining an empire-wide network of granaries to mitigate food shortages and control price and supply fluctuations, the high Qing state did more than pay superficial observance to the idea of Confucian benevolent rule. Its highly interventionist spirit aimed to support rather than supersede market forces and in turn worked to ensure some kind of subsistence net for disaster victims.

What happened to this highly effectual state enterprise during the nineteenth century and into the twentieth has generally been understood as part of a broader devolutionary process. Struggling against diminished resources and bureaucratic inertia, not to mention increased corruption, the ability of the Qing state to address subsistence crises was increasingly handicapped. The formal demise of the Qing and the formation of a Republican government in 1912 did little to alter the shift in power away from a centralized state apparatus. In its place, historians have observed the rise of local elite activism—sometimes working in cooperation with official sponsorship, other times independently—thus shifting the composition and content of famine relief throughout the nineteenth century and into the twentieth.

The story, then, of state and society relations as viewed through famine administration appears to be one of inverse correspondence. Closer consideration of relief initiatives during the post-imperial period, especially during the tenure of the Nanjing government, however, complicates any clear depiction of state-society relations as simply being an increase of local and regional power at the expense of the central state.[65] Indeed, the emergence of a distinctly technocratic and scientific cast to private and public relief campaigns, as well as the intermixing of professional elites in state- and non-state-sponsored programs, highlights the complex interrelations knitting state efforts, however ineffectual, to a broader national consciousness in the form of Chinese nationalism. New scientific knowledge and technical expertise rearticulated human and natural disasters as less an expected part of the natural and political order than a critical component of the national struggle for a modern Chinese nation.[66]

When we consider the nutritional activism of the Refugee Children's Committee, it becomes apparent that this twentieth-century relief program operated according to distinctly different presuppositions about the constitution of hunger than those encompassed by the high Qing model of famine relief or late imperial philanthropic work on the part of trade guilds, native place associations, and local elites. In the first place, strict distinction between state and society actors fails to capture the fluid ways in which a dense, multilayered social network of elite philanthropists had developed during the Republican period. The Chinese involved in the Refugee Children's Committee rarely occupied a single social position, for example, either a state or government official or a member of the local elite, and instead often represented multiple private- and public-sector identities. This characteristic of "wearing many hats" afforded the Nationalist government the luxury of attaching itself to nonstate activism without bearing the burden of financial support. The Refugee Children's Committee received the bulk of its funding from international donors, namely China Child Welfare and, after 1944, United China Relief. Neither funding agency was a state-sponsored enterprise, and yet both maintained direct ties to the Nationalist government in ways that insured a complementarity of interests.[67] With the China Nutritional Aid Council especially, this connection to the Nationalist government became more prominent when Dr. Arthur N. Young, financial advisor to the Chinese government (1929–46), became president of the council and Dr. P. Z.

King (Jin Baoshan), the director of the National Health Administration, the honorary president of the council in 1942.

The increasing levels of international involvement in local relief efforts and the Chinese state's growing insistence on claiming political authority through its adherence to international norms and protocols valorized scientific knowledge as the foundation for modern relief work. For the many physicians, medical researchers, and public health workers active in these organizations, the emphasis upon science was deliberate. Scientific modernization and national salvation were the two paramount social imperatives of their time, and nutritional activism married the two imperatives within a single endeavor.[68]

That the Refugee Children's Committee depended on the participation of elite scientific professionals with pluralistic identities and who often possessed ties to the international community makes more sense when we recognize the coterminous conceptual transformation taking place with respect to the idea of hunger and malnutrition. As the historian Michael Worboys has argued, malnutrition was not a subject of systematic scientific investigation before the 1920s, and when colonial officials and scientists turned their attention to the problem, they increasingly viewed malnutrition as an economical-agricultural problem requiring scientific-technical interventions.[69] Colonial science tended to construe malnutrition in terms of diet and economic productivity. Whether one's political disposition emphasized poverty and British economic policy or the role of culture and "native 'ignorance,'" a biological conception of malnutrition—one that rendered hunger epistemologically equivalent to malnutrition—eclipsed older understandings of the relationship that might obtain between health and diet as well as articulations of power linking diet and the state.[70] Hunger, which had once been assumed to be inevitable or even natural, became socially and politically unacceptable for modern states and populations. Once biomedical science defined hunger as malnutrition and introduced a variety of new concepts, including the calorie and vitamins, new metrics by which to identify, control, manage, and prevent its occurrence arose and became part of a broader language of foreign policy and modern statehood.[71]

Distributing food relief or provisioning a local population with basic grains was a baseline measure—one contiguous to the high Qing model of famine relief and local elite philanthropic works. For the Refugee Children's Committee, this method of food distribution was untenable, because it did not include or address ideas about national health and vitality as measured

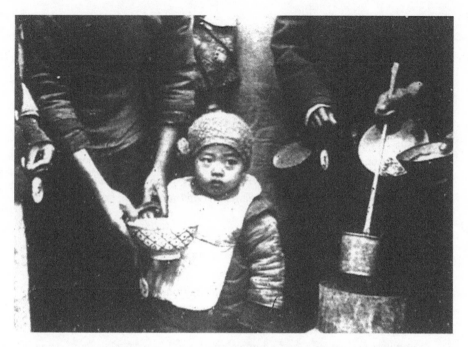

FIGURE 6.3. "Children over three years of age receive one pound of soya bean milk daily." Original caption from *China Quarterly* (Winter 1937–38).

through nutritional indices. Combating malnutrition—one of the primary goals of nutritional activism—becomes a priority once hunger has been reconceptualized in standard, biological terms. This commitment to a scientific model of hunger was not limited to the work of the Refugee Children's Committee and the China Nutritional Aid Council (figure 6.3). In January 1944, the Nationalist government drew up a plan of nutritional improvement, and it couched its recommended courses of action entirely in the language of nutrition science.[72]

Would it not have been more beneficial to the Chinese public had these organizations concentrated their efforts less upon providing specific nutrients (e.g., protein, vitamin B, and calcium) and instead marshaled basic grains to stave off starvation? The question was certainly raised when medical professionals met in April 1942 for the Conference on Child Welfare Problems in China held under the auspices of the United China Relief. Dr. Marion Yang (Yang Chongrui), famous for her role in professionalizing Chinese midwifery, pointed out that most refugees just needed something to eat to avoid starvation.[73] Her assessment highlights the persistent tension underlining nutritional activism during wartime. In a country that continued to be haunted by the appellation "land of famine," concerns about avitaminosis could be construed as misplaced and myopic. In other words, Was China's problem one involving food or health? Nutrition science did not necessarily divorce the two, but when harnessed to the social relief projects of the Refugee Children's Committee and the China Nutritional Aid Council, it privileged health as the most important arena for scientific intervention.

CONCLUSION

War had transformed Shanghai into one massive sea of human swells and uncertainties, and even the most fundamental of tasks, the provision of food, became impossibly implicated in the movement of troops, military strategies, and geopolitical objectives. For the members of the Refugee Children's Committee, making food, any food, available was insufficient. The task they set for themselves was something much less transparent and rather more intangible. Their target was "nutritional health," and their method was the transformation of the simple soybean into a modern, scientific foodstuff. This combination of form and function substantiated a mode of social-scientific inquiry that valorized the possibility of optimal health through social engineering. The Refugee Children's Committee, and its successor, the China Nutritional Aid Council, represented one of the first organized attempts in China at nutritional activism through its application of principles of nutrition science to the social world. Its program—the development of a specific foodstuff to insure sufficient nutritional coverage and its distribution to the youngest, most vulnerable subset of the population, children—became a model for other grassroots efforts to combat nutritional deficiencies.

The success of the Refugee Children's Committee's nutritional work, however, blinded nutritional activists to the exceptional circumstances that allowed them contact with large groups of people in reasonably controlled settings. Distributing soybean milk and espousing its virtues to a captive population within the confines of a refugee camp was not the same as distributing it among communities whose cast and kind fluctuated according to wartime conditions and who, however constrained, maintained private discretion about how best to use their available funds to feed themselves and their families. When the China Nutritional Aid Council attempted to pick up where the Refugee Children's Committee had ended, nutritional activists like

Nellie Lee and Hou Xiangchuan soon discovered the messiness in attempting to tinker with people's social and eating habits. Categories and practices that seemed to work within Shanghai refugee camps became less dependable and efficacious in the backwaters of Southwestern China (see chapter 7).

And yet the conviction in the power of nutrition science, scientific relief, and the soybean persisted. The Refugee Children's Committee had embarked upon a project that situated nutrition as the crucial site for the dissemination of modern knowledge and values. Like the images taken in *China Quarterly*, their work signified order, calm, and scientific virtue. This sensibility would not be forgone, even when challenges arose and despair began to nibble at their confidence. Health, when reconfigured in terms of nutrition science—with its emphases on calories, proteins, and the chemical composition of popular foodstuffs, and its characterizations of healthy bodies according to regulatory principles, numerical assessments, and empirical testing—could and should be bottled and distributed.

CHAPTER 7

The Gospel of Soy

Local Realities and the Tension between Profit and Relief

I N September 1941, Nellie Lee (1909–1994), an American-born Chinese who was in the throes of self-invention, confided in her former college mentor. Having left the cosmopolitan and urbane cityscape of Shanghai, with its streetlights, movie theaters, and paved roads, Lee confronted a very different world in what must have felt like the backwaters of Sichuan. Lee had lived in the United States, where she received her university education. When she returned to China in the 1930s, war loomed large upon the horizon. Whatever proverbial delights of urban living there may have been for Lee in Shanghai, it was all a distant memory made dimmer by the lack of electricity and mud floors in her newly settled home of Chongqing. Gone were the marbled steps and towering buildings of the Bund, the commercial delights of Nanjing Road; in their place, Lee found herself in and between dugouts and mud huts. She wrote: "Rice has been up at almost $3.00 a catty while salaries have been lagging way behind, so nutrition is a big problem. Everybody is more or less undernourished as compared with the pre-war standard, with eggs at .50 a piece and pork $4.00 a catty. My work is very timely and is met with good response, except that it has been terribly difficult to get things done what with the air raids, poor general health of the people which result[s] in frequent illnesses, and the poor transportation which make[s] any movement a big event."[1] Having helped complete what was by all accounts a successful experiment in combatting malnutrition among refugee children in Shanghai, Nellie Lee had, in her own words, "initiated the movement to spread the use of [soy]bean milk and [soy]bean residue cakes in the interior."[2] Her purpose in Chongqing was clear, but the attendant realities muddled her sense of enthusiasm.

War necessitated self-invention, and the Second Sino-Japanese War provided both opportunity and peril for enterprising individuals. For Nellie Lee and her scientific counterpart in Shanghai, Hou Xiangchuan, war became the pretext for undertaking a national initiative for spreading the gospel of soybean and nutritional health. Hou, a senior researcher in the Division of Physiological Sciences at the Henry Lester Institute of Medical Research, had returned to Shanghai's International Settlement after accompanying a research team from St. John's University on retreat to Kunming in 1939.[3] How and why he did so is unclear, but in the relative safety afforded by international Shanghai—a town "conquered but not yet occupied by its conquerors"—Hou began playing a more prominent role in advancing soybean science and blurring the distinctions between advocacy and regulation.[4]

Motivated by a sense of humanitarian paternalism that expressed itself through their efforts to teach poor people how to eat better, nutritional activists like Lee and Hou believed that a solution to the problem of the Chinese diet could be found in the pursuit of new habits appropriate to a modern identity. The habits they sought to instill were all connected with the soybean, which represented an indigenous, economical foodstuff that was somehow misunderstood or improperly used by the Chinese people. Both Lee and Hou sought to reimagine what the soybean could be, how it was used, and the extent to which proper eating was the first step toward engineering a modern Chinese future.

The wartime experiences of Nellie Lee and Hou Xiangchuan demonstrate how strong the will to change how the Chinese people ate was, but the actual circumstances in which these two worked mired their idealism in the gritty mess of local realities. The apparent success they experienced with the Shanghai Refugee Children's Nutritional Aid Committee (see chapter 6) colored their expectations that knowledge of the nutritional value of the soybean could trump any difficulties they encountered. Without recognizing the state of exception that shaped their work among Shanghai refugees, Lee and Hou proceeded as if the local communities of Kunming, Chongqing, and even Shanghai could be managed and instructed through careful guidance and commercial appeal. They integrated public health techniques into their soybean campaigns and adopted commercial strategies in a bid to transform popular Chinese understanding and consumption practices.

CROSSING PROFESSIONAL LINES

Nellie Lee was a young Chinese woman who led the way in promoting soybean milk as an indigenous yet modern and scientific foodstuff that could improve the lives of Chinese children through the war-torn decades of the 1930s and 1940s. Socially, she straddled a number of different societies. Born in New York City, she had nonetheless spent some time at a preparatory school called Pooi To Academy in Canton before matriculating at Mount Holyoke College. She returned to China in 1934 and worked for a handful of new institutions redefining educational and career opportunities for Chinese women. She was a medical social worker in the pediatrics department of the Peking Union Medical College (PUMC). She served as secretary for the agronomist Dr. J. Lossing Buck at the University of Nanjing from 1936 to 1938 and then joined the Refugee Children's Committee. As the on-site manager, Lee oversaw the managerial side of the refugee soybean milk and soybean cake operation. She worked with local businesses to obtain the necessary ingredients and secure premises for the milk and cake production; she organized and coordinated the distribution depots, the delivery routes, and the necessary personnel; and at the end of each month, she delivered a monthly expense report documenting the highs and lows of production, changes in protocol, and a regular summary of scientific investigations undertaken by nutrition scientists, like Hou Xiangchuan, working with the Refugee Children's Committee.

Nellie's affiliation with universities, hospitals, and health demonstration centers was not a coincidence but rather a telling characteristic of the seismic shifts affecting Chinese society in the first half of the twentieth century. By the 1850s, foreign missionaries had begun setting up schools offering the first formalized education for Chinese girls; by the final years of the Qing dynasty, private individuals had created local schools that "combined the values of the [Chinese] classics and family instruction manuals with examples of foreign women."[5] As Chinese women became more visible in public spaces where they had not formerly been, their presence spurred debate about what kinds of roles Chinese women were to play in the new republic. As several scholars have shown, education institutions provided sites where Chinese men and women could reimagine and rearticulate their relationship to the state, their conception of citizenship, and their embodiment of modern values and practices.[6]

Older conceptions of family and home, in which multigenerational households were sustained by a moral and physical order that separated men and women into distinct spheres, were similarly targeted and reinscribed with nationalist values. Chinese intellectuals increasingly linked the fate of the nation to the way in which women enacted their roles as wives and mothers and conducted their "inner sphere" (*nei*) duties. Household management classes that instructed women in the physical practices of keeping the house in order, bearing and raising good children, and cleaning and cooking went hand in hand with the establishment of female education. As the historian Helen Schneider has argued, "Twentieth-century domestic reformers radically re-imagined the home as a place where habits of citizenship were formed, and they believed that opening up the domestic, 'inner' sphere to public scrutiny and to careful management were central parts of becoming modern."[7] But as women increasingly moved into outer (*wai*) domains, home economics as preparatory material for fashioning "good wives, wise mothers" (*liangqi xianmu*) also provided a foundation and practical skills that women could translate into professional careers outside the home.[8] Women like Florence Pen Ho and Chen Peilan did not just study home economics; they went on to help establish university departments and support Nationalist projects in social improvement.

Although not a direct beneficiary of the home economics movement in China, Nellie Lee's own experiences reflect these changing dynamics. A middling student who studiously avoided any science classes, Lee graduated from Mount Holyoke College in 1932 with fairly clear preferences regarding prospective jobs. While open to teaching and secretarial work, her primary interests lay in library work, social work, YWCA work, statistical work, and business. Her subsequent trajectory skittered along these various interest points—graduate studies in social work, a one-year stint as a medical social worker, secretarial work—until she had the good fortune of becoming the logistical supervisor for "the making and delivery of [soy]bean milk to thousands of refugee children" (see chapter 6).[9] Although she was not formally trained in home economics or related sciences, her soybean work brought her into increased contact with other Chinese women who had graduated from home economic or nutrition-related fields, and together these women played a formative role in the growth of nutritional activism during wartime. The scientific mentality and emphasis on rationalizing Chinese everyday life also made sense to Lee, but her lack of proper credentials, especially in the sciences, would ultimately compromise her tenure as program organizer and administrator by the time war with Japan ended.

In the spring of 1939, Nellie Lee approached Julean Arnold, the commercial attaché of the US consulate in Shanghai and a vocal proponent for the development of soybean products, about the possibility of expanding the Refugee Children's Committee's work into the interior. She proposed establishing children's nutritional aid centers in "strategic places in China." In conveying her ideas to J. A. Mackay of China Child Welfare, an American-sponsored aid organization dedicated to child-centered welfare work that provided the bulk of the Refugee Children's Committee's finances, Arnold wrote, "She expressed a desire to pioneer in this work in the interior. Her idea is to set up a model station in Kunming and after having developed this to a proper degree of perfection, then spread the idea for the building up of similar stations in other interior places where they can be advantageously developed."[10]

With published surveys of the beneficial effects of soybean milk and almost two years' experience in production and distribution, the challenge and potential reward in spreading scientific soybean milk in nonemergency settings was great. In Arnold's estimation,

> As our Committee in Shanghai made very commendable progress in the manufacture and distribution of soybean milk and soybean cakes for children in the refugee camps, this presents an excellent opportunity for carrying this work into the interior of the country and making it a permanent factor in the rural economy of China. Thus, it would seem that we could make of this a valuable contribution, not only in emergency relief work for nutrition for refugee children, but at the same time educate the Chinese to the greater appreciation of the possibilities of the use of the soybean for nutritive purposes among the children of the country.[11]

It did not strike Arnold—nor indeed Nellie Lee—as strange that these ambitions for the soybean were predicated on the idea that rural Chinese were somehow ignorant of the soybean's economic and food-related values. Whatever role soybeans may have played in local dietaries was secondary to the message that Arnold and Lee sought to convey. As Lee described it, "While bean milk has been proved to be a satisfactory substitute for cow's milk, this information has been left in the hands of the laboratory. In a land where soybean is grown almost universally, where children grow up without cow's milk, a staple food considered most essential to children's diet, this knowledge of science should be brought to the people."[12] Therein lay the key. It was not the soybean per se but the scientific translation of the soybean that underlay Lee's dedication and enthusiasm.

Nutritional Relief

From 1939 through the end of 1942, with the outbreak of full-scale war in the Pacific, the China Nutritional Aid Council (Zhonghua Yingyang Cujinhui), the successor organization to the Refugee Children's Committee, expanded its nutritional activities in Southwest China across four provinces: Guangxi, Guizhou, Yunnan, and Sichuan.[13] In each of these four provinces, Lee led the initiative to establish local committees under whose directions day-to-day nutritional activities were formulated and implemented. Although the social composition of each committee was made up primarily of Western-trained medical professionals and Christian missionaries, the overall development and programmatic success achieved by each committee was in no way uniform or predictable. Like the Refugee Children's Committee, many, if not most, of the members serving on the branch committees of the China Nutritional Aid Council possessed medical expertise. Dr. T. F Huang, who authored the Chinese Medical Association report on minimum nutritional requirements for Chinese people in 1938, headed the Kunming committee. Dr. C. K. Chu, who served as the director of the Public Health Personnel Training Institute, helped initiate the Guiyang branch committee. The Chengdu branch committee represented a veritable treasure trove of Chinese scientific elite, with several members active in the public health, pediatric, biochemistry, and pharmacy departments of West China Union University. The most prominent member of the Chengdu committee was Dr. C. C. Chen, formerly of the Peking Union Medical College and the rural health experimental center at Dingxian.

As an emergency relief organization, the Refugee Children's Committee knew exactly who should receive its assistance and under what conditions such assistance should be given. But once Nellie Lee began working with different local communities to establish a regular, non-emergency-related nutrition program, questions about to whom and to what extent such aid should be given (and what kind of aid) arose front and center for deliberation. In addition, although nutrition science remained the primary language through which the China Nutritional Aid Council articulated its goals and justified its activities, organized experiments or clinical trials were more difficult to implement given the precarious nature of life during wartime. War in Shanghai had produced a concentrated and confined population available for nutritional intervention; war in the southwest provinces tended to disperse the local population and obscure clear distinctions between the needy and the not so needy. Thus, Lee and the branch committees had to adapt their understanding of nutritional activism to fit local circumstances.

The experience of the branch committee in Kunming (Kunming Ertong Yingyang Weiyuanhui), established in February 1940, provides a good case study for how nutritional activism had to adapt to address the particularities of local circumstance. In general, branch committees broadened the scope of nutritional activism beyond the production and distribution of nutritional supplements to include educational outreach in local communities. They continued to adhere to the nutritional standards set forth by the China Nutritional Aid Council headquartered in Shanghai (henceforth "the Shanghai committee"), but they also recognized that each locale needed to make accommodations to reflect local contingencies. In practice, this resulted in slightly different soybean milk recipes. The Kunming branch committee, for example, added potassium iodide to the standard milk formula twice a month to combat goiter.[14]

Children were the obvious target recipients, but whereas the Refugee Children's Committee had identified its child recipients within the refugee camp structure and organized them by age (those under six receiving milk, those over six but not older than fourteen receiving the soybean residue cake), the Kunming committee needed to reevaluate who exactly counted as children and what kinds of children. Organizing and differentiating within the general category of children—"undernourished street children," "underprivileged children," "malnutritioned children and infants," or "normal children"—meant reassigning meanings to commonplace associations.[15] Was it age that demarcated one group of children from another? Was it a child's ability to pay money for whatever services she received that separated "street children" from "normal children"? Or was medical expertise required to identify physiological signs in the "undernourished" as opposed to "malnutritioned" child? Each of these questions generated both confusion and the desire to know with greater clarity who did and did not count as a child recipient for nutritional work. The Kunming committee did not resolve all these questions, but they did attempt to expand the range of people who counted as "children." While most of their efforts focused on children under the age of twelve, the Kunming committee was not doctrinaire, including "students" within its working definition. This permitted greater institutional flexibility to participate in the development of a "bean milk cooperative" for undernourished students of Southwestern University.[16]

Clarifying who ought to be beneficiaries of nutritional relief was not the only difficulty. Kunming, in contrast to Shanghai's International Settlement, was a much less developed city, and it lacked much of the health infrastructure the Refugee Children's Committee had depended upon to carry out its work. Once Japan had secured control of Indochina in September 1940, Japanese air raids against Kunming increased and further hindered the branch committee's work. Buildings that might have been serviceable as distribution and production centers were destroyed, roads were damaged, and the population scattered for fear of the next round of Japanese attacks.

The Nationalist government's state health system, which had partitioned the country into a hierarchy of provincial and municipal health departments, county health centers with hospitals, district health stations, rural health substations, and village health workers, had by 1937 only succeeded in establishing three health centers in the entire province of Yunnan.[17] By 1941, there were 77 health centers. This investment of human and material resources into building the local health infrastructure came about in conjunction with the infusion of new people and talents, but the superficial improvement in number should not obscure the real hardships faced by those engaged in the effort. Faced with a lack of development in local infrastructure, inflation, and the high cost of drugs, health personnel often had to make do with what little they had. In the words of Sze Szeming of the Chinese Medical Association, the people lived "very close to the good earth."[18]

In terms of the administration of nutritional relief, the Kunming committee had to forge its own path. City residents were not bound to a specific area like a refugee camp, and children ranging in age from infancy to twelve years were not likely to be found all in the same place at the same time. To reach children in the community, the Kunming committee divided the city into four districts with seven distribution centers (five churches, one hospital, and one clinic). Due to the city's poor infrastructure and the committee's limited personnel, the Kunming committee voted in favor of a decentralized system, with each center producing its own milk for distribution. This setup was considered more advantageous, because "a small unit . . . can be an example to be copied in any small district or even in homes, and thereby help to facilitate the spread of bean milk."[19]

Identifying locations from which to produce and distribute soybean milk satisfied the basic question on the supply side, but not the demand side. To pique public interest and spur attendance, the Kunming committee had to find ways in which to build connections and establish relations with local communities—an issue that did not arise at all in the Shanghai refugee camps. Prior to the opening of each station, Nellie Lee and her staff visited the homes of the surrounding neighborhoods to raise awareness of their program, register the number and ages of children in the area, and request the attendance of children under the age of twelve.

Contrary to expectations, this strategy produced neither high nor consistent results. According to the committee's Four Months' Report for December 1939–March 1940, "The general attendance was much less than expected; the most that came at one time seldom exceeded 150. Many were street children, too poor to go to school, but in some centers, more than half were school children. The attendance is very mobile, there is a constant change, for instance in one center, of the 371 children registered, only 13 reappeared the following month." The variable attendance resulted in part because of the philanthropic policy adopted by the committee. In choosing to first provide the milk free, the committee had hoped to acquaint the children with the nutritional significance of soybean milk and cultivate a taste for it. As Lee explained, "The original plan was to give free milk to all as an advertisement, then ask for payment from those who can pay after two months of free milk." The Kunming committee created a graduated pay scheme, which they failed to implement, largely on account of difficulties encountered when opening each distribution center. The pay scheme was attentive to the difficult economic straits facing the larger community. Milk would continue to be free for the "destitute," half free for the poor, at cost for "those who are better off," and slightly above cost ("a little profit") for those with higher incomes. The problem with this approach became apparent when the free trial period had expired. "It was found," Lee wrote, "quite to the contrary as expected, [that] those who took free milk for a period of time instead of being willing were reluctant to pay while new comers are more willing to pay."[20]

Willingness to pay was only one of the possible explanations for low attendance. Lee also proposed, "With the little charity work done in this province, people are suspicious of the motives of giving something for nothing." Later, she surmised, "It takes intelligence to learn and accept new things. The children who come for bean milk are largely from the poor and ignorant class who are generally indifferent to new things. Many well intended plans to help the poor are often not profited by those who need it most, like for instance the Birth Control Movement."[21] Lee and the Kunming committee had hoped that bodily practice in the form of drinking soybean milk would provide sufficient empirical knowledge of the milk's nutritional benefits. So long as they found ways to attract the children to the centers, the milk itself would be its own best advertisement. Nutritional value and commercial value were assumed by the committee to be comparable and easily comprehensible. Surely, they reasoned, local consumers would pay for that which they deemed self-beneficial. When they did not, the default rationale advanced by Lee expressed classist disdain for the moral and educational prospects of the poor.

But as attendance diminished and reluctance manifested itself, what became apparent was the inequivalence and incomprehension surrounding the various activities. For Lee and the committee, their soybean milk was produced precisely because it satisfied the biomedical criteria of being nutritious: it was high in protein, B vitamins, and iron, and it was fortified with calcium lactate.[22] They chose distribution centers at hospitals, clinics, and churches in order to "give people the confidence that bean milk is good for children" and convey the scientific and nutritional authority of their work.[23] Home visits too were meant to communicate a personal assurance of the good the child would receive were he or she to visit the center for milk, while also helping to create a social network in which actions were accounted for and recorded. Lee also sought assistance from locals, with the expectation that local residents speaking local dialects would better translate the nutritional value of adding soybean milk to a child's daily diet.[24] Echoing earlier efforts by the Refugee Children's Committee, Lee and the Kunming committee also attempted to institute their own clinical studies on the nutritional benefits of soybean milk for malnourished infants in the hopes that positive, empirical results would help persuade the hesitant and the skeptical to send their children for milk.

Each of these measures served to reassure organizers that their work as nutritional activists upheld the highest standards of science and modernity. The committee's attempts to build a social network of relations that thereby enabled their intervention into the daily dietaries of local residents rested upon claims of superior knowledge and transparency. But insofar as soybean milk was a tool for instilling greater nutritional consciousness among the people, these details were neither obvious nor particularly comprehensible to the child recipient. Children neither recognized nor understood the nutritional value of soybean milk. "Children were drawn by the novelty rather than real understanding of [soybean milk's] value."[25] Their parents evinced similar incomprehension. Nutritional value as represented by the soybean milk drink did not lend itself to easy translation and comprehension, because in actual practice, it failed to communicate with the exigencies of day-to-day living.

And yet, even in the face of adversity and apparent failure, the branch committees did not abandon their commitment to the idea that experimental research was essential for modern relief work. Moreover, they continued to pursue strategies that blended social and scientific praxis. Community work was always paired with experimental work, however rudimentary or schematic: physical examinations, height and weight surveys, and limited feeding trials to assess the nutritional benefits of giving soybean milk to malnourished infants. The Jiangxi branch committee cooperated with the Jiangxi Provincial Medical College and the Jiangxi Provincial War Orphanage Number Two in a three-month survey of the diet, growth, and overall health of orphans.[26] Dr. P. S. Tang of the Tsinghua University Physiological Laboratory joined the Kunming committee for the express purpose of conducting experiments and related laboratory work. The extent to which Tang actually gained research material is unclear based on extant records. At the very least, he assisted the other physicians on the committee in devising alternate soybean milk formulas for normal and malnourished children and clarifying specific feeding directions for the different infant cases encountered at the distribution centers.[27]

The branch committees of the China Nutritional Aid Council had to reconfigure their nutritional activities in Southwest China to meet local circumstances and incorporate various forms of education into their campaign. In Ganxian, Guangxi, the branch committee established a "nutritional restaurant" that sold soybean milk, soybean residue cakes (*douzha bing*), bread, and a "simple meal of balanced diet at $3 per person."[28] In Chengdu and Chongqing, the branch committees experimented with specialized food shops, tearooms, and diet kitchens that provided public demonstrations of "proper cooking." Branch committees conducted educational campaigns and published pamphlets on dietary habits, the fundamentals of good nutrition, and the benefits of soybean-based diets. They placed articles in local papers, arranged for broadcast times on radio stations, and scheduled lectures by physician and nurse members of the committee. In addition, they entertained plans for retraining local bean makers in the ways of scientific soybean milk, and they worked with schools to integrate soybean milk into the daily schedule. They made accommodations for those too poor to pay for milk, and they added other nutritional supplements as circumstances permitted.[29]

NUTRITIONAL ENDORSEMENT

From 1940 until Japan's attack on Pearl Harbor on December 7, 1941, the Shanghai committee was the de facto headquarters of national operations for the China Nutritional Aid Council. The Shanghai committee was intended to function as a "clearinghouse," to coordinate the work on soybean milk and accessory products in the interior, "so as to prevent unnecessary duplication and secure a wide spread utilization of the work and studies thus far accomplished."[30] In theory, it would expedite, correlate, and give "intelligent aid and direction" to the branch offices. It would oversee the allocation of available funds, especially from American funding agencies like China Child Welfare and United China Relief; gather together the available literature on soybeans and other relevant nutritional topics in China and abroad; and help prepare educational materials for distribution at local nutritional centers. In practice, its work was rather more localized and reflective of its situation in Shanghai. Its committee members emerged from the same pool of highly specialized and distinguished medical clinicians and researchers as had defined the Refugee Children's Committee.

Nellie Lee's counterpart in the endeavor to spread soybean nutrition could be found in Hou Xiangchuan. A graduate of St. John's University in Shanghai and PUMC in Beijing and a specialist in deficiency diseases, Hou was representative of a new generation of Chinese nutrition scientists who had been primarily trained at science programs in China during the 1920s and 1930s. His interest in the soybean derived from his general sense that the absence of dairy in the Chinese diet rendered the application of Western nutritional standards impractical, if not quixotic. Instead, he argued that "the use of soybeans and soybean products should be encouraged since the proteins most approximate animal proteins, closer than any other common plant proteins."[31]

Hou's crossover into nutritional activism occurred in the aftermath of the outbreak of war between China and Japan. The influx of refugees into Shanghai in late 1937 posed an incredible challenge in terms of feeding so many people. But for someone like Hou, it also afforded an unusual opportunity for combining science and relief work. He and the other physicians who volunteered time and provided medical care to the camps "became alarmed at the conditions" prevailing there.[32] Overcrowding, an insufficient water supply, damp and dirty quarters, little attention to the spread of infectious diseases—all of these problems emerged in one form or another at the refugee camps in Shanghai. But change for the better was possible, and for Hou, who also served as the chairman of the Refugee Health Committee of the Shanghai International Red Cross, the Refugee Children's Committee was aptly situated to make a unique contribution to the general refugee social relief efforts taking place in the International Settlement. By focusing on children, and in particular their diet, it played a key role in helping to alleviate the inequities and uncertainties of camp life. Hou, for his part, provided the scientific know-how and experimental temperament to transform the China Nutritional Aid Council's work from simply emergency refugee relief into a scientific enterprise fit for a burgeoning capitalist economy.

Hou argued for strong scientific representation and pushed for the inclusion of specialists in the ranks of the China Nutritional Aid Council's membership—men like Wu Xian, the eminent biochemist and chairman of the Chinese Medical Association's Committee on Nutrition, which had published its recommendations for minimum nutritional standards for the Chinese in 1938; Bernard E. Read, director of the Division of the Physiological Sciences at the Lester Institute; Dr. T. F. Huang, Professor of Public Health at the National Medical College, Kunming; Dr. H. Y. Yao, director of the Provincial Health Department of Yunnan and former graduate of PUMC; and Dr. Robert Lim, director of the Chinese Red Cross Relief Unit and professor of physiology at PUMC.

The extent to which any of these men became involved with the China Nutritional Aid Council varied. Wu Xian, H. Y. Yao, and Robert Lim appear to have expended little, if any, attention on the organization. T. F. Huang headed the Kunming branch committee, and Bernard Read took up various nutrition initiatives for the Council after Japan's surrender in 1945. For its part, the Shanghai committee did attract the involvement of Dr. Ernest Tso, professor of pediatrics at PUMC, who first came up with a recipe for feeding fresh soymilk to infants; Dr. Sao-ke Alfred Sze, who having retired from the diplomatic service in 1937, settled in Shanghai and become active with the International Relief Committee and the Anti-Tuberculosis Association, which he founded; and Dr. Szeming Sze, eldest son of Dr. Sze, who later went on to play a major role in establishing the World Health Organization as a specialized agency of the United Nations. And in contrast to its early incarnation, the China Nutritional Aid Council also attracted the participation of prominent business and industry figures from companies like the China Cotton Manufacturing Company, the Yee Tsoong Tobacco Company, Percy Kwok & Co., China Chemical Works, Ltd., and the Henningsen Produce Company.

The Shanghai committee was committed to the goal of improving the general nutritional health of the Chinese people, but it defined the concept of nutritional health rather differently than other branch offices. From the very beginning, the Shanghai committee directed its efforts toward the "popularization of the soybean and bean cakes."[33] The reason behind the selection of the soybean as a kind of proto-superfood stemmed from the China Nutritional Aid Council's commitment to "economical nutrition," which Julean Arnold defined as "the utilization of the country's agricultural resources to the best possible extent in meeting the needs of its masses."[34] Rather than devote resources toward the sole purpose of creating and running nutritional aid stations in Shanghai, the Shanghai committee focused on expanding experimental research with soybeans and building relationships with the commercial sector. It emphasized the importance of devising production methods and equipment that could be easily used, could be moved about, and was cost efficient. One of the main projects enacted by the Shanghai committee involved the creation of a model unit for the production of soybean milk that could be distributed to commercial sites.

The Shanghai committee actively sought relations with the commercial sector in the hopes that private companies could be persuaded to manufacture and sell soybean milk in Shanghai. The committee would provide interested companies the "correct formula" for making soybean milk, as well as the equipment with which to make the milk. This brand of nutritional activism conceived of social awareness and nutritional knowledge in commercial terms. To help inculcate a notion of good health—to develop and spread "soybean milk conscious[ness]"—the Shanghai committee began with the assumption of the public as consumer. To change dietary habits meant changing, or at least influencing, consumption patterns.

Within months of its formation, the Shanghai committee sought to establish a model unit for the production of soybean milk in Shanghai.[35] With the financial backing of P. Y. Tang of the China Cotton Manufacturing Company, the Shanghai committee solicited proposals and designs from its members on plant administration and soybean milk production. There were four considerations influencing work on the model equipment: "(a) that the materials of the whole plant should be all procurable from the interior of China, (b) that the materials should be serviceable but not expensive, (c) [that] the equipment should be power-saving and (d) that the plant should be unitary."[36] Tang allocated space in his cotton mill for the model equipment, and by May 1940, several trial runs had been made. The process was not without several hiccups. The trial runs conducted at Tang's mill revealed a number of problems with the designed equipment:

(1) It would be impossible to combine and inter-change the motor or power driving with the driving of manual labor into one device; and therefore it is necessary to design two models separately for local convenience and adoption, (2) The presser as originally designed was found to be a failure as the bean-residues so pressed would be subjected to too much handling and therefore makes [sic] the milk rancid, (3) The cooker proved quite satisfactory but upon the suggestion of other members of the Council, it was thought wise to design a new one for three purposes, (a) boiling of milk, (b) sterilization of utensils and (c) baking of soybean residue cakes.[37]

To test the economic efficiency of its model plant, the Shanghai committee approached the Shanghai Municipal Council's jail authorities in spring 1940 about the possibilities of setting up a model plant with an experimental laboratory at the Ward Road Jail. Although hardly "consumers" in the traditional sense, because inmate diets had to adhere to predetermined budgetary constraints, the Shanghai committee argued that the Ward Road Jail would be the ideal setting in which to evaluate "our idea of giving adequate nutrition at economized finances." Negotiations with jail representatives quickly revealed a number of obstacles forestalling the adoption and implementation of the plan. The initial setup costs were estimated to be at least $2,000—far exceeding the jail's budgetary allocations. Moreover, jail authorities were concerned that too much tinkering with the inmates' diet might result in violent dissatisfaction. As the jail rations already included two ounces of soybean per inmate per day, an additional allotment of soybean milk seemed both excessive and unnecessary.[38] When those plans fell through, the Shanghai committee shifted course toward the commercial sector and decided that the model equipment designed and then tested on the premises of Tang's cotton mill "has now [arrived] at a stage when the equipment should be properly installed and run on [a] business basis."[39]

In pursuing commercial ties, the Shanghai committee hoped to "encourage such enterprising merchant[s] like the Fresh Fruit Drinks, Inc., to manufacture and sell soybean milk in Shanghai according to the Council's formula so as to popularize and make the Shanghai people soybean milk conscious."[40] For an organization dedicated to promoting the well-being and good health of the Chinese people "by educating them to make wider use of the soybean and its products," the Shanghai committee had adopted a rather novel approach. The novelty lay not so much in its attempts to draw upon commercial enterprises to produce and market soybean milk for sale but rather in its decision to position the organization as an official arbiter of scientific soybean milk. By stressing the necessity that local companies like Fresh Fruit Drinks adopt "the Council's formula," the Shanghai committee blurred the lines between social advocacy and commercial profit and recast the value of scientific research as testimony of the efficacy of nutritional relief.

The Shanghai committee continued to include charitable giving in its repertoire of activities, but the purpose of providing free milk shifted from nutritional aid to experimental testing of different soybean milk formulas. Hou Xiangchuan argued in 1940 that an existing feeding program at the Refugee Children Camp at 181 Jessfield Road could serve as testing grounds for a new soybean milk powder mixture Hou was developing.[41] Lack of funding had halted soybean milk distribution to the 400 children at the camp, but Hou proposed that since the camp was well run, "it should serve as a good place for a large experimental trial of the soybean powder mixture. By feeding 200 children with the powder and others not, it will be possible to observe the effect of the soybean powder supplement." Funding for the experiment was obtained from China Child Welfare ($1,900) and other sources ($500), and on July 15, 1940, Hou initiated the experiment. He expected that "results of the experiment will be known after another two and half months' time."[42]

The tensions between running a business venture and serving the public interest were apparent from the beginning. Could an organization that claimed to serve the cause of social welfare also support private economic ventures? The executive secretary, K. H. Fu, seemed to be of two minds when he wrote, "Of course, I realize that neither the Sun Company project nor the Green Spot project conforms to our original aim, which was for the nutrition of the common masses. I am, therefore, investigating at present whether it would be possible to start a center at . . . Robinson Road where the working class congests."[43] The agreement with the Sun Company gained the Shanghai committee not only a site for the manufacture of soymilk and soybean residue cakes—the model equipment developed by the Shanghai committee was transferred and installed at the Sun Company's East Nanjing Road building—but also three separate counter spaces, one in the basement, another on the ground floor, and the third adjacent to the soda fountain, for the sale of the products. With its reputation as one of Shanghai's big department stores, the Sun Company afforded the Shanghai committee a unique opportunity to reach the commercial masses. But so long as that engagement was framed as a commercial activity, it remained open to debate the extent to which the Shanghai committee could also help educate the public about good nutrition, and the soybean's role therein. Fu's proposal that a nutritional clinic be set up to attend to the working class demonstrates an awareness of the possible conflicts of interest facing the Shanghai committee. "If the Sun Company project can make people to drink [sic] soya bean milk as a fashion and the Robinson Road project will make people to drink [sic] soya bean milk as a matter of good nutrition, then I believe that the two projects will supplement instead of defeating each other."[44]

There was one further obfuscation enacted through the Shanghai committee's decision to become an arbiter for scientific soybean milk. By seeking to take on the role of arbiter, the Shanghai committee challenged the jurisdictional authority of existing governmental agencies and attempted to reposition itself as a nonprofit aid organization and a long-term mediator between profit and social good. Hou had been keenly involved in the development of a soybean milk formula that satisfied scientific standards and carried the China Nutritional Aid Council's seal of approval, and for this reason, he played a key role in adjudicating commercial requests for endorsement.

This attempt to transfer scientific authority through a form of commercial credentialing may have seemed an optimal way in which the China Nutritional Aid Council could exert its influence over the manufacture of commercial soybean milk, but in practice, it generated a web of knotty problems. Despite having agreed-upon minimum nutritional standards that commercial soybean milks had to meet, questions persisted about the frequency of testing, whose financial responsibility it was to bear the costs of chemical testing, the duration of the Council's endorsement, and even the potential contamination of value that might occur with the mixing of science and advertising.

In 1940, Pure Fruit Drinks Inc. submitted a request for an endorsement of their soybean milk product, "Vito-Milk." As the chairman of the Committee on Regulations, Standards, and Inspections for the China Nutritional Aid Council, Hou led an inspection of the plant where Vito-Milk was produced and reviewed the chemical analysis of a Vito-Milk sample. In recommending to the chairman of the China Nutritional Aid Council the endorsement of Pure Fruit Drinks' project, Hou stipulated that the "calcium content of the milk should be increased to not less than 0.06%" while nonetheless preserving the other "values of the [existing] chemical analysis."[45]

Hou's recommendation seemed slightly premature to another member of the same committee, one H. Pedersen, a veterinary scientist also employed by the SMC's Public Health Department. Pedersen pointed out that as Vito-Milk's "calcium content is below the minimum standard laid down by the [China] Nutritional Aid Council, . . . we would not be working in the best interest of the Nutritional Aid Council if we made such a precedent." Moreover, as chemical analyses of any food sample were expensive, Pedersen believed it only fair that the cost of the analysis be borne by the manufacturers. The sampling would be performed by members of the China Nutritional Aid Council or the SMC's Public Health Department, but the attendant fees would be charged to the soybean milk manufacturers. Pedersen may have been indirectly sharing the internal concerns of members of the SMC's Public Health Department. When Pure Fruit Drinks contacted the China Nutritional Aid Council for its endorsement, it also sent a letter to J. H. Jordan, Commissioner of the Public Health Department, in which it detailed its efforts to produce a "soybean milk . . . [that] meet[s] the requirements of a part of the people in Shanghai as advised by Drs. W. S. Fu, H. C. Hou, and Ernest Tso" and expressed hope that such efforts demonstrated the sincerity and thoroughness of their endeavor. The company's primary objective was to obtain the requisite license for proper marking and labeling of products sold in the International Settlement.

Hou countered Pedersen's concerns by pointing out that multiple samples had been analyzed, and the lower-than-desired calcium content was found in only one of the samples. Pure Fruit Drinks, in pursuing the endorsement of the China Nutritional Aid Council, had acceded to the stipulation that it make its product available for analysis "from time to time" and accept "constant supervision of the China Nutritional Aid Council as well as abide with any instruction of the Council for improvement." In Hou's opinion, this willingness amounted to a good-faith effort. Moreover, as the Council's endorsement was conditional upon the maintenance of requisite scientific standards, he remained convinced that Pure Fruit Drinks' request warranted approval, because they could always revoke the endorsement in the future.

What Hou was unaware of was the parallel discussion of nutritional standards taking place at the SMC Public Health Department. Hou had conceded that that calcium content was less than desired, but he made no mention of the vitamin profile of Pure Fruit Drinks' Vito-Milk. In contrast, Pedersen and his Public Health Department colleagues fixated on both the name "Vito-Milk" and the vitamin content of the drink. Pedersen communicated to his Public Health colleagues, "this word 'Vito' either indicates full of vitamins or strength, and with a little propaganda by the dealers, the consumer would never know of the make-up of the contents." For this reason, he felt it imperative that the company add the Chinese characters for "bean milk" (*dounai*) to its labels. For even greater clarity, he insisted that "bean milk" in English be clearly marked both on the hood and cap of each bottle.[46] "Vito," it was further reasoned, connotes vitamins, and based on the in-house analysis, Pure Fruit Drinks' Vito-Milk lacked vitamin A, and what little vitamin D it contained had been "added . . . in a manner not recommended by the League of Nations."[47]

Despite the difference of opinions and the skepticism voiced by the SMC Public Health Department, the issue was ultimately resolved in favor of granting a China Nutritional Aid Council endorsement to Pure Fruit Drinks' Vito-Milk.[48] When the company launched its product in the Shanghai market in the summer of 1941, it emphasized the scientific authorities backing the venture. "This new product has been tested and approved by the Shanghai Municipal Council, the French Municipal Council, and the China Nutritional Aid Council as a food drink for young and old."[49] Uncontaminated by "tubercular bacteria" and the "equivalent to cows' milk," the product was further distinguished as "entirely done by machinery" and more superior to "ordinary soya bean milk, as peanuts, walnuts, and almonds are added to enrich the milk and add to its flavor."[50] The public response was enthusiastic. In response to these claims, the company announced that 13,000 new subscribers had placed orders within a fortnight of the launching of their advertising campaign. The demand caught the company off guard, and "the original staff, equipment and delivery facilities have become jammed."[51]

Such advertising gusto could hardly have dampened concerns that conferring endorsements would compromise the mission and integrity of the China Nutritional Aid Council. Indeed, when another company, Welly

Nourishing Food Products Co., placed a full-page advertisement for Welly Soya Milk (*Weili dounai*) in the October 8, 1941, issue of *Shenbao*, it included a complete reprint, with Chinese translation, of the letter of endorsement sent from the China Nutritional Aid Council (figure 7.1). That the SMC Public Health Department had previously rejected Welly's application for a license did little to improve relations between the department and the China Nutritional Aid Council. The latter's attempt to position itself as a scientific arbiter of commercial soybean milk challenged existing power relations without necessarily reconciling the ongoing tensions between profit and social good. The China Nutritional Aid Council's ability to even broker such a position highlights the highly factionalized nature of politics in wartime Shanghai.

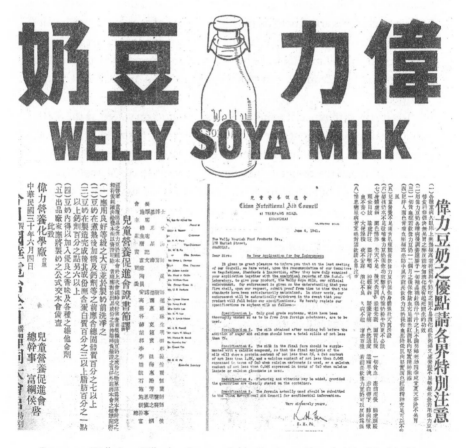

FIGURE 7.1. Welly Soya Milk advertisement. Folder U1-16-1745, Shanghai Municipal Archives.

CONCLUSION

Adapting to local contingencies reflected both necessity and innovation under difficult circumstances. Incorporating commercial strategies to sell soybean nutrition provided a seemingly straightforward approach that reconciled, in part, the vastly more variegated population the China Nutritional Aid Council sought to reach. For Nellie Lee, pioneering soybean work in the interior meant devising new approaches and making choices without a lot of guidance or prior consultation. A young woman of Cantonese extraction now attempting to mobilize local resources with neither the local dialect nor an established community upon which to depend, Lee faced considerable odds. She relied on Christian contacts and whenever possible deferred to "local" experts, who, like her, were in many instances recently transplanted migrants who had followed the Nationalist retreat to the southwestern provinces. Lee often found herself shorthanded, alone, and without a clear path forward. The fortitude required came in spurts as she battled long bouts of despondency and frustration. In November 1942, Lee sent a long letter to Julean Arnold in Shanghai. After first apologizing for the absence of formal and regular correspondence regarding her work in the interior, Lee wrote, "There are reasons for my silence. Man prefers to be alone in sorrow. Ever since I came into the interior, there has been a succession of frustration, feeling most of the time lonesome in my struggle."[52]

The documentary trail for Hou Xiangchuan does not allow one such a candid glimpse of the personal travails attendant to propagating soybean nutrition. That such work was difficult, especially with regards to its determined intent to change people's food habits, cannot be overstated. It required endless negotiation with all sorts of actors, including but not limited to the young child who had previously received free milk, the newly trained nurse whose fluency in the local dialect and perhaps familial connections gained her some advantage when setting off to establish a rural soybean milk station, the enterprising salesman of a newly founded soybean milk company, and the steely-eyed bureaucrat who prided himself on knowing and enforcing a separation between scientific objectivity and commercial profit.

What tied the work of these people together was the conviction that food mattered. Food mattered, not simply because it sustained life. It mattered, because through food—especially certain foods—twentieth-century reformers could reimagine the Chinese nation as strong, productive, and resourceful. As part of a larger campaign to improve the nutritional health of Chinese children, Lee and Hou embarked upon a project that situated nutrition as the crucial site for the dissemination of modern knowledge and values. Health, when reconfigured in terms of nutrition science, became fertile grounds for entrepreneurial experimentation and self-invention. The soybean, with its endless adaptability, could nourish and help reinvent the Chinese nation as a nation of doers who built rural clinics, set up soybean milk distribution programs at local schools, and redefined the terrain of scientific expertise beyond the university and government. Children fed soybean milk could grow up strong and healthy; parents attuned to the nutritional value of foods might willingly accept the authority and expertise of outsiders on all matters, including how and what one should eat. Broad-minded and rational, the Chinese people could imbibe modernity one sip at a time.

But as compelling as this vision may have been, it was rooted in exceptional circumstances. Refugee children and refugee camps afforded opportunities and advantages that could not be replicated when the campaign to promote soybean nutrition moved beyond Shanghai. Questions abounded about who was a proper recipient, whether or not a fee should be charged (and how much and to whom), where distribution should take place, and how the specific act of consumption would lead to broader educational transformations, that is, the nurturing of soybean consciousness among the Chinese people. This is not to suggest that there were no minor victories and successes as Nellie Lee and Hou Xiangchuan plied their efforts in Southwest China and Shanghai, respectively. But adapting to local contingencies meant rethinking the boundaries of both their work and their positions. Both of them diversified the meaning of soybean nutrition to include quasi-commercial ventures, and both attempted to expand the bounds of professional influence upon daily habits and local governance.

Their efforts, however, were ultimately unsuccessful and nondurable. After Pearl Harbor, Japan dismantled Shanghai's foreign concessions and imposed its authority through the establishment of a Chinese puppet government. The modest degree of freedom the China Nutritional Aid Council had enjoyed under the auspices of the International Settlement evaporated. In light of the political change of government, the Council moved inland to Chongqing, and Dr. Arthur N. Young, the American financial adviser to the Nationalist government, assumed directorship of the organization. Hou's attempts to position the Council as the arbiter of scientific soybean milk ended once its headquarters relocated to Chongqing. And yet, the influence of his endorsement program can be seen in measures undertaken by the occupation government in 1943 to craft a set of scientific standards for soybean milk that would presumably bring regulatory order to soybean milk's commercial production in Shanghai.

As for Nellie Lee, she began in late 1944 to petition China Child Welfare, which had been absorbed into United China Relief, for a scholarship that would allow her to travel to the United States and obtain a graduate degree in nutrition. Her reason was to bolster her credentials so as to defuse local challenges she had encountered out in the field. Lee argued that local elites had been antagonistic toward her when she attempted to create nutrition centers and reach out to local mothers and their children because she lacked a specialized degree. She insisted upon attending a program in New York, partly because she had family in the city, and partly because the prestige of New York universities would be better received.[53]

The scholarship program officers at United China Relief were doubtful but attributed many of their doubts to Nellie Lee's previous lack of training in the sciences. For them, a graduate degree in nutrition required extensive work in biology, biochemistry, and chemistry—all courses she had not taken as an undergraduate. Moreover, her request for placement in New York did not fit their understanding of the most suitable nutrition programs for her line of work. For them, a land-grant institution like the University of Minnesota or the University of Tennessee would be a better fit. Before reaching a decision, the program officers contacted a number of specialists, including the agronomist J. Lossing Buck and biochemist Leonard A. Maynard, to determine whether there were potential gains in sending Lee to the United States for graduate studies. In the end, Lee was granted permission, and she matriculated at the nutrition program at the University of Tennessee at Knoxville. When she left for the United States in April 1945, her position at the China Nutritional Aid Council was quickly filled by a rotation of young Chinese women who had recently received degrees in chemistry or nutrition science.

Lee's time in Knoxville proved difficult. In a confidential letter from Dr. Florence L. Macleod, head of the Nutrition Department and assistant director of the Agricultural Experiment Station in charge of home economics research, Macleod described Lee as "a square peg trying to squeeze into a round hole. She seemed to lack personal enthusiasm and sympathetic understanding of people." Lee did not participate in class discussions, she did not take an active role in the "field work of community nutrition" (e.g., extension programs at mills, factories, well-baby and prenatal clinics), and she dipped into and out of classes with alarming regularity. A more negative assessment could hardly have been written about Nellie Lee. Her time and labor as an administrator for the China Nutritional Aid Council was belittled, and her complaint that "she was not receiving what she wanted" from the courses and the fieldwork in Knoxville was dismissed as poor manners.

There is, however, another interpretation. Given her experiences in Southwest China during the previous five years, what she encountered in the classrooms of the University of Tennessee exposed too great a disjunction. If there was a single lesson she had learned, it was that context mattered. Nutrition science was value laden and context specific. However much her studies in Tennessee insisted that there existed a universal basis for nutrition science, one that rendered all human bodies a composite of specific nutritional needs and efficiencies and all communities a permutation upon those living in and around Knoxville, Nellie Lee knew better. Educating the Chinese "to the greater appreciation of the possibilities of the use of the soybean for nutritive purposes" was neither simple nor straightforward. To build a new, modern consciousness of the value and worth of soybean milk required the creation and elaboration of a sociotechnical system in which bricolage, negotiation, and creative compromise dominated. It required young Chinese reformers to remake themselves as they endeavored to remake the communities around them. That her American teachers and peers could not sympathize with her struggles may have betrayed a limit in their own topography of everyday experience, not hers.

Epilogue

Negotiating Past and Future through the Soybean

A MONG the various ephemera I encountered during research for this book was a postcard produced by the China Nutritional Aid Council (figure E.1). A piece of memorabilia without practical intent—the unsent postcard had been kept pristine among the papers of Julean Arnold, the former commercial attaché of the US consulate in Shanghai, who became one of the strongest proponents of soybeans in Republican China—it gestures to a world eerily familiar yet nonetheless unrecognizable. In a scene both playful and violent, a soybean family led by a well-heeled soybean "granny" and armed with sticks chases a dairy cow toward the gate of a museum. Architecturally, the museum appears to possess both Chinese and Western design elements, with its bilaterally symmetrical gate and winged roof tiles fronting the Georgian-style building behind them. The convergence of these visual details challenges easy assumptions about China and the West and the common temporal assignation of China and things Chinese to the past. After all, the museum as a repository of the past (presumably for public consumption) was itself a new and modern construct in Republican China. Its pastiche of stylistic elements and tone underscores a vision of Chinese nutrition that positions the soybean as the main protagonist in a tale weaving together food, family, and the nation. Looking at this postcard, it is impossible not to wonder about the world it is referencing.

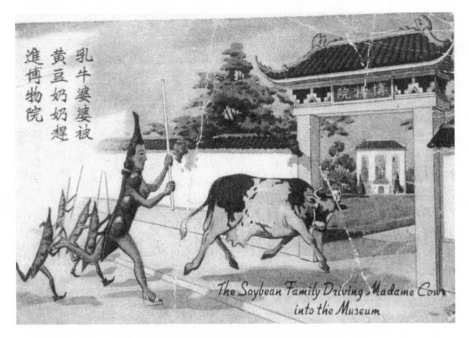

乳牛婆婆被
黄豆奶奶趕
進博物院

The Soybean Family Driving Madame Cow
into the Museum

FIGURE E.1. Postcard issued by the China Nutritional Aid Council. Julean Herbert Arnold
Papers, Box 13, Folder "Soy Protein," Hoover Institution Archives.

To understand the how and why behind the visual semantics of this postcard, we need to revisit the implicit stakes raised by the notion of the Chinese diet and the role specific foods should play therein. In 1926, when the
biochemist Wu Xian raised the question of whether the Chinese diet was
adequate in light of our modern knowledge of nutrition, he sought to challenge the implicit assumptions and cultural prerogatives that might lead the
Chinese people to tacitly, complacently accept food as sustenance or survival.
He was responding to the formation of a globalized world in which national
diets seemed both a prerequisite and a natural consequence of modern life.
In such a world, agricultural goods were increasingly entangled in industrial
chains that stretched from local village to urban metropolis, in and outside
of China. The very meaning of food was being rewritten by scientific elites
in terms of analytic categories that stressed the universalism of the biochemistry of life and mass production. Against this backdrop in which global
capitalism and science were steadily transforming the political economy of
food around the world, the issue of dietary adequacy channeled fears about
Chinese fitness (bodily and geopolitically).

For someone such as the Chinese anarchist/later Nationalist statesman Li Shizeng, whose advocacy of the soybean began a good decade prior to Wu Xian's expression of nutritional concern and pivoted on the crop's fungibility in the service of an emerging technoscientific order, the soybean represented not the inadequacy of the Chinese diet but its potential to change. If Li was less concerned about the extent to which the Chinese diet was adequate according to modern nutritional knowledge, he was nonetheless convinced that nutrition science was the language in which to communicate how certain foods common to local dietaries could be reinvented for the modern age. The key to transforming the soybean into a modern agro-industrial commodity did not require a disavowal of its former meanings (i.e., famine food, animal feed, and fertilizer); rather, an intellectual shift among the Chinese thinking classes was needed. If the Chinese embraced agricultural science and actively cultivated its native technologies for hidden advantages, then China could dictate its own rules of participation in the emerging global order of industrial modernity.

In contrast, for Wu, the Chinese diet was a conceptual category backed by a growing body of scientific research and plagued by the specter of deficiency, whose functions extended beyond the individual to the nation writ large. It was a discursive entity made manifest through everyday actions that could nonetheless be rendered accountable to the dictates of science and the demands of the modern age. The Chinese diet was never just what Chinese people ate; it derived from the accretion of social, environmental, and historical forces. It marked out the alimentary terrain that had constituted the Chinese nation and established Chinese standing in relation to other nations in clear, discrete units of analysis. If one could not reasonably conclude that the Chinese diet was adequate in light of modern nutritional knowledge, then the Chinese diet had to be changed, adjusted, manipulated, and adapted, because the Chinese path toward modernity entailed nothing less than the steadfast will to introspection and willingness to grapple with self-perceived Chinese deficiencies. The soybean was an important—but temporary—solution to improve Chinese protein intake, because the long-term trajectory to achieve dietary optimality required deep structural changes to the country's agricultural economy and people's everyday eating habits.

On these points, Wu's scientific colleagues agreed. But for men such as Hou Xiangchuan, Luo Dengyi, and Ernest Tso, the soybean was more than a stopgap measure for fixing the Chinese diet. They, like Li Shizeng, were dazzled by the transformative possibilities of the soybean to make seemingly universal, but largely Western-inspired, dietary notions about milk and protein, growth and development meaningful and practicable for a modern China. The Chinese diet may indeed be inadequate, they argued, but the means for change lay close at hand. With the soybean, one had the basis for creating a vegetal milk whose nutritive properties equaled—or even exceeded—those of cow's milk, that modern elixir of progress and development that had nurtured the rise of the West. Scientifically testable, standardizable, and locally available, soybean milk represented indigenous creativity in the face of adversity. It could be served to infants, children, and students. It could be packaged and sold through subscriptions that were then delivered by bicycles. It could be centrally produced and distributed as a fortified nutritional supplement. It was hygienic, because it could be industrially produced and was uncontaminated by distressed or diseased animals. And it was affordable, for Chinese and Westerners alike. The soybean, it could be said, was a classic example of Chinese frugality: a seemingly indigestible and not very palatable legume that nonetheless sustained one through times of travail and uncertainty, a food more commonly associated with the poorer side of life that could nonetheless spur invention and innovation, and not just for some preindustrial form of subsistence living.

If the Chinese people needed, as the China Nutritional Aid Council suggested, greater soybean consciousness (greater understanding of the scientific and nutritional value of the soybean to improve Chinese dietary practices), then a variety of programs could be instituted to enlighten the masses. Few would have asked for the exigencies of war as the platform on which to launch broader social change, and yet war had nonetheless afforded an incomparable opportunity with which to begin restructuring everyday habits. The Shanghai Refugee Children's Nutritional Aid Committee recognized this, as did the China Nutritional Aid Council. Refugee children served as the first target of reform, but as with all matters of conscience, the end goal encompassed a wide swathe of common people, from children up through their parents. Under the banner of national survival, scientific soybean milk could be presented as both an emergency nutritional supplement and an everyday solution to endemic nutritional deficiencies. An army of young professional women like Nellie Lee took up the cause of raising soybean consciousness in the rural hinterland of Southwest China. She and her fellow nutritional activists canvassed local households to encourage turnout and increase awareness. They struggled with the practical and ethical ambiguities associated with translating abstract categories into workable programs. Their work, as Lee's experience shows, was fraught, precisely because they had to directly confront the tensions between what the historian Joan Judge has called the "everyday" and "epic" agendas, "agendas focused on disseminating knowledge derived from and necessary for the conduct of daily life, and agendas driven by broader global and national concerns."[1] Scientific soybean milk was designed to be a habituated form of nutritional enlightenment. Getting people to drink it with such elevated recognition, however, required fortitude and perseverance and not a little bit of wishful thinking.

This narrative of change and transformation, of self-initiative and invention rings no less true in sentiment today than it did at the beginning of the twentieth century, even as the terms of engagement have radically shifted. Indeed, if there exists any semblance of continuity, it lies with the ongoing perception of the soybean's adaptability, even flexibility, to accommodate new social and economic imaginaries while still retaining ties to the past. In the early twentieth century, introspection and fear of inadequacy had motivated Chinese scientific elites to set the terms by which nutrition science could be integrated into the Chinese everyday. Their advocacy for rationalizing the Chinese diet to make it conform with international standards of growth and development arose from a deeper impulse to reevaluate all aspects of Chinese culture and tradition. This process of examination was neither straightforward nor predictable, and while the adoption of nutrition science might suggest an outright embrace of all things Western and foreign, in practice the ways in which nutrition science and the soybean reproduced themselves in everyday life were more variegated and layered. Older understandings were never eliminated; rather, a pastiche of meanings surfaced in new forms and helped enliven new realities. In this way, it was possible for the soybean to operate in multiple registers, for there to be ongoing traffic between the values embodied by scientific soybean milk and *doujiang*, between tradition and modernity. The ties with the past had to be managed, if not reinterpreted, but if one could lead the public to scientific soybean milk through more familiar paths, expediency prevailed. Scientific soybean milk represented a particular path by which China could incorporate itself into the modern world on terms of its own devising and interpretation. The imaginative possibilities created by soybean milk articulated a future defined by progress, wealth, and power, but in ways not completely divorced from the past. After all, scientific soybean milk was the rationalized, modernized incarnation of a more common and customary food, *doujiang* or *doufujiang*.

This sense of the soybean's generative potential in crafting a Chinese future is less apparent today. Indeed even as the importance of the soybean as an agro-industrial crop grows, the popular conception of the soybean is increasingly delimited by its most common culinary manifestation, tofu, and in ways that harken back to a glorified Chinese past. Consider how the 2012 food-centric documentary *A Bite of China* (Shejian shang de Zhongguo), which made its debut on CCTV China's official state broadcaster in 2012, introduced and discussed tofu.[2] With its high production value and lush visuals, the original seven-episode series explored a different theme in each episode—preserving by salt, pickling, or wind; staple foods; fermentation; the "gifts of nature"—with particular attention paid to the human dimensions of food production, such as the mother-daughter relationship involved in making Anhui's famous hairy tofu or the anxiety felt by a young Yunnanese woman at the matsutake counting. Audience response to the series was overwhelming, with some 100 million mainland viewers. During the original airing, the first five episodes spurred over 5.3 million Chinese to search online for the regional specialties shown on the program.[3] And the reviews, at home and abroad, have been glowing. The *Guardian* journalist Oliver Thring called the series "the best TV show I've ever seen about food."[4] A second series was produced and released in 2014, and a third has already begun production.[5]

For many, the material, visual, and affective delights evoked by *A Bite of China* affirm a sense of Chineseness that transcends time and geography and blurs the divisions wrought by class, ethnicity, gender, age, and other social markers.[6] Chinese food as lovingly presented on the program is both distinctively local (the product of a diverse range of factors including climate, geography, and customary practices) yet essentially national (inclusive of Uighur flatbreads, Inner Mongolian *nai doufu* [milk tofu], and other ethnic minority cuisines) in ways that can be read as either political propaganda or an expansive embrace of Chinese culinary diversity. Indeed, the title itself foregrounds the importance of the geopolitical body of the People's Republic of China (PRC) to this culinary envisioning of China as a multiethnic nation.[7]

There is another kind of performative glossing in operation in *A Bite of China*—one that takes us back to the soybean, and tofu specifically, in both expected and surprising ways. Whether or not explicitly intended as such, technology is implicitly cast as both the "midwife and child of the modern industrial world."[8] Nearly all the food production shown tends to emphasize the kind of embodied knowledge characteristic of preindustrial production, in which "customary procedures for the transformation of matter . . . are routinized yet flexible," resistant to translation into either words or numbers, and largely under threat from the advance of a more globalized industrial economy.[9] By focusing on the producers of local foods, the audience is welcomed into a world of artisanal production where technical skill is intertwined with ecologically sensitive understanding. Weathered hands and faces all speak to the delicate balance of forces competing, surely, but also cooperating to forge the rich traditions of food and community.

To take just one example, an episode featuring specialty tofu dishes found in Yunnan, Anhui, and Zhejiang celebrates tofu as an enchanting spectacle of human innovation enacted through microbial fermentation. The episode's title, "Inspiration for Change" (Zhuanhua de linggan), posits transformation (*zhuanhua*) as the governing motif.[10] Echoing sentiments expressed by Lin Yutang, the opening lines intoned by the narrator emphasize how the Chinese have always been guided by taste to such a degree that they have never limited themselves to a simple list of existing foods. In pursuit of taste, they have endlessly experimented and innovated, seeking inspiration from subtle and not-so-subtle processes of transformation. Tofu, in its myriad forms, serves as the quintessential example of such transformation. To explain why the Chinese expended such effort in experimenting with tofu, the narrator highlights the long-standing place occupied by the soybean in Chinese agricultural history. Among the various beans known to man, the soybean has the highest protein content and is the most economical. The digestive challenges posed by soybeans—boiled soybeans are not especially tasty and can cause gas—spurred the Chinese search for better methods of preparation, and over the centuries, the fruits of this endeavor have yielded a diverse range of regionally inflected food products whose implicit role in local dietaries has solved both nutritional and gastronomic concerns. What makes tofu so remarkable and a quintessentially Chinese food, the program asserts, is how local experimentations with processing transformed the humble soybean into a gastronomic delight. Tofu's generous nature (*baorong de gexing*) when combined with Chinese cooking techniques expanded the horizon of Chinese gastronomy, and in ways highly enjoyable and palatable to the mouth and stomach, tofu represents the best kind of culinary invention: a food that is tasty and good for you—a highly efficient, superior form of nutriment for satisfying one's protein needs.

The nutritionist rationale for why ancient Chinese expended effort in making the soybean palatable is clearly a post facto reconstruction that appeals to a contemporary audience, but this kind of reasoning only makes sense for those familiar with the benefits of modern nutritional analysis and for whom the ideology of nutritionism has, to various degrees, become commonplace. To celebrate the soybean's protein and vitamin profile—that "a pound of ordinary dry soybeans contains twice the protein of a pound of beefsteak, that it is high in vitamin A, calcium, thiamine, riboflavin, and other B-complex vitamins, but low in calories and cholesterol"[11]—exposes our modern proclivities, not those of past Chinese who appreciated the virtues of the soybean along different registers. That this line of reasoning should appear in a popular documentary celebrating Chinese culinary heritage seems a fitting nod to Republican-period efforts to introduce nutrition science into the popular consciousness. It is as if *A Bite of China* has identified a from-the-future response to the *Shenbao* writer who had previously appropriated Zhu Ziqing's tofu to highlight the nutritive value of soyfoods.

That the importance of protein should be invoked when showcasing the diverse ways in which tofu has been prepared signals the domestication of nutrition science as a paradigmatic way in which Chinese today navigate meanings of food, health, and nation. For Republican scientists like Wu Xian and Hou Xiangchuan, popular recognition of the importance of protein and greater attention to the nutritional composition of everyday foods would all have been received as positive signs of the emergence of a modern Chinese sensibility—one that understood the importance of Chinese dietary choices and properly assessed foods according to their nutritional values. At the base of these ideas is a concept of the Chinese diet as a socially and politically meaningful object of investigation, adaptation, innovation, and transformation. As a discursive category, the Chinese diet bears within its epistemological boundaries the tension between what Chinese people eat and what they ought to eat. The notion that Chinese people have been eating tofu and drinking soybean milk for centuries is powerful not because it is historically proven; it is powerful because it neutralizes this tension in ways that reaffirm the conceptual integrity of the Chinese diet and its role in arbitrating the value of different kinds of foods for the Chinese nation. Rather than querying the reductive focus on the nutrient composition of foods as the best means for understanding their healthfulness, we have the satisfaction of having been proven retrospectively correct for making and eating something nutrition science has confirmed to be healthful.

For Republican nutrition scientists, Chinese dietary inadequacy represented the singular problem of their times. They engaged in a complex dance in which universalist presumptions about the inherent similarities of human bodies and their nutritional needs (matched with a progressivist understanding of national development) and political languages of power and wealth built on hierarchies of difference came together and separated in alternating bars. At turns, they argued that the Chinese diet was inadequate because it lacked animal-derived proteins and was too vegetarian in nature, or because the country lacked the economic infrastructure to build dairies and encourage the proper growth and development of the nation's children, or because the common people did not understand the true value of the foods they sought out and ate. Driven by hunger or status, the Chinese people did not eat well, because they ate for the wrong reasons. All of these reasons for explaining the inadequacy of the Chinese diet arose in conjunction with the emergence of modern *yingyang* as both a foundation and a toolset for diagnosing and curing China's maladies.

For the twenty-first century observer, the most striking difference between *A Bite of China*'s and the *Shenbao* writer's reference to protein lies in the general context shaping how Chinese people eat. Republican scientists and soybean promoters were modernizing elites who sought to dispel older dietetic ideas and customs from the popular consciousness in favor of science-based, health-oriented knowledge. They did so against an increasingly self-assimilated yet pernicious Western construction of the Chinese diet as a reflection of the inherent inadequacy of China's place within a modern global order. Their tactics and strategies varied by degrees, but all were in agreement that the primary virtue of the soybean was its adaptability, its flexible nature that could be reshaped to suit new, modern pursuits. It was with this newfound faith that the Chinese anarchist Li Shizeng sought to reinterpret Chinese vegetarianism as a form of modern hygiene and promote the soybean and its derived foods as Chinese technological innovations that could compete with and trump the West's dedication to the cow.[12] Even the biochemist Wu Xian, who tended to evince greater skepticism about the soybean's prospects as a permanent replacement for animal-derived protein, nonetheless recognized the adaptive ways in which soybeans could be used in local Chinese dietaries to ensure the proper growth and development of the Chinese people. Faith in the power of the soybean to transform the bodies of Chinese children was the keystone of wartime efforts to produce and distribute a fortified soybean milk to Chinese infants and children. Whether serving the functional roles of meat or dairy, the soybean in its early twentieth-century reinvention represented Chinese ingenuity in the face of adversity.

Protein continues to signify wealth and power—indeed, the modernist idea of meat-as-progress remains as strong today as it did in the early twentieth century—but today's PRC lacks little when it comes to the provisioning and consumption of meat and dairy. Deng Xiaoping's economic reforms dating from 1978 have transformed the Chinese diet from one rich in grains and vegetables to one laden with meat, sugar, and edible oils. The privation and rationing that typified the Maoist era has largely disappeared as income growth, urbanization, and the establishment of a market economy have radically altered the contemporary food landscape.[13] From the late 1970s through the early 2000s, the Chinese population has experienced a dramatic dietary transition toward a more animal-based, westernized diet.[14] Total energy intake has risen: from 1,724 calories in 1952 to 2,386 calories per capita per day in 2000.[15] The proportion of energy from animal foods has been increasing. Based on data from the China Health and Nutrition Survey in 2002, animal foods contributed 12.6 percent of daily energy intake, 25.1 percent of daily protein intake, and 39.2 percent of daily fat intake.[16] The general shift toward a Western dietary pattern, with high intake of red meat and other high-energy-dense foods, has raised concerns of a growing epidemic of obesity and other diet-related chronic diseases.[17] It has also stoked debate about food security, food safety, and the environmental consequences of agro-industrial expansion in the service of more meat-intensive diets and the PRC's goal for food self-sufficiency.[18]

The soybean today occupies a demonstrably less commanding position within the Chinese imagination. It does not fuel visions of a Chinese modernity in which the nutritional and physiological goals set by cow's milk are equally matched by soybean milk, nor does it serve as an essential nutriment to feed the poor and comfort the displaced. Moreover, despite the importance of soybeans as a global agro-industrial commodity in our contemporary world—the quintessential flex crop—few people today associate soybeans with Chineseness.[19] The United States has been the world's leading soybean producer since 1941, and by 1956, the center of world production too shifted to the Western Hemisphere, when the United States passed Asia in total production.[20] In 1990, the United States produced 50 percent of the world's soybeans. Since then, deconcentration of soybean production has split world production between the Americas, with the United States constituting

31 percent, Brazil 31 percent, and Argentina 19 percent of the total (circa 2014).[21]

Today, China has emerged as the world's largest importer of soybeans. According to the General Administration of Customs, China imported 95.53 million tons of soybeans in 2017.[22] Between 1991 and 2014, Chinese share of global soybean production declined from 9 percent to 4 percent.[23] While striking, especially when compared to the early twentieth century, when the northeast (Heilongjiang, Jilin, and Liaoning) represented the historic site of soybean cultivation as well as the primary site for the production of exports to Japan and Europe, these statistics may not fully reflect the complex ways in which the trajectories of soy development have unfolded in the post-1978 PRC. Soybeans have become the PRC's most important import crop, traded primarily for the industrial livestock sector. While more soy is consumed in China than any other place in the world, the importance of soybean as livestock feed has grown as Chinese per capita meat consumption has quadrupled since 1980 (FAOSTAT). Available meat sources (e.g., beef, poultry, pork, seafood, etc.) have also diversified, but the meat of preference continues to be pork. Half of the world's pigs, half of the world's pork production, and half of the world's pork consumption occur in China.[24] For the PRC, modernizing the Chinese diet has entailed a strategically managed set of policies, discourses, relations, and resources aimed at massively increasing meat consumption for the urban middle and upper classes. This "industrial meat regime" necessitated the redefinition of soybean as an *industrial*, as opposed to agricultural, commodity and the establishment of a Chinese feed industry, of which soybean crushing constitutes a central component.[25]

Thus even as China dominates the world in soybean consumption, the form in which soybeans are consumed has shifted dramatically since the Republican period. Tofu, soybean milk, and soy sauce remain common fixtures of Chinese cooking and diets, but increasingly, Chinese people now consume soybeans indirectly via pork and chicken and as cooking oil.[26]

Given the trajectory of soy development in the PRC, it may be less surprising that a documentary like *A Bite of China* minimizes attention on the soybean itself in favor of the diverse local foods that can be made from it. Li Shizeng's paean to the soybean's flexible nature has been outshined by gastronomic celebration of tofu as the quintessentially Chinese food whose own adaptive nature can be seen in its various regional manifestations. The crop itself is little more than raw material whose high protein value infuses and justifies the resulting food inventions. Indeed, there is nothing especially

Chinese about the soybean per se. Chineseness, if we continue with the theme of the *A Bite of China* episode, becomes entangled with the soybean only when we pause to appreciate the inventiveness with which Chinese people have developed their culinary arts. Be it through the skillful application of microbial fermentation or the transposition of techniques from one food to another—whether deliberately or as a consequence of migration—Chinese people have over the centuries experimented and identified new paths by which to transform seemingly indigestible raw materials into gastronomical delights. Tofu, the program insists, rewrote the soybean's destiny. In the words of the narrator, "With great flexibility, tofu offered a huge space for the imagination of the Chinese, well known for its culinary skills. The disadvantages of soybean were eliminated by reason or unconsciously. As the ancient Chinese transformed soybeans into tofu, the value of soybean protein to the human body reached a climax with the invention of tofu. Chinese cooks' understanding of tofu will often take you by surprise. Maybe it's also correct to say that the Chinese are showing their adaptability through tofu."[27]

Soybean milk as *doujiang* has not disappeared, but its potential role in strengthening young Chinese bodies and uplifting a nation has largely been vacated. In the early twentieth century, soybean milk was a curiosity for much of the world outside of East Asia; today, it has become a staple item in grocery stores around the world. It is alternatively seen as a dairy alternative for the lactose intolerant, a health food, and a traditional Chinese food that reanimates lost ties to home and belonging, but also as a potential cancer agent.[28] Among these various social and cultural resonances, the one that dominated the imaginations of Republican scientists and social reformers— soybean milk as a scientific and Chinese alternative for cow's milk for nourishing the nation's young and supporting enhanced physical growth—is absent. Scientific soybean milk was treated in the first half of the twentieth century as a symbol of national growth and development on Chinese terms, and the extent to which it could nutritionally compete against cow's milk staked out precious ideological terrain for mapping out China's relationship to global modernity and imperialism.

Such concerns no longer resound in contemporary China. With the rapid rise of per capita incomes, the growing Chinese middle class increasingly associate cow's milk with economic success and the high-tech trappings of modernity.[29] Moreover, the idea that children ought to drink cow's milk— an idea that has been promoted by the dairy industry, governments, health officials, dieticians, and nutritionists—has become normative in the twenty-first century.[30] Although China has historically lacked a prominent dairying culture, cow's milk has nonetheless achieved official status as a growth- and strength-promoting food. The Chinese food pagoda, which visually expresses dietary guidelines for Chinese residents, recommends a daily consumption of 300 grams of milk and milk products.[31] (In comparison, the recommended daily amount of soybean and nuts amounts to 25 to 30 grams.)[32] Speaking at Chongqing's Guangda Milk Technology Park in 2006, then-Premier Wen Jiaobao said, "I have a dream to provide every Chinese, especially children, sufficient milk each day."[33] His sentiment was matched by increased governmental support for the development of the Chinese dairy industry and increased consumption of dairy among the Chinese population from the mid-1990s through the 2000s.

Republican efforts to espouse the wonders of soybean nutrition to the Chinese people represented a project of self-invention in which modern *yingyang* refashioned the soybean as both Chinese and modern. It was a project that relied heavily upon a conception of the Chinese diet as inadequate to the needs of the modern world yet amenable to engineering, and the soybean's fungible, adaptable nature proffered material opportunities with which to change both what and how Chinese people ate. It was a project deeply attuned to the goal of national rejuvenation through nutritional uplift. Such visions are no longer accorded to the soybean—certainly not in present-day China, which in 2012 became the world's third largest producer of fresh cow's milk.[34] But it is worth remembering this earlier project as an alternative vision of Chinese nutritional modernity. Promoting soybean nutrition was a way to reassert Chinese identity and Chinese prerogative. As the China Nutritional Aid Council postcard suggests, the Chinese soybean family, led by an energetic and strong soybean granny, are playing for keeps, and Madame Cow best keep running along.

Chinese Character Glossary

Bali Doufu Gongsi (Usine Caséo-Sojaïne) 巴黎豆腐公司
bunao zhenjing 補腦振精
buyao 補藥

caichan 財產
Chen Daming (Harry Chan) 陳達明
Chen Sanli 陳三立
Chen Yingning 陳櫻寧
chuxuli 儲蓄力

danbaizhi 蛋白質
Ding Fubao 丁福保
dongji bupin 冬季補品
doufan 豆飯
doujiang 豆漿
dounai 豆奶
douru 豆乳
douzha bing 豆渣餅
douzhi 豆汁

Ertong Yingyang Cujinhui 兒童營養促進會

fada shenti 發達身體
Fan Bingqing 樊炳清
fan dou 飯豆
fayu 發育
fazhan 發展
fuqiang 富強
fuwu shehui 服務社會

Gainaisheng 鈣奶生
Gainaisheng Yingyangfen 鈣奶生營養粉
gezhi 格致
guohuo 國貨
guohuo yundong 國貨運動
guomin zhi mu 國民之母

Hou Xiangchuan (H. S. Hou) 侯祥川
huangzheng 荒政
Huashang lianhebao 華商聯合報
Hubei shangwubao 湖北商務報
Hujita Toyobachi 藤田豐八

jiang 醬
jianshen qiangzhong 健身強種
Jin Baoshan (P. Z. King) 金寶善
Jin Shuchu (Sohtsu G. King) 金叔初
jindai yingyangxue 近代營養學
jing qi shen 精氣神
jingli 精力
jueju 絕句

kexue fangfa 科學方法
Kojyo Teikichi 古城貞吉
Kunming Ertong Yingyang Weiyuanhui 昆明兒童營養委員會

Li Hongzhang 李鴻章
Li Jinghan 李景漢
Li Shizeng 李石增
aka Li Yuying 李煜瀛
liangqi xianmu 良妻賢母
Luo Dengyi 羅登義
Luo Zhenyu 羅振玉

maifan 麥飯
minsheng 民生
minzu 民族

neidan 內丹
Ni Zhangqi (T. G. Ni) 倪章其
nianlao zhe 年老者

nong wei bang ben 農為邦本
Nongbaoguan 農報館
Nongxuebao 農學報
Nongxue congshu 農學叢書
Nongxueshe 農學社

qingnian 青年
qixue 氣血
qiuji bupin 秋季補品

ranliao 燃料
rengong yingyangfa 人工營養法
rulao 乳酪
rutang 乳糖

Shanghai Nanmin Ertong Yingyang Weiyuanhui 上海難民兒童營養委員會
Shangwubao 商務報
shanshi 膳食
shao xiandu 少限度
Shen Tong 沈同
shenghuo jineng 生活機能
Shengsheng Douru Gongsi 生生豆乳公司
shi 豉
shi yao 石藥
Shi Zhaoji (Sao-ke Alfred Sze) 施肇基
shijin 食禁
shiwu 食物
Sun Simiao 孫思邈
Sun Zhongshan (Sun Yat-sen) 孫中山

Taizo Kawai 河相大三
tanshui huahewu 碳水化合物
Tao Menghe (L. K. Tao) 陶孟和
tianran 天然
tonghua 同化

Wang Guowei 王國維
wangfei 枉費
Weili dounai 偉力豆奶
wenming bing 文明病
wenming guguo 文明古國

wu fu huo 無浮火

Wu Xian (Wu Hsien) 吳憲

wugu 五穀

wuwei 五味

wuxing 五行

xixue dongjian 西學東漸

xinchen daixie 新陳代謝

xue 血

Yang Chongrui (Marion Yang) 楊崇瑞

yangmin 養民

yangsheng 養生

yilao 遺老

yinghai 嬰孩

yingyang 營養

yingyang biaozhun 營養標準

yingyang wenti 營養問題

yingyang zhuanjia 營養專家

yinshi 飲食

Youyi Douru Gongsi 有益豆乳公司

yuanliao 原料

yuying wenti 育嬰問題

Zhang Jian 張謇

Zhang Zhidong 張之洞

Zheng Ji 鄭集

Zheng Zhenwen 鄭貞文

zhengdang zhi yangliao 正當之養料

zhifang 脂肪

Zhongguo dadou wenti 中國大豆問題

Zhonghua Yingyang Cujinhui 中華營養促進會

Zhu Bolu 朱伯盧

Zhu Shenzhi (Ernest Tso) 祝愼之

Zhu Zhenjun 朱振鈞

Zhu Ziqing 朱自清

zhuangnian 壯年

ziyang geng wei fengfu 滋養更為豐富

zui shiyi yishizhu 最適宜衣食住

Notes

Introduction

1   Pollard, "Zhu Ziqing (1898–1948)," 216–17; Finnane, "Food and Place."

2   Zhu Ziqing, "Dongtian," in *Zhu Ziqing sanwen xuan*, 126.

3   See the first page of Lillian M. Li's introduction to *Fighting Famine in North China* for the origins of this phrase.

4   "Doufu he doufujiang," *Shenbao*, 5 January 1939.

5   "Doufu he doufujiang," *Shenbao*, 5 January 1939. *Doujiang*, which we commonly translate into English as soybean milk, is the base liquid to which coagulants are added to make tofu.

6   Huters, "Culture, Capital, and Temptations of the Imagined Market," 41.

7   My translation of Chen Sanli's poem is deeply indebted to David "Andy" Knight and Shengqing Wu, who both kindly assisted me in identifying the poem's various allusions. For a sensitive and nuanced analysis of Chen's poetic opus, see Wu, *Modern Archaics*, 108–64. For an introduction to Chen Sanli's biography and literary accomplishments, see Ma and Dong, *Chen Sanli nianpu*.

8   Lu and Needham, "Contribution to the History of Chinese Dietetics," 19. This article was originally submitted for publication in 1939 but was not published on account of war conditions until 1951.

9   See, for example, Ji, "Ding Fubao he Zhongguo jindai yingyang weisheng kexue"; Seung-joon Lee, "Patriot's Scientific Diet"; and Swislocki, "Feast and Famine in Republican Shanghai," 67–108, and "Nutritional Governmentality," 9–35.

10 Ji, "Jindai yixue he yingyangxue," 44.

11 For the history of dietetics in the West, see also Shapin, "Philosopher and the Chicken" and "How to Eat Like a Gentleman," in *Never Pure?*, 237–58, 259–86.

12 Ji, "Jindai yixue he yingyangxue," 45.

13 See Sivin, *Traditional Medicine in Contemporary China*, 152–64.

14   Ji, "Jindai yixue he yingyangxue," 47. Known initially in English as the *Chinese Scientific Magazine*, the *Gezhi Huibian* ran from 1876 until 1892. It was the earliest scientific journal to reach Chinese readers in the treaty ports in 1876.

15   Grace Shen, "Murky Waters," 590.

16   Daston, *Biographies of Scientific Objects*, 1–14.

17   For a general introduction to the history of nutrition, see Gratzer, *Terrors of the Table*; and Levenstein, *Revolution at the Table*. For nutrition as ideology, see Huff, "Corporeal Economies"; Kamminga and Cunningham, *Science and Culture of Nutrition*; Mudry, *Measured Meals*; and Scrinis, *Nutritionism*.

18   Heather Paxson makes this point brilliantly; see "Rethinking Food and Its Eaters," 269.

19   Seung-joon Lee makes a similar point by emphasizing the public agency in shaping the popularization of nutrition science in Republican China; see "Patriot's Scientific Diet." Contemporary anthropological analysis affirms this point. See, for example, Farquhar, *Appetites*, 47–78; and Farquhar and Zhang, *Ten Thousand Things*.

20   Swislocki, "Feast and Famine in Republican Shanghai," 67. I share Swislocki's interest in examining nutrition research findings in Republican-era medical journals, but whereas Swislocki did so largely as nutritional, economic, and regional aspects of urban food culture in Shanghai, my analysis seeks to understand scientific research in nutrition as part of Chinese attempts to grapple with a new material world shaped by modern science and industry in their everyday lives.

21   Andrews, *Making of Modern Chinese Medicine, 1850–1960*; Lei, *Neither Donkey nor Horse*. The significance of Andrews's and Lei's respective works lies in their insistence that the epistemological integrity of Chinese medicine was not a completed project in the early twentieth century but rather one forged through its engagement and active assimilation of some aspects of Western medicine, which itself was "a changing assemblage of theories, technologies, and practices that defies easy definition." Andrews, *Making of Modern Chinese Medicine, 1850–1960*, 7. As will become evident, this book pursues a parallel course for the science of nutritional knowledge, but one that also insists that we take seriously the incompleteness of global science and its perambulations around the world.

22   For an examination of colonial dynamics in matters of food, diet, and cuisine, see Jayanta Sengupta, "Nation on a Platter."

23   Although not a direct offspring, the modern term for nutrition shares semantic terrain with the Chinese term *weisheng*, which Ruth Rogaski has shown to indicate a range of private, culturally sanctioned activities intended to "protect or guard life"—like breath training, gymnastics, and dietary therapy—before becoming increasingly associated with state management

of the health of public spaces and citizens' bodies. The importance of Chinese translations of Japanese scientific and medical works to this process cannot be overstated. Rogaski, *Hygienic Modernity*. For further discussion of the transposition of medical concern from the wealthy to the poor, see Swislocki, "Nutritional Governmentality," 12.

24 Elman, *On Their Own Terms*.

25 Elman, *On Their Own Terms*, part 5. In terms of scholarship, this disparagement of nineteenth-century Qing efforts in science and technology has to some degree blinded us to the actual work conducted on the ground. That is to say, earlier scholarship, like Kwok's *Scientism in Chinese Thought*, has tended to emphasize how Chinese intellectuals talked about "science" to the exclusion of how Chinese scientists articulated and practiced science. Starting in the 1990s, there were several important studies that shifted focus to more productive areas in which science practitioners occupy the foreground. See Reardon-Anderson, *Study of Change*; Schneider, *Biology and Revolution in Twentieth-Century China*; and Hu, *China and Albert Einstein*. Complementary to this shift has been the growing number of studies that explore scientific bodies like the Science Society of China, Academia Sinica, and other institutions in Republican China. Such scholarship has deepened our understanding of scientific production as a real and concerted enterprise that shaped Nationalist state-building efforts during the 1930s and 1940s. See, for example, Shiwei Chen, "Government and Academy in Republican China; Neushul and Wang, "Between the Devil and the Deep Sea"; Zhang Jian, *Kexue shetuan zai jindai Zhongguo de mingyun*; Zuoyue Wang, "Saving China through Science"; and Kirby, "Technocratic Organization and Technological Development in China."

26 Elman, *On Their Own Terms*, 396.

27 Shellen Wu, *Empires of Coal*, 67.

28 See Lydia Liu, *Translingual Practice*, appendix B; and Masini, *Formation of Modern Chinese Lexicon*. Technically speaking, there were two ideographs associated with *eiyō*: 栄養 and 営養, both of which entered modern Chinese as linguistic equivalents for "nutrition." The latter ideograph achieved translingual stability in the Chinese context, as it came to reference both the scientific discipline and the physiological objective. In contrast, in Japanese there appears to have been a divergence in semantic reference, with the former adopted by home economics and the latter by scientific disciplines. For a detailed discussion of the appearance of these ideographs in Japanese, see Ehara, "Changes of Terms about Food in Household Textbooks" (in Japanese), 533–42.

29 Ji Hongkun, "Zheng Zhenwen he tade 'Yingyang huaxue,'" 42–45.

30 See Huters, "Culture, Capital, and Temptations of the Imagined Market," 27–50. For a more targeted analysis of the role of editing and publishing in

shaping, indeed authenticating, science in the public imagination, see Lean, "Proofreading Science," 185–208.

31 Culp, "Mass Production of Knowledge," 207–41.

32 Barona, *Problem of Nutrition*; Levenstein, *Paradox of Plenty*; Kamminga and Cunningham, *Science and Culture of Nutrition*.

33 Will, *Bureaucracy and Famine in Eighteenth-Century China*; Will and Wong, with Lee, *Nourish the People*; Lillian M. Li, *Fighting Famine in North China*.

34 For a related discussion of the rise of *suzhi* (quality) discourse in post-Mao China, see Anagnost, "Corporeal Politics of Quality (*Suzhi*)"; Murphy, "Turning Peasants into Modern Chinese Citizens"; Jacko, "Cultivating Citizens"; and Sigley, "*Suzhi*, the Body, and the Fortunes of Technoscientific Reasoning."

35 Jin Shuchu's preface in Zheng Ji, "Zhongguoren zhi yingyang gaikuang," 25–34.

36 Quoted in Platt, "Soya Bean in Human Nutrition," 834.

37 See, for example, Fuller et al., "Got Milk?"; Gerth, *As China Goes, So Goes the World*, chapter 7; Schneider, "Developing the Meat Grab"; and Watson, "Meat." For a visual celebration of tofu and other soybean-derived foods emblematic of the diversity of traditional Chinese cuisine, see episode 3, "Spirit of Transformation" (Zhuanhua de linggan) of the Chinese documentary series, *A Bite of China* (Shejianshang de Zhongguo).

38 I have drawn inspiration from Francesca Bray's thoughtful and penetrating insights into the intellectual value and imperative of global histories. Bray et al., *Rice*, 3.

39 Henriot, "Rice, Power, and People"; Seung-joon Lee, *Gourmets in the Land of Famine*; Swislocki, "Feast and Famine in Republican Shanghai," 109–37.

40 Swislocki, "Feast and Famine in Republican Shanghai," 113.

41 Tsing, "Worlding the Matsutake Diaspora," 58.

42 The "five grains" (*wugu*), a common expression found in classical texts, designated the main cereal crops as well as field crops like hemp or beans, which were also cultivated for their grains. The expression was understood to comprise *ji* (setaria millet), *shu* (panicum millet), *dao* (rice), *mai* (wheat and barley), and *shu* (legumes, including soybeans). Bray et al., *Rice*, 21; Bray, *Agriculture*, 432.

43 H. T. Huang, *Fermentations and Food Science*, and "Early Uses of Soybean in Chinese History."

44 H. T. Huang, "Early Uses of Soybean in Chinese History," 45–55.

45 H. T. Huang, "Early Uses of Soybean in Chinese History," 52.

46 Du Bois, Tan, and Mintz, *World of Soy*.

47 Prodöhl, "'A Miracle Bean,'" and "Versatile and Cheap"; Shuang Wen, "Mediated Imaginations," esp. the chapter "Ubiquitous Yet Invisible."

48 Du Bois, Tan, and Mintz, *World of Soy*, 6.

Chapter 1: The Romance of the Bean

1   "Chinese Factory in France," *North-China Herald*, 3 February 1911.

2   The Shanghai Municipal Council was the governing body for the International Settlement, the American and British foreign concessions in Shanghai that had been awarded after the Qings' defeat in the First Opium War (1839–1842).

3   "Japan's Foreign Policy," *North-China Herald*, 3 February 1911.

4   "Paris and the Bean," *Christian Science Monitor*, 24 January 1911.

5   "Paris and the Bean," *Christian Science Monitor*, 24 January 1911.

6   For more details on the Chinese relationships Li Shizeng drew upon in establishing his factory and its connections to Li's work-study initiatives, see Zhao and Wang, "Buli cun liufa gongyi xuexiao," 101–8.

7   "Soya Bean," *The Times*, 19 July 1910.

8   Adachi, *Manchuria*, 160.

9   H. T. Huang, "Early Uses of Soybean in Chinese History," 45–46.

10 Quoted in H. T. Huang, "Early Uses of Soybean in Chinese History," 47.

11 Bray, *Agriculture*, 514.

12 For further details, see H. T. Huang, *Fermentations and Food Science*, 293.

13 H. T. Huang, "Early Uses of Soybean in Chinese History," 48.

14 On the early history of fermented soy products in the Han dynasty, see Yü, "Han."

15 Bray, *Agriculture*, 514.

16 Bray, *Agriculture*, 514.

17 Isett, *State, Peasant, and Merchant in Qing Manchuria*, 235–37.

18 Pomeranz, *Great Divergence*, 226–27.

19 Xue, "'Fertilizer Revolution'?," 198, 209–10.

20 Xue, "'Fertilizer Revolution'?," 198.

21 The issue of how much Manchurian beancake entered the Lower Yangzi or the Jiangnan region relates to a broader question about agricultural productivity/stagnancy and the environmental factors (exogenous and endogenous) helping to drive the divergence between Chinese and English/European development. See Pomeranz, *Great Divergence*; and Huang's rebuttal, "Development or Involution." For a more detailed discussion about the proportion of soybeans to grains in Manchurian exports, see Isett, 228–34.

22 See Pomeranz, *Great Divergence*, 226; Muzumdar, *Sugar and Society in China*; Isett, "Sugar Manufacture and the Agrarian Economy of Nineteenth-Century Taiwan"; and Isett, *State, Peasant, and Merchant in Qing Manchuria*, 234–48.

23 The Imperial Maritime Customs, which was renamed the Maritime Customs Services after the collapse of the Qing dynasty in 1912, was established in 1854

to collect taxes on maritime trade when Qing officials were unable to do so during the Taiping Rebellion. Staffed by an international, through predominantly British, bureaucracy under the supervision of successive Chinese governments, the office became responsible for significantly more than maritime tax collection. Its functions grew to include domestic customs administration, postal administration, harbor and waterway management, weather reporting, and antismuggling operations. Shaw, *Soya Bean of Manchuria*, 15.

24 Xue suggests that as much as 90 percent of the soybean trade was captured by foreign vessels in the 1890s. Xue, "A 'Fertilizer Revolution'?," 223, footnote 7. In contrast, foreign attempts to dominate the market for soybean processing (i.e., production of oil and beancake) encountered significant difficulties in the pre-1895 period. See Brown, "Cakes and Oil"; and Hsien-chun Wang, "Revising the Niuzhuang Oil Mill (1868–1870)."

25 Xue, "'Fertilizer Revolution'?," 213–15.

26 Howell, *Capitalism From Within*.

27 Howell defines "protoindustrialization" as the development of rural regions in which the majority of the population lived entirely, or to a considerable extent, on industrial mass production for interregional and international markets. Howell, "Proto-Industrial Origins of Japanese Capitalism," 269.

28 Manchuria, or the region the Chinese call "the Northeast" (*Dongbei*), currently consists of three provinces: Liaoning, Jilin, and Heilongjiang.

29 Elliott, *Manchu Way*.

30 Hoshino, *Economic History of Manchuria*, 13.

31 Hoshino, *Economic History of Manchuria*, 14.

32 Reardon-Anderson, *Reluctant Pioneers*, 71–84.

33 Manchuria's population increase during the eighteenth and early nineteenth centuries was spectacular. The Shengjing Military Region, which had been the most populated area of Manchuria at the beginning of the Qing dynasty, had a population of 360,000 in 1741, but almost 1.8 million by 1820. For a more detailed discussion of the breakdown of the manorial system and its replacement by competitive markets in land, labor, and other resources, see Reardon-Anderson, *Reluctant Pioneers*, 46–70.

34 Gottschang, "Economic Change, Disasters, and Migration," 461. See also Gottschang and Lary, *Swallows and Settlers*.

35 McKeown, *Melancholy Order*, 49–51.

36 Reardon-Anderson, *Reluctant Pioneers*, 179.

37 Reardon-Anderson, *Reluctant Pioneers*, 198, footnote 63.

38 Piper and Morse, "Soybean," 4–5.

39 Piper and Morse, "Soybean," 5.

40 Hoshino, *Economic History of Manchuria*, 27.

41   Adachi, *Manchuria*, 78.

42   Adachi, *Manchuria*, 77.

43   The importance of the soybean to Japanese and Russian imperial competition was evident during the Russo-Japanese War. Both sides set up laboratories to adapt and transform soybeans into practical necessities such as soap, axles, artillery lubricants, and animal fodder to reduce the importation of war material from European Russia and Japan. Wolff, "Bean There," 245.

44   Matsusaka, *Making of Japanese Manchuria*, 61–85, 103–48. For economic concerns driving Japanese imperialism into China, see Duus, "Economic Dimensions of Meiji Imperialism," 128–71; and Wray, "Japan's Big-Three Service Enterprises."

45   Reardon-Anderson, *Reluctant Pioneers*, 208–17.

46   According to William Joseph Morse (W. J. Morse, 1884–1959), who began his career in 1907 as a scientific assistant to Dr. C. V. Piper of the Office of Forage Crops, US Department of Agriculture, the German botanist Englebert Kaempfer introduced the soybean to Europeans in the seventeenth century. Kaempfer had spent two years, 1691–92, in Japan working as a medical officer of the Dutch East India Company. The soybean plant found its way into botanic gardens in France as early as 1740 and at Kew, England, in 1790. Piper and Morse, "Soybean," 1.

47   Hymowitz, "Dorsett-Morse Soybean Collection Trip," 378.

48   See, for example, Schlegel, "Chinese Bean-Curd," 144–45; and "Use of 'Soy Bean' as a Food in Diabetes," 1844–45. See also Friedenwald and Ruhräh, *Diet in Health and Disease*. "Soya bread" was included as one of the permissible foods private nurses were instructed to give diabetics. McIsaac, "Practical Points on Private Nursing," 122.

49   Prodöhl, "Miracle Bean," 119.

50   Shaw, *Soya Bean of Manchuria*, 1.

51   Prodöhl, "Miracle Bean," 119.

52   Shaw, *Soya Bean of Manchuria*, 13.

53   Reardon-Anderson, *Reluctant Pioneers*, 210–12.

54   Elman, "From Pre-modern Chinese Natural Studies to Modern Science," 25–74, and *On Their Own Terms*, especially chapters 10–11.

55   Vittinghoff, "Social Actors in the Field of Learning," 516.

56   Yue, "Hybrid Science versus Modernity," 13–52.

57   Amelung, "*The Complete Compilation of New Knowledge*," 97. For a discussion of Chinese agricultural writing, see Bray, "Towards a Critical History of Non-Western Technology," 158–209, and "Agricultural Illustrations," 521–68.

58   Elman, "Toward a History of Modern Science," 24.

59   Elman, *On Their Own Terms*, chapters 6–7.

60   The numbers of Chinese students in Japan declined after 1906 on account of increasing government restrictions. Bailey, *Reform the People*, 228.

61   Elman, "Toward a History of Modern Science," 27; Wang Yangzhong, "1850 niandai zhi 1910 nian Zhongguo yu Riben," 144–45; Reynolds, *China 1898–1912*, 58–61.

62   To suggest that Luo Zhenyu occupies a vexed place in modern Chinese history would be an understatement. An antiquarian, scholar, collector, art dealer, and agriculture and education reformer, Luo was an important *yilao*, a "relict" of the preceding Qing dynasty. His loyalty to the Qing after the dynasty's demise and his willingness to serve the Japanese puppet state of Manchukuo led to his portrayal as a traitor to the Chinese nation twice over. More recent scholarship has sought to shed greater light on the position of Qing loyalists, and Luo Zhenyu specifically, in the cultural history of the Republican period. See Chen Hsiu-ching, "Qingmo shangzhan xia de shanghai 'Wunonghui'"; and Yang and Whitfield, *Lost Generation*.

63   Cited in Lü, *Qingmo Zhong Ri jiaoyu wenhua jiaoliu zhi yanjiu*, 78.

64   See Li Yongfang, "Qingmo nonghui shulun," 1–16; and Wang Yejian, "Jindai Zhongguo nongye de chengzhang ji qi weiji," 355–70.

65   What led to Luo's interest in agriculture is unclear, although Lü suggests that the Shanghai-based newspaper *Current Affairs* (Shiwubao) played a key role in shaping Luo's intellectual interests. Created by Huang Zunxian and edited by Liang Qichao, *Shiwubao* became the newspaper that was read and shared by reform-minded literati. Lü, *Qingmo Zhong Ri jiaoyu wenhua jiaoliu zhi yanjiu*, 76–77; Yoon, "Literati-Journalists of the *Chinese Progress*," 48–76.

66   Stross, *Stubborn Earth*, 45. For a reassessment of Zhang Zhidong's reformism, see Hon, "Zhang Zhidong's Proposal for Reform."

67   In the beginning, Luo Zhenyu employed the expertise of two Japanese sinologists, Kojyo Teikichi (1866–1949) and Hujita Toyobachi (1869–1929), in the translation of Japanese material for his journal. *Agricultural News*'s subscription sales enabled Luo to establish a Japanese study society, with Hujita serving as an instructor. The study society nurtured the talents of Wang Guowei, Fan Bingqing, and Shen Hong, who were among the most prolific and preeminent Chinese translators of Japanese. Lü, *Qingmo Zhong Ri jiaoyu wenhua jiaoliu zhi yanjiu*, 79.

68   Kawai, *Nyugyu oyobi seinyu shinsho*.

69   Shen Hong, "Niuru xinshu xia."

70   See "Nongchan zhizaoxue," *Nongxuebao* in issues 115, 116, and 117.

71   Shen Hong, "Nongchan zhizaoxue," *Nongxuebao* 116 (1900), 43.

72   During the nineteenth century, Niuzhuang served as the principal link connecting agricultural producers in the Liao River basin and the port cities of eastern China. Its prominence in the Manchurian soybean trade was later

eclipsed by the port city of Dairen during the early twentieth century. "Shangqing: bensheng, huangdou xiaochang," 1; Reardon-Anderson, *Reluctant Pioneers*, 204–17.

73   "Bensheng shangqing: huangdou zhangjia," *Hubei shangwubao* 25 (1899): 10–11.

74   See, for example, "Niuzhuang dadou doubing shangqing: yi *Zhongwai shangye xinbao*," *Hubei shangwubao* 30 (1899): 10. Chugai Commercial Paper is now the *Nikkei*.

75   For a more nuanced exploration of the soybean's agro-industrial entanglements in the economic development of imperial peripheries of Manchuria and Egypt, see Wen, Shuang, "Chinese-Arab Interactions in the Age of Late Imperial Capitalism," book manuscript under preparation.

76   Sheng Yin, "Manzhou dadou zhi xinshichang," *Tongwen bao* 416 (1910): 7.

77   Sheng Yin, "Manzhou dadou zhi xinshichang," *Tongwen bao* 416 (1910): 7. For similar sentiments, see also "Jinsan nianjian shuru zhi Yingguo zhi dadou lei," *Huashang lianhehui* (1910); and Li Shangyue, "Dadou zhi gailiang," *Fengtian quanye bao* (1910), 6.

78   For a more complete biography, see Bailey, "Cultural Connections in a New Global Space" and "Sino-French Connection."

79   Li Shizeng, "Ershier sui chuyou sihai," 74; see also "Xinhai geming qianhou de Li Shizeng xiansheng," reprinted in Zhu Chuanyu, *Li Shizeng zhuanji ziliao*, 47–49.

80   Li Shizeng, "Le soja," 178.

81   Lemarié, "Les sojas du Japan," 493–98.

82   Li Yuying. Vegetable Milk and Its Derivatives. British Patent 30275. Li was incredibly active in patenting his various soybean-related products and techniques. Alongside this application for "vegetable milk," Li also applied and received British patents for "sauce consisting chiefly of soja grains" and "soja flour and its derivatives," as well as French patents for soybean-made meats and cold cuts and chocolate.

83   For references to his presentation to the French Society of Agriculture, see Hitier, "Société Nationale d'Agriculture de France: Le soja," 24–25; and Blin, "Le soja ou fève de Mandchourie," 141–422, both cited in Shurleff and Aoyagi, *Li Yu-ying (Li Shizeng)*, 17, 21.

84   US Department of Agriculture, *The International Dairy Federation and International Dairy Congresses*, 9–10.

85   "Bulletin agricole et horticole: Le congrès international de laiterie," 719; Fédération Internationale de Laiterie, *2e Congrès International de Laiterie Paris, 16–19 Octobre 1905*, 387–89.

86   De Chaou, "Une curieuse plante," 7.

87   De Chaou, "Une curieuse plante," 7.

88 Fédération Internationale de Laiterie, *2e Congrès International de Laiterie Paris*, 389. See also, Zhao and Wang, "Buli cun liufa gongyi xuexiao," 101.

89 "Exposition de la Meunerie et Salon de l'Alimentation," 760.

90 "Franco-Chinese Industry," *North-China Herald*, 15 April 1911.

91 Cited in Yi Ren, "Bali doufu gongsi yu liufa qingong jianxue," 35.

92 Quoted in Yi Ren, "Bali doufu gongsi yu liufa qingong jianxue," 35.

93 See Lydia Liu, *Translingual Practice*, 77–102; Zhou Gang, *Placing the Modern Chinese Vernacular in Transnational Literature*, 115; and Leo Ou-fan Lee, *Shanghai Modern*, 47–52.

94 Li Shizeng, "Xinzhishi: lun dadou gongyi," 29–38.

95 Li Shizeng, "Xinzhishi: lun dadou gongyi," 29–30.

96 Li Shizeng, "Xinzhishi: lun dadou gongyi," 30.

97 Li Shizeng, "Xinzhishi: lun dadou gongyi," 31.

98 Bailey, "Cultural Connections in a New Global Space."

99 See Li Shizeng, "Dadou shipin zhi gongyong"; "Lun dadou gongyi wei Zhongguo zhizi zhi techang"; and *Da Dou*. Li was also prolific in espousing the virtues of soybeans in French. He wrote a series of essays on the state of past and current scientific research on soybeans that appeared in the French journal *L'Agriculture pratique des pays chauds (Bulletin du Jardin Colonial)* in 1911 and 1912. He also republished an extended version of *Da Dou* in French in 1912. For more detailed account of his soybean-related publications, see Shurtleff and Aoyagi, *Li Yu-Ying (Li Shizeng)*.

100 Huang Shirong, "Da dou de gongyong," in *Wei tui ju suibi*.

101 "Douru yu niuru zhi bijiao." Whether the author realized it, he had overstated Li's success. As the historian Angela Leung has noted, Li's factory was unprofitable and quickly became reliant on French government subsidies for making soya products for Chinese soldiers fighting for the French government during World War I. Leung, "To Build or to Transform Vegetarian China," note 28.

102 See, for example, Hu Chengdian, "Dadou zhi zhizaopin ji qi gongyong"; Cang Shui, "Tebie diaocha: Huangdou yu douyou doubing zhi shuchu gaikuang"; and "Guowai yaowen: Bali doufu gongsi gaikuang."

CHAPTER 2: THE LIGHT OF MODERN KNOWLEDGE

1 Sun Yat-sen opened his August 17, 1924, lecture, "The Problem of Food," with the saying, "The nation looks upon the people as its foundation, and the people look upon food as their heaven" (*Guo yi min wei ben, min yi shi wei tian*).

2 Seung-joon Lee, "Patriot's Scientific Diet," 1813–15.

3 Following the Boxer Uprising of 1900, the Qing government agreed to pay an indemnity of 450 million taels of silver over the course of thirty-nine years to

the eight nations involved in the suppression of the Boxers. Because the Qing made payments according to the exchange rates at the time (i.e., with interest), the total amount expended far exceeded the original indemnity amount. The United States agreed to use its proportional difference to establish a scholarship program to bring Chinese students to the States.

4   Wu first gave this lecture to students of biochemistry at Peking Union Medical College in April 1926. His lecture was transcribed by Zhu Liqing and published twice in Chinese. See Wu Xian, "Zhongguo shiwu zhi xiandai yingyang zhishi" (1927) and "Zhongguo shiwu zhi xiandai yingyang zhishi" (1928). Wu later published an English version, from which all quotes have been taken. Wu Xian, "Chinese Diet," 56.

5   For an analysis of the rhetorical history of the discourse of quantification in shaping American understandings and relationships to food, see Mudry, *Measured Meals*.

6   Swislocki, *Culinary Nostalgia*.

7   Anderson, *Food and Environment in Early Medieval China*, 44.

8   H. T. Huang, "Early Uses of Soybean in Chinese History," 45–55.

9   The classic formulation of this can be found in K. C. Chang, *Food in Chinese Culture*, 11.

10 For the role of foodways in China's religious traditions, see Sterckx, *Of Tripod and Palate*.

11 Sterckx, "Food and Philosophy in Early China," 49–51.

12 Waley-Cohen, "The Quest for Perfect Balance," 99–134.

13 Waley-Cohen, "The Quest for Perfect Balance," 108.

14 Medical historians have preferred to translate *wu wei* as "sapors" rather than "flavors" to emphasize the medical rather than culinary virtues of the term. Some, like Nathan Sivin, have argued that the functional role of the five flavors in Chinese medicine has long since been divorced from the neuro-physiological experiences of taste, such that "sweet" or "bitter" refer to concepts, not simple and direct sensations.

15 Lo, "Pleasure, Prohibition, and Pain," 163–64.

16 Quoted from Lo, "Pleasure, Prohibition, and Pain," 165.

17 Engelhardt, "Dietetics in Tang China."

18 Hu Sihui was a court nutritionist apparently of Turkic linguistic background. He wrote *Yinshan zhengyao* as a dietary and nutritional manual that included recipes for over 200 dishes, with detailed instructions regarding measurements of ingredients and cooking methods. Françoise Sabban has described the text as a Chinese "refinement" of Middle Eastern culinary style and ingredients overlaid with Chinese cooking methods and medical values. Sabban, "Court Cuisine," 161–70.

19 Hou, "Dietary Principles in Ancient Chinese Medicine," 349–50.

20   Shen Tong, *Yingyang xinlun*, 1.

21   For discussion of Wu Xian as a "returned student," see Bullock, *American Transplant*, 108–9. For Boxer students and their role in the formation of the Science Society, see Zuoyue Wang, "Saving China Through Science."

22   Luo, "Zhongguo shiwu lun," 880.

23   Zheng Ji, "Shiwu yu jiankang," 1557.

24   Zheng Ji, "Shiwu yu jiankang," 1560–1.

25   Zheng Ji, "Zhongguoren de shanshi wenti," 885.

26   Lin Yutang, *My Country and My People*, 320.

27   Hayford, "The Several Worlds of Lin Yutang's Gastronomy," 232–51.

28   Medhurst, *China*, 40–1.

29   Roberts, *China to Chinatown*, esp. chapters 1–5.

30   Quoted in Roberts, *China to Chinatown*, 28.

31   Fascination mixed with disgust toward Chinese consumption of cats and dogs persisted over the course of the nineteenth century and into the twentieth. John L. Stoddard's travelogue, *China*, which was reprinted three times after its initial publication in 1897, reveled in spectator disgust when describing Canton cat or dog restaurant owners haggling for "cadaverous kittens" and "coolies, each with a plate and spoon, devouring the canine stew as eagerly as travelers eat sandwiches at a railway restaurant after the warning bell has rung." Stoddard, *China*, 66–67.

32   Lawrence Wang, "Beyond *Xin Da Ya*," 240–41.

33   Bickers, "Walter H. Medhurst (1796–1857)."

34   Bays, *A New History of Christianity in China*, chapters 2–3.

35   Laudan, *Cuisine and Empire*, chapter 7.

36   Medhurst, *China*, 40.

37   Medhurst, *China*, 43.

38   Reinders, "Blessed Are the Meat Eaters."

39   The "Northern Provinces" in question here were the southeastern provinces north of Guangdong. Fortune, *Three Years' Wandering*, 27; Rose, *For All the Tea in China*.

40   Fortune, *Three Years' Wandering*, 110.

41   Fortune, *A Residence among the Chinese*, 42–43.

42   Wilson and Charles Denby, who had been appointed the American Minister to China in 1885, were both railroad enthusiasts keen to develop American railroad concessions in China. Li, a leading figure in the self-strengthening movement and whose political influence dominated Chinese politics and international affairs from the late 1860s until his death in 1901, endeavored to build a military industrial complex that would enable China to reduce or even abjure altogether its reliance on foreign aid. Wilson, *China*; Pletcher, *Diplomacy of Involvement*, 141–42.

43 LaFeber, *Cambridge History of American Foreign Relations*, 98.

44 Wilson, *China*, 71.

45 Wilson, *China*, 71–2.

46 Wilson, *China*, 73, 306.

47 Wilson, *China*, 78.

48 Wilson, *China*, 67.

49 Smith's most famous book, *Chinese Characteristics*, which had first been published as a series of essays in the *North China Daily News* of Shanghai in 1889, was translated into Japanese in 1896 and then into classical Chinese in 1903. Lydia Liu, *Translingual Practice*, 51–52.

50 Arthur Smith, *Chinese Characteristics* (1897), 330.

51 Hayford points out that though Smith and his colleagues insisted upon their living as "natives," the process was not without its contradictions. In contrast to Catholic priests, Protestant missionaries came as families with middle-class proclivities that necessarily demarcated their station from both their converts and the surrounding community. Hayford, "Chinese and American Characteristics," 153–76.

52 Hayford, "Chinese and American Characteristics," 153. For a discussion of the background and impact of Smith's work, see Lydia Liu, *Translingual Practice*, 51–60.

53 Lam, *A Passion for Facts*, chapter 1.

54 The 1890 edition printed in Shanghai contains thirty-nine chapters, one for each characteristic. In contrast, the 1897 edition narrowed the list from thirty-nine to twenty-seven, changed the order in which the characteristics appeared, and specifically eliminated the chapter titled "Eating."

55 Arthur Smith, *Chinese Characteristics* (1890), 23, 26.

56 Arthur Smith, *Chinese Characteristics* (1890), 26, 27.

57 Arthur Smith, *Chinese Characteristics* (1897), 21.

58 Arthur Smith, *Chinese Characteristics* (1890), 22–23.

59 Arthur Smith, *Chinese Characteristics* (1897), 19.

60 Arthur Smith, *Chinese Characteristics* (1890), 23.

61 Dupuis advances a provocative analysis that situates Gilded Age American fascination with and revulsion at the Chinese diet in terms of the white working class, free labor, and the right to eat meat. She highlights how integral criticism of the Chinese diet was in defending white free labor from Chinese "coolie" labor in the United States. *Dangerous Digestion*, 69–72.

62 Lam, *Passion for Facts*, 40.

63 Lam, *Passion for Facts*, 40.

64 Hsiao, "From Europe to North American," 130–46; Arkush, *Fei Xiaotong and Sociology in Revolutionary China*, 25–31; Janet Chen, *Guilty of Indigence*, 48–53; Chiang, *Social Engineering and the Social Sciences in China*.

65 Lam, *Passion for Facts*, 142–49.

66 Sidney Gamble, one of the heirs of the Proctor & Gamble fortune, was "*the center of social research in Peking*" during the late 1910s and early 1920s. He conducted several surveys in cities and towns in North China, offered fellowships for students of the Sociology Department at Yanjing University, and financed several others. Chiang, *Social Engineering and the Social Sciences in China*, 242.

67 Gamble, *Peking*, 28.

68 Lam, *Passion for Facts*, 149.

69 For other important studies, see Meng and Gamble, "Prices, Wages and Standards of Living in Peking, 1900–1924"; Tao, *Livelihood in Peking*; Yang and Tao, *Study of the Standard of Living of the Working Families in Shanghai*; and Li, *Dingxian*.

70 For a discussion of the different scales devised to measure the demand for food, see Williams and Zimmerman, "Studies of Family Living in the United States and Other Countries," 49–55.

71 Tao, *Livelihood in Peking*, 77.

72 Tao, *Livelihood in Peking*, 77.

73 In explaining this divergence, Tao surmised that since mutton was relatively less expensive and more flavorful, it was also preferable to pork. Sidney Gamble, whose 1933 study *How Chinese Families Live in Peking* provided numerical support for the characterization of the Chinese as a "pork-eating race," suggested that the difference may have originated in the high proportion of "Mohammedan" households making up Tao's sample.

74 Tao, *Livelihood in Peking*, 89.

75 Tao, *Livelihood in Peking*, 100–1.

76 Quoted in Janet Chen, *Guilty of Indigence*, 49.

77 Lam, *Passion for Facts*, 151.

78 Lam, *Passion for Facts*, 152–53. For some perspective on these percentages, Lam notes that between 1927 and 1935, 9,027 surveys were undertaken in China, most of which were led by Chinese social scientists.

79 Tao had obtained all the data he cited on food values from Wu Xian, and although we have no reason to assume that Tao was among those in the lecture hall when Wu gave his lecture on the Chinese diet in 1926, the two men operated within the same intellectual circles and responded to each other's scientific work as it applied to contemporary social and political issues.

80 S. D. Wilson, "Study of Chinese Foods," 503–8.

81 Maynard, "Wilbur O. Atwater," 3–9.

82 Embrey and Wang, "Analyses of Some Chinese Foods," 247.

83 Daisy Yen Wu, *Hsien Wu, 1893–1959*, 3.

84 Shang-Jen Li, "Eating Well in China," 119–23.

85 China's inclusion within "the tropics" by Westerners served as a way "of defining something culturally and politically alien, as well as environmentally distinct, from Europe and other parts of the temperate zone." Arnold, *Warm Climates and Western Medicine*, 6.

86 Shang-Jen Li, "Eating Well in China," 119–23.

87 Quoted in Shang-Jen Li, "Eating Well in China," 121.

88 Quoted in Shang-Jen Li, "Eating Well in China," 116.

89 Jin Shuchu's preface to Zheng Ji, "Zhongguoren zhi yingyang gaikuang," 25. Jin Shuchu (Sohtsu G. King) was a wealthy businessman who had also been a serious student of natural history. He was an active member of the Geological Society of China and a key financial contributor to the Geological Survey's establishment of a fuel laboratory in 1930.

90 Worboys, "Discovery of Colonial Malnutrition," 222.

91 Wu Xian, "Chinese Diet," 63–74. For a more detailed exposition of how Wu and his colleagues constructed a narrative of deficiency for the Chinese diet, please see chapter 3.

92 Wu Xian, "Chinese Diet," 81. Wu's lecture was delivered in English and translated into Chinese by Zhu Liqing. Zhu translated "minimum" as *shao xiandu* and "optimality" as *zui shiyi yishizhu*. See Wu Xian, "Zhongguo shiwu zhi xiandai yingyangxue zhishi," 97.

CHAPTER 3: OF QUALITY AND PROTEIN

1 Luo, "Zhongguo shiwu lun," 879.

2 Although it was unattributed, Luo took the quote from a Chinese version of Wu Xian, "Chinese Diet."

3 By the time of his essay, Luo had taught at Chengdu University and then Peking University until 1935, when he left China to obtain his master's in agricultural biochemistry from the University of Minnesota. He returned to China in 1937 just before the outbreak of war with Japan.

4 See, for example, Gamble, *How Chinese Families Live in Peiping*, 44–108.

5 Li Jinghan obtained a master's in sociology under the direction of F. H. Giddings at Columbia. He served as the Director of Social Research for the China Foundation and taught at Yenching University before joining James Yen's Mass Education Movement to investigate rural life in North China. For the origins of Li's work in Dingxian, see Hayford, *To the People*, 92–97.

6 In contrast to urban diets, Dingxian diets included little oil and only a bit of salt. Pork, though popular, was not eaten on a regular basis. Most families had 45 eggs during the year, and, Li stressed, most of those eggs were used for entertaining family and friends. Li, *Dingxian*, 260–66.

7 According to the nutritional knowledge of the time, an adequate diet should contain sufficient calories to meet bodily requirements, sufficient amount of proteins "of the proper kind," sufficient coverage of vitamins, and proper amounts of mineral elements like calcium, phosphorus, and iron. For a literate but nonspecialist discussion of the criteria to determine the Chinese diet's nutritional adequacy, see Luo, "Zhongguo shiwu lun."

8 For the association between a bread-and-beef diet and imperial power, see Laudan, *Cuisine and Empire*, chapter 7.

9 Guoqin Xu, *Strangers on the Western Front*.

10 Tsu, *Failure, Nationalism, and Literature*, chapters 3–4.

11 Tsu, *Failure, Nationalism, and Literature*, 99–105.

12 Dikötter, *Discourse of Race in Modern China*; Rogaski, *Hygienic Modernity*; Yip, *Health and National Reconstruction in Nationalist China*.

13 Morris, *Marrow of the Nation*.

14 See, for example, Luo, "Zhongguo shiwu lun," "Shanshi zhidao lun," and "Shanshi biaozhun lun"; Mao, "Lun Zhongguo shanshi you gailiang zhi biyao"; and Long, "Gailiang Zhongguo shanshi fangfa."

15 For Zheng's educational experiences, see Zheng Ji, "Qingnian zeye wenti taolun." For the biology program at National Central University, see Schneider, *Biology and Revolution in Twentieth Century China*, 33–63.

16 Zheng, "Zhongguoren zhi yingyang gaikuang."

17 Zheng, "Zhongguoren zhi yingyang gaikuang," 26.

18 Wu Xian, "Woguoren zhi chifan wenti."

19 "Lun Zhongguo shanshi you gailiang zhi biyao," *Yixuezazhi*, 11.

20 Mao, "Lun Zhongguo shanshi you gailiang zhi biyao," 2.

21 Wu Xian, "Chinese Diet," 74–75.

22 Wu Xian, "Chinese Diet," 75.

23 Wu Xian, "Chinese Diet," 74.

24 Schwartz, *In the Search of Wealth and Power*, 239.

25 Schwartz, *In the Search of Wealth and Power*, 240.

26 Zheng, "Guan shijie bolanhui hou zhi kexue shijie duzhe," 742.

27 Tuberculosis and trachoma (*shayan*) were oft-cited maladies consequent of China's poor diet. Wu Xian included a chart of Chinese mortality rates juxtaposed with figures from other countries, including Japan, Spain, France, the United States, and India, in the third edition of his popular textbook on nutrition science, *Yingyang gailun* (131). Based on that chart, China had a mortality rate of 30 deaths per 1,000 people in 1931.

28 Zheng, "Zhongguoren zhi yingyang gaikuang," 26.

29 Fu, "Measuring Up."

30 See, for example, Stevenson, "Collected Anthropometric Data on the Chinese"; Wang, Jimin, "Zhongguo yinghai tige zhi di'er ci baogao";

Chen-lung Tung, "Physical Measurements in Chinese"; Xu and Wu, "Shang-hai shi xueling ertong shenchang tizhong zhi cubu yanjiu"; Li Xizhen, "Jieshao yige Zhongguo ertong zhi shenchang tizhong biao"; Lin Ziyang, "Huaren shenchang tizhong zhi tongji"; and Ni Zhangqi (T. G. Ni), "Height-Weight Measurements of Shanghai School Children."

31 Stevenson, "Collected Anthropometric Data on the Chinese."

32 For comparative studies of Cantonese children living in and outside China, see Appleton, "Growth of Kwangtung Chinese in Hawaii" and "Growth of Chinese Children in Hawaii and in China." For studies of variation in basal metabolism, see Wang and Hawks, "Basal Metabolism of Twenty-One Chinese Children"; C. C. Wang, "Basal Metabolism of American-born Chinese Girls and of American Girls"; and Earle, "Basal Metabolism of Chinese and Westerners."

33 Ni Zhangqi (T. G. Ni), "Height-Weight Measurements of Shanghai School Children," 59.

34 Mar, "Physical Measurements of Cantonese School Boys in Shanghai," 47–58.

35 Wu Xiang, "Guoren shengli shuizhun zhi yanjiu," 32.

36 McCollum's phrase, "the newer knowledge of nutrition," was intended to bracket the conceptual revolution ushered in by the discovery of vitamins.

37 Cited in Gratzer, *Terrors of the Table*, 162.

38 See, for example, the work of the PUMC chemist Embrey, "Investigation of Chinese Foods," 422.

39 Luo, "Jinshi yingyang huaxueshang danbaizhi yanjiu zhi fazhan," 791.

40 The other two foundational elements of nutrition were carbohydrates and fats. Levenstein, *Revolution at the Table*, 90.

41 Wu and Wu, "Growth of Rats on Vegetarian Diets," 173. Chinese translations of this and other related publications appeared in 1934. See, for example, Wan, "Sushi shu yu hunshi shu qiguan liang du zhi bijiao."

42 Wu and Wu, "Growth of Rats on Vegetarian Diets," 174.

43 The question of how to understand the social and political significance of Chinese vegetarianism was a contested field for Republican intellectuals. An early generation of late Qing and Republican political figures such as Wu Tingfang, Li Shizeng, and Sun Yat-sen saw in vegetarianism, if properly understood and practiced according to scientific principles, "a moral food choice for a modernizing Asian nation" that acknowledged and advanced the natural strengths of China's agricultural and dietetic traditions. See Leung, "To Build or to Transform Vegetarian China?," 4.

44 Wu and Wu, "Growth of Rats on Vegetarian Diets," 174.

45 Wu and Chen, "Growth and Reproduction of Rats on Vegetarian Diets," 157.

46 Wu Xian, "Danbaizhilei zhi shengli de jiazhi."

47 The other three physiological functions of food were reproduction, lactation, and maintenance. Xu Pengcheng, "Yingyang de shengli jichu," 56.

48 The distinction between "energy-bearing" and "protective" expanded, even as it also retraced, a nineteenth-century chemical conception of the healthy diet as requiring only nitrogenous and carbonaceous foods (that is, proteins and fats), some minerals, and water.

49 Columbia University professor of chemistry Henry C. Sherman authored a popular textbook on chemistry that set forth nutritional standards often repeated in Chinese scientific circles. That he supervised a number of those same scientists, for example, Daisy Yen Wu, helps account for his popularity. Zheng, Tao, and Zhu, "Nanjing dongji shanshi diaocha"; Ge, "Zhongxuesheng shanshi yingyang chubu yanjiu"; Guy and Yeh, "Peking Diets."

50 *Report on the Physiological Bases of Nutrition*, 16.

51 *Report on the Physiological Bases of Nutrition*, 16.

52 For a more extensive discussion of the role of milk in the Chinese diet, see chapter 4.

53 McCollum, *Newer Knowledge of Nutrition*, 67; and Valenze, *Milk*, 239.

54 *Report on the Physiological Bases of Nutrition*, 15.

55 Adolph, "Protein Problem of China," 2.

56 Milles, "Working Capacity and Calorie Consumption," 77.

57 Carpenter, *Protein and Energy*, 89.

58 Carpenter points out a telling terminological sleight of hand performed by von Voit in his attempt in 1889 to understand how a vegetarian test subject of his managed to maintain his health and vigor without any animal protein in his diet. Although his vegetarian test subject was also a working man, von Voit refers to him as the "vegetarian" in contradistinction to the "worker," who served as von Voit's point of comparison. Carpenter suggests that the "worker," whom von Voit put on a vegetarian diet and had described as "no lover of vegetable foods," may have been the same man whose normal diet included cheese, sausage, meat dumplings, bread, and beer, thereby yielding some 120 grams of protein daily. Carpenter, *Protein and Energy*, 89, 95; Levenstein, *Revolution at the Table*, 89.

59 Carpenter, *Protein and Energy*, 105.

60 Benedict, "Nutritive Requirements of the Body," 416.

61 Carpenter, 112–18.

62 Benedict draws on the work of the Italian economist Francesco Nitti, who argued that individual and national states of nourishment directly translated to greater or lesser physical strength for the individual and greater or lesser productive energy for the nation. See Nitti, "Food and Labor-Power of Nations"; and Benedict, "Nutritive Requirements of the Body," 427–28.

63 Wu Xian, "Danbaizhilei zhi shengli de jiazhi," 1050.

64 Wu Xian, "Woguoren zhi chifan wenti," 15.

65 Wu Xian, "Woguoren zhi chifan wenti," 15.

66 Wu Xian, "Woguoren zhi chifan wenti," 15.

67 Adolph, "A Study of North China Dietaries."

68 Wu and Wu, "Study of Dietaries in Peking," 142–43.

69 Zhu Zhenjun, "Shanghai ren zhi shanshi," 1187.

70 *Xiao baicai* can refer to either bok choy (*Brassica campestris* subsp. *chinensis*) or Chinese/Napa cabbage (*Brassica campestris* subsp. *pekinensis*, both variant cultivars or subspecies of the turnip. Napa cabbage, which originated in the Beijing region, is the vegetable more likely to have been used in Wu's study. Wu initially identified *xiao baicai* as young cabbage (*Brassica oleracea*), but later corrected himself when new research indicated it was an entirely different plant.

71 The normal rate of growth had been obtained from rats raised on Sherman's Diet No. 13, which consisted of two-thirds ground whole wheat and one-third whole milk powder (Klim).

72 Wu and Wu, "Growth of Rats on Vegetarian Diets," 188.

73 Wu Xian, "Chinese Diet," 59.

74 Wu Xian, "Chinese Diet," 59.

75 Wu Xian, "Chinese Diet," 59.

76 Wu and Wu, "Growth of Rats on Vegetarian Diets," 192. Although less appreciated by Wu and his contemporaries (Chinese or otherwise), the growth rate of a young rat as opposed to that of child of four to five years of age is not actually comparable with respect to body size. A young rat weighing 50 to 60 grams will gain five to six grams per day, yielding a rate of about ten percent of his body weight per day. Physiologically, this means the process of growth in a rat results "in a great dilution of the body stores of nutrients," and for researchers, "makes it very easy to produce a variety of nutritional deficiencies." A young child will also gain five to six grams per day, but on average weighs significantly more, such that her growth rate is negligible compared to body size. Hegsted, "Relevance of Animal Studies to Human Disease," 3537–39; for the correlation between the age of laboratory rats and humans and its relevance to rats as the preeminent model mammalian system, see Pallav Sengupta, "Laboratory Rat," 624–30.

77 Luo, "Shushi lun," 59. For the spread of population-level thinking for enacting changes in the economy, see Thompson, "Foucault, Fields of Governability, and the Population-Family-Economy Nexus in China."

78 Zheng Ji, "Zhongguo zhi yingyang yanjiu wenti," 348–51.

CHAPTER 4: WHICH MILK?

1 During the Tang period, milk products formed a significant part of the diet of the upper classes, but the long-term effects of this dietary practice remained

tied to the dynasty itself. See Chang, *Food in Chinese Culture*, especially Schafer's chapter on the Tang.

2 Sabban, "Session 4: To Each His Own Milk."

3 For further discussion of Li Shizeng's soybean-related enterprises, please see chapter 1.

4 Gerrit Jan Mulder, physician and professor of chemistry at Utrecht, coined the term "protein" in 1838.

5 Quoted in Valenze, *Milk*, 164.

6 Quoted in Dupuis, *Nature's Perfect Food*, 31.

7 Dupuis, *Nature's Perfect Food*, 35.

8 Quoted in Valenze, *Milk*, 249.

9 Quoted in Apple, *Mothers and Medicine*, 7.

10 Mendenhall, *Milk*, 14. For more on the development of American pediatrics and its relationship to the broader children's health and public health movements in the United States, see Markel, "For the Welfare of Children."

11 Valenze, *Milk*, 251.

12 McCollum, *Newer Knowledge of Nutrition*, 150–51.

13 Such associations were not limited to scientific discourse. Andrea Wiley recounts nearly identical ideas in Samuel Crumbine and James Tobey's 1929 book, *The Most Nearly Perfect Food: The Story of Milk*, which further highlighted milk's contributions to the "virility of the white races." Wiley, "Cow's Milk as Children's Food," 236.

14 Valenze, *Milk*, 249. For further discussion of McCollum's role in popularizing milk through his editorial work at *McCall's* magazine and interviews in the *Saturday Evening Post* and the *New York Times*, see Valenze, *Milk*, 249–51.

15 DuPuis, *Dangerous Digestion*, 87–94.

16 League of Nations, *The Problem of Nutrition*, 60–64.

17 The cross-national studies were published in the League of Nation's 1936 "Report on the Physiological Bases of Nutrition" in the multivolume book, *The Problem of Nutrition*. For an assessment of those earlier studies and their reliance on faulty methodology, see Brantley, "Kikiyu-Maasai Nutrition and Colonial Science."

18 Sabban, "The Taste for Milk," 194; Glosser, "Milk for Health, Milk for Profit," 208–11.

19 Li Zhongping, "Cong jindai niuru guanggao kan Zhongguo de xiandaixing," 107, footnote 4.

20 Glosser, *Chinese Visions of Family and State*, chapter 3.

21 In the United States, this idea developed alongside the emergence of nutrition science and the medical specialty of pediatrics in the early twentieth century. See Halpern, *American Pediatrics* and Levenstein, *Revolution at the Table*.

22 Surprisingly little has been written about these new sciences of the child in Republican-period China, but a good foundation can be obtained from the following: Bai, *Shaping the Ideal Child*; Fernsebner, "A People's Playthings"; Plum, "Orphans in the Family"; and Tillman, "Precocious Politics."

23 "National Child Welfare Association of China," 1928, Box 4, Folder 8, China Child Welfare, Manuscripts, Archives and Rare Books Division, New York Public Library.

24 "National Child Welfare Association of China," 1928, Box 4, Folder 8, China Child Welfare, Manuscripts, Archives and Rare Books Division, New York Public Library.

25 The Shanghai branch of the National Child Welfare Association launched the first Children's Day on March 7, 1931, and it petitioned the Ministry of Education to adopt the calendrical designation for the entire country. Jia, Wei, and Liu, "Ertong jie jinian de qingxing ji banfa."

26 Chen Chun, "Yingyangsu yu ertong jianquan fayu zhi guanxi," 16.

27 Xu Yizhe, "Ertong shiwu yingyang wenti."

28 Zhu Zuoting, *Xiaoxue ertong yingyang zhi yanjiu*, 5.

29 Chen Chun, "Yingyangsu yu ertong jianquan fayu zhi guanxi," 16.

30 "Yingyang bu liang," *Xuexiao yu jiating* 6 (1934): 28.

31 Zhu Zuoting, *Xiaoxue ertong yinyang zhi yanjiu*, 5.

32 Lu Yongchun, "Yingyang de wenti," 48.

33 "Ni youmeiyou liuxin dao ni haizi de shanshi?," *Jiating yu funü* 3, no. 6 (1940): 224.

34 Wu Xian, *Yingyang gailun*, 105.

35 Lu Yongchun, "Yingyang wenti," 49. *Douzhi* can refer to either soybean milk or a fermented drink made from ground mung beans, which is especially popular in the Beijing area. It seems likely that Lu is referring to the fermented mung bean drink. Not everyone agreed that infants and children could, without consequence, consume protein amounts in excess of their physiological needs. Some commentators pointed out the digestive difficulties associated with casein, the primary protein found in cow's milk and cheeses, and encouraged mothers to limit cow's milk to one and half *liang* (roughly 75 cubic centimeters). "Ni youmeiyou liuxin dao ni haizi de shanshi?," *Jiating yu funü* 3, no. 6 (1940): 224.

36 Zhu Zuoting, *Xiaoxue ertong yingyang zhi yanjiu*.

37 Sheng Keyou, "Ertong yingyang wenti," 30.

38 See, for example, Xie Baoling, "Ertong yingyang wenti," *Jiankang jiaoyu* 2, no. 3 (1937): 1.

39 Chen Chun, "Ertong yingyang wenti," 1.

40 Zhu Zuoting, *Xiaoxue ertong yingyang zhi yanjiu*, 1. Another variation of this sentiment can be found in Xu Yizhe, "Ertong shiwu yingyang wenti," 974.

41   Li Suizhi, "Xueling ertong yu yingyang wenti," 108.

42   Xu Yizhe, "Ertong shiwu yingyang wenti," 975.

43   Sheng Keyou, "Ertong yingyang wenti," 29.

44   Zhu Zuoting, *Xiaoxue ertong yingyang zhi yanjiu*, 8.

45   Zhu Zuoting, *Xiaoxue ertong yingyang zhi yanjiu*, 9.

46   Hammond and Sheng, "Development and Diet of Chinese Children."

47   Hammond and Sheng relied on Baldwin's *Physical Growth of Children* and Holt's *Standards for Growth and Nutrition*, 359, for the height, weight, and sitting height curves of American boys.

48   Lest one doubt the reliability of their data, Hammond and Sheng wrote, "There can be but little source of error, as the boys have not money, are not allowed to leave the school grounds, and receive no food any other time except at their meals." Hammond and Sheng, 738.

49   Hammond and Sheng, 742.

50   Hammond and Sheng, 731.

51   Hammond and Sheng, 731.

52   Adolph, "4000-Year Experiment," 427.

53   Adolph, "4000-Year Experiment," 427.

54   Adolph, "Chinese Foodstuffs," 13.

55   Adolph, "4000-Year Experiment," 427.

56   Adolph, "4000-Year Experiment," 428.

57   Wu Xian, "Chinese Diet," 81.

58   For a more general discussion of the changing patterns of priority and care for maternal and child health, see Johnson and Wu, "Maternal and Child Health."

59   Glosser, *Chinese Visions of Family and State*, xi. Translated literally, *guomin zhi mu* were "mothers of citizens," and, like the postrevolutionary French and American ideal of republican motherhood, this placed women at the source of the nationalist project, while at the same time constraining their role to a more conservative vision that embodied long-standing cultural norms.

60   Johnson, *Delivering the Nation*, 35–72.

61   Sabban, "Taste for Milk in Modern China," 185.

62   The cost of fresh cow's milk to the consumer was largely prohibitive. Those with the means to afford cow's milk were primarily foreigners, Japanese hospitals, and wealthy Chinese. Other milk products like condensed and evaporated milk were available, but based on anecdotal evidence, consumption of these commodities was limited to wealthier segments of the population, at least until the China National Relief and Rehabilitation Administration (CNRRA) began distributing milk products as part of its food relief. More research, however, remains to be done on this topic.

63   Glosser, "Milk for Health, Milk for Profit."

64 Platt, "Approach to the Problems of Infant Nutrition," 417.

65 Platt and Gin, "Chinese Methods of Infant Feeding and Nursing."

66 Platt and Gin, "Chinese Methods of Infant Feeding and Nursing," 354.

67 Tso, "Development of an Infant," 33. Tso's study was printed in Chinese as "Yong douru bu ying'er zhi chengji."

68 Quoted in Tso, "Development of an Infant," 33–40. The original quote comes from the section titled "No Foods in China and Other Oriental Countries Suitable for Feeding Young Children" in McCollum's *Newer Knowledge of Nutrition* (1922), 399.

69 McCollum, *Newer Knowledge of Nutrition* (1922), 399.

70 Tso, "Development of an Infant," 33.

71 For a comparison with American physicians, see Apple, *Mothers and Medicine*, chapter 2.

72 Platt, "Approach to the Problems of Infant Nutrition," 417.

73 See, for example, "Xiao'er tianran de buru zhi jiazhi," *Shenbao*, 17 May 1923; Aibo, "Ying'er yinshi de wenti"; Shao Wenshan, "Tantan ying'er weisheng de jijian zhongyao wenti"; and Jiang, "Ying'er buyang wenti."

74 Platt, "An Approach to the Problems of Infant Nutrition," 415–16.

75 Laoshao nian, "Ying'er buru wenti."

76 Aibo, "Yin'er yinshi de wenti," 15.

77 Sabban, "Taste for Milk in China," 195. Incidentally, Chinese dairymen also attempted to present their commercial forays into dairying as nationalistic enterprises, such that buying fresh milk could also be construed as supporting China against foreign aggression and imperialism. See Susie Wang, "Buyu Zhongguo," 218.

78 See Hsiung, "To Nurse the Young" and *A Tender Voyage*, 83–90; and Johnson, *Delivering the Nation*, 35–72.

79 Zhang Bufan, "Bu ru'er rengong yingyangfa"; Yun, "Weisheng zhi ying'er burufa."

80 Xu Yizhe, "Ertong shiwu yingyang wenti," 975.

81 There was disagreement about how best to prepare cow's milk for infant consumption. Some Chinese commentators recommended diluting cow's milk with hot water and adding granulated sugar. Others insisted that one should allow the curds and whey to separate and use only the curds (*rulao*) for infant feeding. See, for example, Shao Qiu, "Zai tan ying'er buru wenti"; and Zhou Yunfen, "Ruyou'er zhi fayu ji qi yingyangfa."

82 See, for example, "Yu er fa," *Shenbao*, 23 December 1917; "Yu er fa (zai) (xu)," *Shenbao*, 25 December 1917; "Ying'er tiaoyang fa," *Shenbao*, 17 March 1921; and "Lun jiating jiaoyu," *Shenbao*, 8 January 1922.

83 For other medical studies encouraging the use of soybean milk as infant food, see, for example, Siddal and Chiu, "Feeding Experiment with Soybean

Milk"; Wen Zhongjie, "Huang douru zhi yanjiu"; and "Douru, huashengru, yumi mian yu niurufen yingyang jiazhi zhi bijiao," *Nankai daxue yingyong huaxue yanjiusuo baogaoshu* 3 (1935): 71–76.

84   Tso, "Development of an Infant."

85   See, for example, Adolph and Chen, "Bone Building Properties of Soybean Diets"; Fan, Wu, and Chu, "Metabolic Studies on the Roasted Soybean Meal as an Infant Food"; Guy and Yeh, "Soybean Milk as a Food for Young Infants"; Tso, Yi, and Chen, "Nitrogen, Calcium, and Phosphorous Metabolism in Infant Fed on Soybean Milk"; and Tso and Chang, "Soluble Soybean Milk Powder and Its Adaption to Infant Feeding."

86   Platt, "Approach to the Problems of Infant Nutrition," 419.

87   Su Zufei, *Ertong yingyang*, 16.

88   "Yijie xiaoxi: jingshi weisheng shiwusuo faming doujiang buying," *Guangji yikan* 10, no. 10 (1935): 6.

89   Su Fei, "Dou ji douru"; Leung, "To Build or to Transform China?"

90   "Doujiang ke dai rennai," *Xing hua* 32 (1935): 18–19; "Yong douru bu yinghai zhi chengji," *Weisheng gongbao* 2 (1929): 5.

91   See, for example, "Jishi: sanduo douruchang faxing doufujiang," *Wujiang* 30 (1922): 1; "Zawen: doujiang shangshi," *Qinghua zhoukan* 322 (1924): 24; and "Doujiang zhi fenxi," *Nankai daxue yingyong huaxue yanjiusuo baogaoshu* 1 (1933): 21–22.

92   "Zuo douru de fazi," *Guanhua zhuyin zimu bao* 100 (1920): 20–22; "Shi weisheng shiwusuo faming doujiang buying," *Guangji yikan* 10, no. 10 (1933): 92–93; Ming, "Xinfa zhi doujiang," *Jiaoyu duanbo* (1934): 51.

93   Wen Zhongjie, "Huangdouru zhi yanjiu."

94   Laudan, "Power Cuisines, Dietary Determinism, and Nutritional Crisis"

CHAPTER 5: *DOUJIANG* AS MILK

1   Folder U1-16-1945, Shanghai Municipal Archives.

2   Included among those manufacturers was one China Commercial Bean Curd Milk Company (Zhongguo Gongshang Douru Gongsi) located in the French Concession and another, the Beneficial Soybean Milk Co. (Youyi Douru Gongsi), in Zhabei, a district north of Suzhou Creek under the administration of the Chinese government.

3   Barlow, "Advertising Ephemera and the Angel of History," 113.

4   Barlow, "Advertising Ephemera and the Angel of History," 115–26.

5   Folder U1-16-1745, Shanghai Municipal Archives. The specific term used was *shi yao*, which refers to Daoist alchemical elixirs that use various minerals like gold; see Jin, "'Shennong bencao jing' shiyao tantao," 347–50.

6   Folder U1-16-1745, Shanghai Municipal Archives.

7 Xun Liu, *Daoist Modern*, 151.

8 Folder U1-16-1745, Shanghai Municipal Archives.

9 Folder U1-16-1745, Shanghai Municipal Archives.

10 Folder U1-16-1745, Shanghai Municipal Archives.

11 Many thanks to Eric Karchmer for pointing out the slightly "suspicious" nature of this list of benefits.

12 "Yishi xinwen (neiguo zhi bu) - Shanghai: Shengsheng doujiang zhi fada," *Yixue shijie* 28 (1913): 59; "Sanru zhi gongyong yu jinji: douru, niuru, maru," *Yiyao changshi bao* 2 (1930): 3.

13 Many thanks to Eric Karchmer for helping me work out the contrasting functions involved here.

14 "Sanru zhi gongyong yu jinji: douru, niuru, maru," *Yiyao changshi bao* 2 (1930): 3.

15 Max Huang, "Medical Advertising and Cultural Translation"; and Mittler, *Newspaper for China?*, 318–22.

16 Mittler, *Newspaper for China?*, 319.

17 Anderson and Anderson, "Modern China: South"; Hommel, *China at Work*.

18 Folder U1-16-1745, Shanghai Municipal Archives.

19 *Xueli* is more commonly marketed as a "Korean pear" in the United States. Folder U1-16-1745, Shanghai Municipal Archives.

20 This suggestion that soybean milk's capacity to *bunao* for young people is highly suggestive of an already reconceptualized semantic field that targets the ailments and concerns of modern urbanites. Whereas the traditional Daoist discourse of *bunao* applied to middle-aged and older men whose body (*jing* and qi) are generally regarded as depleted, modern reinterpretation defined *bunao* as the remedy for dealing with mental stress, the lack of sleep or overwork, and other such distress resulting from urban living.

21 Folder U1-16-1745, Shanghai Municipal Archives.

22 For the scientific valorization of cow's milk in the West, see Valenze, *Milk*, especially chapter 8.

23 Shen Tong, *Yingyang xin lun*, 20.

24 Wu Xian, "Vegetarianism," 1–11.

25 Hou, "Diet and Health in China," 416.

26 *Report on the Physiological Bases of Nutrition*, 17.

27 Susie Wang, "Buyu Zhongguo." The imperative of evolutionary advancement and competition reverberated in popular and specialist texts about children's health throughout the Republican period. Although it is not possible to elaborate upon the issue of infant feeding practices, suffice it to say that changing understandings of what constituted appropriate foods for infants was also taking place at this time. Please see chapter four.

28 Li, *World Chinese Biographies*, 23. For information on Chen's father, Chan Tong Ork, see Lai, *Chinatowns*, 217.

29 Li, *World Chinese Biographies*, 23.

30 Chan, "Wet Grinding of Soybean Curtails Value."

31 For an account of his role in shaping American economic perspectives on China, see Robert Yang, "Julean Arnold and American Economic Perspectives."

32 Please see chapter 6 of this book.

33 "The Soybean "Cow" of China," Box 13, Julean Herbert Arnold Papers, Hoover Institution.

34 Glycine advertisements often combined multiple languages: English and Chinese, English and Japanese. Folder U1-16-1745, Shanghai Municipal Archives.

35 Folder U1-16-1745, Shanghai Municipal Archives.

36 Folder U1-16-1745, Shanghai Municipal Archives.

37 Chou, "Xiongbu yu pingbu." For comparison with Japan, see Nakayama, "Nutritional and Moral Responsibilities," forthcoming.

38 Folder U1-16-908, Shanghai Municipal Archives.

39 Folder U1-16-908, Shanghai Municipal Archives.

40 Folder U1-16-908, Shanghai Municipal Archives.

41 In an internal report by one of the analysts working for the SMC's Department of Public Health, Dr. Chan's claims about the nutritive values of Glycine milk was dismissed as a consequence of "sales value" rather than scientific accuracy. Folder U1-16-1745, Shanghai Municipal Archives.

42 Barlow, "Advertising Ephemera," 151.

CHAPTER 6: THE RISE OF SCIENTIFIC SOYBEAN MILK

1 The British-led International Settlements and the French Concession were the two primary foreign concessions in Shanghai. Hongkew (present-day Hongkou), the area of the International Settlements to the north and northeast of the Bund, had by the 1920s become a Japanese-dominated area and an informal Japanese concession. The Chinese administered the parts of Shanghai outside of the International Settlement and the French Concession, which include the present-day day districts of Baoshan, Yangpu, Zhabei, and Nanshi.

2 Henriot, "Shanghai and the Experience of War," 220–21, footnote 11.

3 Ristaino, *Jacquinot Safe Zone*.

4 My use of "biomedical" owes much to the work of medical anthropologists Arthur Kleinman and Margaret Lock. Biomedicine, Kleinman explains, encapsulates "the established institutional structure of the dominant profession of medicine in the West," whose primary knowledge-generating and training system relies upon the scientific paradigm and an extreme

insistence on materialism. Kleinman, "What is Specific to Western Medicine," 15–23.

5   "Monthly Reports," China Child Welfare, Box 4, Folder 12, New York Public Library.

6   For further analysis of the complex yet intimate hand-holding of biomedicine and Chinese state-building during the early twentieth century, see Lei, *Neither Donkey nor Horse*.

7   Duus, *Japanese Informal Empire in China, 1895–1937*, xxiv.

8   The missing soldier returned to base less than half an hour after he disappeared.

9   "Thousands Pour Out of Zhabei," *North-China Herald*, 11 August 1937.

10 "Thousands Pour Out of Zhabei," *North-China Herald*, 11 August 1937.

11 "Peak Reached in Refugees," *North-China Herald*, 1 September 1937.

12 Folder U1-16-1037, Shanghai Municipal Archives, 13.

13 Nagler, "Problem of food and shelter for refugees in Shanghai," 69–70.

14 Yi, Feng, "Élites locales et solidarité."

15 Three main committees—the Shanghai International Relief Committee, the Federation of Shanghai Charity Organizations (Shanghai Cishan Tuanti Lianhe Jiuzaihui), and the Chinese municipality-sponsored Refugee Relief Committee (Nanmin Jiuji Weiyuanhui)—were created to coordinate the multifarious relief initiatives. The Shanghai International Red Cross was also active, but largely in a coordinating capacity. Henriot, "Shanghai and the Experience of War," 227.

16 3 September 1937 letter from J. K. Choy, Vice President, Cantonese Residents Association to Judge C. Franklin, Chairman of the SMC. Folder U1-16-1037, Shanghai Municipal Archives.

17 Folder U1-16-1037, Shanghai Municipal Archives.

18 4 September 1937 memorandum from Acting Commissioner of Public Health to Secretary of SMC, Folder U1-16-1037, Shanghai Municipal Archives.

19 Folder U1-16-1037, Shanghai Municipal Archives.

20 See table I in Henriot, "Shanghai and the Experience of War," 228.

21 Henriot, "Shanghai and the Experience of War," 231–34.

22 Doodha, "Organization of Refugee Camps."

23 Sze, "Medical Care for Shanghai Refugees," 77.

24 The Cantonese Refugees' Relief Committee was composed of members from the Cantonese Residents Association, the Cantonese Guild, and the Cantonese Merchants Association. Folder U1-16-1037, Shanghai Municipal Archives, 35.

25 Folder U1-16-1037, Shanghai Municipal Archives, 16.

26 Folder U1-16-1037, Shanghai Municipal Archives, 21.

27 "New World Camp Made Habitable with Sanitation Improved," *Shanghai Times*, 23 September 1937.

28 Folder U1-16-1037, Shanghai Municipal Archives, 63–64.

29 The Public Health Department of the Shanghai Municipal Council was not
    the only funding source; the Shanghai International Red Cross also provided
    monthly grants to assist in the maintenance and administration of refugee
    clinics. For both agencies, conformance with stipulated requirements was
    necessary to ensure sustained financial support. Sze, "Medical Care for
    Shanghai Refugees," 80.

30 Folder U1-16-1037, Shanghai Municipal Archives, 36–39, 61–62. Social organ-
    izations engaged in the emergency relief effort, particularly native-place
    associations, organized the evacuation of refugees to their home villages as
    part of their work in refugee assistance; see Yi, Feng, "Élites locales et solidar-
    ité," 92–93. These evacuations were not punitive in nature, and it is unclear
    how the Public Health Department would have effectively communicated the
    punitive aspect of their deportation of refugees for lack of compliance.

31 For a general discussion of the SMC Public Health Department's preventative
    public health work, see "Health Department Annual Report," 378.

32 The dissolution of the Shanghai United Epidemiology Committee in
    January 1938 resulted in the reversion of such services to the auspices of the
    Shanghai International Red Cross. See "News and Notes," *Chinese Medical
    Journal*, 397–98.

33 "News and Notes," *Chinese Medical Journal*, 397–98. For a description of
    delousing process, please see Chi and Su, "Delousing in Refugee Camps,"
    271–77.

34 Sze, "Medical Care for Shanghai Refugees," 80.

35 Sze, "Medical Care for Shanghai Refugees," 80.

36 "News and Notes," *Chinese Medical Journal*, 304.

37 "News and Notes," *Chinese Medical Journal*, 303, 397–98.

38 Quoted in Lei, "When Chinese Medicine Encountered the State, 1910–1949," 60.

39 Lei, "When Chinese Medicine Encountered the State, 1910–1949," 60–61,
    119–20.

40 The importance of local physicians in civic life and the extent to which
    the more prominent ones could affect the lives of city residents of all
    socioeconomic levels is testified to by the life and work of the famous
    gynecologist Cai Xiangsun. Wakeman notes that Cai played a major
    leadership role in several Jiangwan associations and was responsible for
    a variety of civic activities, ranging from garbage collection and road
    paving to setting up hospitals and refugee shelters. See Wakeman,
    "Occupied Shanghai," 269.

41 China Child Welfare was established in February 1928 in New York City for
    the primary purpose of raising funds for the relief of children in China,

especially orphans and victims of war and famine. Its operations were merged with the China Aid Council of United China Relief after 1944.

42 "Soya Bean Milk for Refugee Children," China Child Welfare, Box 4, Folder 12, New York Public Library.

43 "July Report," "August Report," China Child Welfare, Box 4, Folder 12, New York Public Library. In December 1938, there were six full-time girls and one half-time girl helping distribute cod liver oil; by March 1939, they too felt the brunt of downsizing.

44 Alumnae Biographical File, Lee Nellie F., Class of 1932, "5 September 1941 letter to Dr. Hackett," Reminisces, 1982, Archives and Special Collections, Mount Holyoke College, South Hadley, MA. A later recollection of her wartime activities with the Refugee Children's Committee, "Bean Milk for China's Refugee Children During the Sino-Japanese War 1937–1945," can also be found in this file.

45 "Beancake for Youngsters," *North-China Herald*, 31 August 1938.

46 "Beancake for Youngsters," *North-China Herald*, 31 August 1938.

47 "Soya Bean Milk for Refugee Children," China Child Welfare, Box 4, Folder 12, New York Public Library.

48 "Soya Bean Milk for Refugee Children," China Child Welfare, Box 4, Folder 12, New York Public Library.

49 Qiao Shumin, "Feichang shiqi zhong zhi yingyang wenti."

50 Hou, *Nutritional Studies in Shanghai*, 1.

51 Hou, *Nutritional Studies in Shanghai*, 1.

52 Hou, *Meeting of Members of the Commission and Other Nutrition Experts*, 5.

53 Ristaino, *Jacquinot Safe Zone*, 52–53; Henriot, "Shanghai and the Experience of War," 226–27.

54 Mitchell derives the phrase from Georg Simmel and uses it to highlight the effect of distance created between the expert and the object calculated. Such effects form the basis of modern forms of expertise that purports to be a detached rationality that can be applied regardless of local contingencies and diverging social orders. Mitchell, *Rule of Experts*, chapter 3.

55 Folder U1-16-908, Shanghai Municipal Archives.

56 Hou, *Nutritional Studies in Shanghai*, 14.

57 Hou, *Nutritional Studies in Shanghai*, 16.

58 Should calcium lactate be unavailable or for reasons of economy, Hou advised substituting finely ground bone meal, calcium carbonate, or calcium hydroxide (slaked lime).

59 Folder U1-16-908, Shanghai Municipal Archives.

60 Hou, *Nutritional Studies in Shanghai*.

61 Hou, *Nutritional Studies in Shanghai*, 43.

62 Hou, *Nutritional Studies in Shanghai*, 38.

63 Lillian M. Li, *Fighting Famine in North China*, 2.

64 Will, *Bureaucracy and Famine in Eighteenth Century China*; Will and Wong, with Lee, *Nourish the People*; Lillian M. Li, *Fighting Famine in North China*.

65 Seung-joon Lee, "Taste in Numbers"; Dillon, "Politics of Philanthropy"; Henriot, "Rice, Power and People."

66 Lillian Li links the increasing levels of international participation in famine relief in the early twentieth century to a paradigm shift in how the Chinese public perceived famines. Li, *Fighting Famine in North China*, 283–309.

67 Mitter, "Classifying Citizens in Nationalist China."

68 For a related examination of the links between scientific modernization and national salvation, see Watt, *Public Medicine in Wartime China*.

69 Worboys, "Discovery of Colonial Malnutrition."

70 Mark Swislocki makes an important distinction in how we think about the categories of hunger and malnutrition. Defining hunger as malnutrition was a "modern" enterprise, but this scientific and cultural recoding should not blind us to "the medical prehistory of new concepts of *malnutrition*," which for China entailed class-based and regionally specific conceptions of nutritional health, as well as differing state priorities regarding food, hunger, and malnutrition. Swislocki, "Nutritional Governmentality"; Vernon, *Hunger*.

71 Cullather, "Foreign Policy of the Calorie."

72 Folder 372-342, Second Historical Archives of China, Nanjing.

73 "Summary of the Proceedings of a Conference on Child Welfare Problems in China held under the auspices of United China Relief, Hotel Shelton, New York City, 11 April 1942," United Service to China MC #135, Box 9, Folder 4, Princeton University Library.

CHAPTER 7: THE GOSPEL OF SOY

1 Alumnae Biographical File, Lee Nellie F., Class of 1932, "5 September 1941 letter to Dr. Hackett," Reminisces, 1982, Archives and Special Collections, Mount Holyoke College, South Hadley, MA.

2 Alumnae Biographical File, Lee Nellie F., Class of 1932, "5 September 1941 letter to Dr. Hackett," Reminisces, 1982, Archives and Special Collections, Mount Holyoke College, South Hadley, MA.

3 Michael Shiyung Liu, email to author, January 18, 2015.

4 The description comes from Auden and Isherwood, *Journey to a War*, 252.

5 Schneider, *Keeping the Nation's House*, 11.

6 See Bailey, *Gender and Education in China*; Cong, *Teachers' Schools*; Culp, *Articulating Citizenship*; Edwards, *Gender, Politics, and Democracy*; Goodman

and Larson, "Introduction" in *Gender in Motion*; and Judge, "Meng Mu meets the Modern."

7   Schneider, *Keeping the Nation's House*, 2–3.

8   See Schneider, *Keeping the Nation's House*, chapters 4–5.

9   Alumnae Biographical File, Lee Nellie F., Class of 1932, Reminisces, 1982, Archives and Special Collections, Mount Holyoke College, South Hadley, MA.

10 Julean Arnold to J. A. Mackay, 6 October 1939, China Child Welfare, Box 4, Folder 12, New York Public Library.

11 Julean Arnold to J. A. Mackay, 6 October 1939, China Child Welfare, Box 4, Folder 12, New York Public Library.

12 "The Report of the Children's Nutrition Committee, Kunming Branch, 1940," Folder U1-16-908, Shanghai Municipal Archives.

13 The China Nutritional Aid Council also identified itself as the Ertong Yingyang Cujinhui.

14 "Minutes of the First Medical Sub-Committee Meeting Children's Nutrition Committee," China Child Welfare, Box 4, Folder 12, New York Public Library.

15 "Field Worker's Report of Trip to Kunming and Kweiyang, July 10–Oct. 9, 1942," China Child Welfare, Box 4, Folder 2, New York Public Library.

16 As part of the Nationalist retreat into the interior, the Ministry of Education ordered the consolidation of Nankai University, National Peking University, and Tsinghua University to form first the Temporary University at Changsha, Hunan, and then from 1938 Southwestern University (National Southwest Associated University).

17 Yip, *Health and National Reconstruction in Nationalist China*.

18 Cited in Yip, *Health and National Reconstruction in Nationalist China*, 176.

19 "[Kunming] Children's Nutrition Committee: A Four Months Report, December 1939–March 1940," China Child Welfare, Box 4, Folder 2, New York Public Library.

20 "[Kunming] Children's Nutrition Committee: A Four Months Report, December 1939–March 1940," China Child Welfare, Box Folder 2, New York Public Library.

21 "[Kunming] Children's Nutrition Committee: A Four Months Report, December 1939–March 1940," China Child Welfare, Box Folder 2, New York Public Library.

22 The specific formula, which called for the proportion of soybean to milk to be one to nine pounds, yielding a solid content of 5.5 percent and the calcium lactate added at 1/3 of a gram per pound of milk, was also testament to its scientific quality.

23 "Minutes of the First Meeting of the Kunming Children's Nutrition Committee," 28 November 1939, China Child Welfare, Box 4, Folder 2, New York Public Library.

24 "[Kunming] Children's Nutrition Committee: February 1940 Report," China Child Welfare, Box 4, Folder 2, New York Public Library.

25 "The Report of the Children's Nutrition Committee, Kunming Branch, 1940," Folder U1-16-908, Shanghai Municipal Archives.

26 Letter from Chang Fu-liang to Arthur Young, 3 July 1942, China Child Welfare, Box 4, Folder 12, New York Public Library.

27 "Minutes of the Second General Meeting of the Kunming Children's Nutrition Committee," China Child Welfare, Box 4, Folder 12, New York Public Library.

28 China Child Welfare, Box 4, Folder 2, New York Public Library.

29 Both the Kunming and Guangxi branch committees dabbled with the complementary distribution of cod liver oil and vegetable soup, but the former had to be imported, and the latter depended upon available monies and local prices.

30 Arnold to Mackay, 15 February 1940, China Child Welfare, Box 4, Folder 12, New York Public Library. Interestingly, the initial name for the committee drawn up by Julean Arnold was the National Committee for Promotion of Soybean Food Products—a title rather more flavored by economic possibilities and particularly suggestive given the direction of the Nutritional Council's development.

31 "Dr. H. C. Hou Lectures on Diet," *China Press*, 23 December 1936.

32 Internal report: "Soya Bean Milk for Refugee Children: A Shanghai Experiment," Box 4, Folder 12, New York Public Library. Hou and his colleague Peter Mar, both associates at the Henry Lester Institute of Medical Research, volunteered their services at area camps. Folder U1-16-1037, Shanghai Municipal Archives.

33 Arnold to Mackay, 15 February 1940, China Child Welfare, Box 4, Folder 12, NY Public Library.

34 Arnold to Mackay, 15 February 1940, China Child Welfare, Box 4, Folder 12, NY Public Library.

35 Folder U1-16-908, Shanghai Municipal Archives.

36 Folder U1-16-908, Shanghai Municipal Archives.

37 Folder U1-16-908, Shanghai Municipal Archives.

38 Folder U1-16-908, Shanghai Municipal Archives.

39 Folder U1-16-908, Shanghai Municipal Archives.

40 Folder U1-16-908, Shanghai Municipal Archives.

41 Folder U1-16-908, Shanghai Municipal Archives.

42 Folder U1-16-908, Shanghai Municipal Archives.

43 K. H. Fu to Julean Arnold, 16 October 1940, China Child Welfare, Box 4, Folder 1, NY Public Library.

44 K. H. Fu to Julean Arnold, 16 October 1940, China Child Welfare, Box 4, Folder 1, NY Public Library.

45 H. C. Hou to Major A. Bassett, 31 March 1941, Folder U1-16-908, Shanghai Municipal Archives; *Missouri Historical Review*, 614.

46 Memo from Dr. H. Pedersen, 14 October 1940, Folder U1-16-1745, Shanghai Municipal Archives.

47 Apparently, the company increased the vitamin D content through irradiation, a process that influenced the other chemical elements in the food (e.g., carbohydrates, proteins, amino acids, and fats) as well as destroyed existing amounts of vitamin A. Letter from J. H. Jordan to the Secretary and Commissioner General of the Shanghai Municipal Council, 15 October 1940, Folder U1-16-1745, Shanghai Municipal Archives.

48 The Public Health Department's reservations about granting a license were sufficiently strong that the department sought legal advice regarding a possible charge of fraudulent misrepresentation. See correspondence of 17 October 1940 and 22 October 1940, Folder U1-16-1745, Shanghai Municipal Archives, 168–70.

49 News clipping from *China Press*, "Vito-Milk is Placed on Local Market," 10 June 1941, Folder U1-16-1745, Shanghai Municipal Archives.

50 News clipping from *China Press*, "Vito-Milk is Placed on Local Market," 10 June 1941, Folder U1-16-1745, Shanghai Municipal Archives.

51 "Pure Fruit Drinks Co.," *China Press*, 17 June 1941; "13,000 Order Vito-Milk," *North-China Herald*, 18 June 1941.

52 Nellie Lee to Julean Arnold, 17 November 1942, China Child Welfare, Box 4, Folder 1, New York Public Library.

53 "China Nutritional Aid Council," Box 103, Arthur N. Young Papers, Hoover Institution Archives.

Epilogue

1 Judge, *Republican Lens*, 8.

2 For the program's official website as well as the entire first season, see *A Bite of China*, http://english.cntv.cn/special/a_bite_of_china/homepage/index .shtml. A quick search through YouTube will yield other English-subtitled versions of the documentary.

3 Chow, "CCTV's 'Bite of China' Takes Off."

4 Oliver Thring, "A Bite of China: The Finest Food TV Ever?" *Guardian*, 12 September 2012.

5 Han, "A Bite of China to Return with Worldview."

6 Blum, "A Bite of China."

7 My reading of the political stakes raised by *A Bite of China* has been shaped by Michelle King's unpublished paper, "Nation, Regions, Culture, Cuisine: What is Chinese Food?"

8   Bray, *Technology, Gender, and History in Imperial China*, 19.

9   Bray defines such procedures as "techniques." *Technology, Gender, and History in Imperial China*, 178.

10   "Inspiration for China" is the CCTV's English title for episode 3.

11   *A Bite of China*, episode 3, "Inspiration for Change," directed by Chen Xiaoqing, aired May 2012 on CCTV.

12   For contemporary reexaminations of Buddhism, vegetarianism, and traditional Chinese purity rules, see Goossaert and Palmer, *Religious Question in Modern China*, 271–313; and Klein, "Buddhist Vegetarian Restaurants."

13   Huang and Scott, "Market Development and Food Demand in Rural China"; Gould and Hector, "An Assessment of the Current Structure of Food Demand in Urban China."

14   He et al., "Consumption of Meat and Dairy Products in China"; Kearney, "Food Consumption Trends and Drivers"; Popkin, "Synthesis and Implications"; Min et al., "Demographics, Societal Aging, and Meat Consumption in China"; Zhai et al., "Prospective Study on Nutrition Transition in China."

15   Du et al., "New Stage of Nutrition Transition in China."

16   He et al., "Consumption of Meat and Dairy Products in China," 385.

17   Yang et al., "Rapid Health Transition in China 1990–2010."

18   See, for example, Norse and Ju, "Environmental Costs of China's Food Security"; Yu, "Meat Consumption in China and Its Impact on International Food Security"; and Schneider, "Wasting the Rural."

19   A flex crop is one that can be used for food, feed, fuel, or industrial material. See Franco et al., "Towards Understanding the Politics of Flex Crops and Commodities."

20   The US was not the world's leading soybean producer in 1947. Since 2006, the United States has been locked, with some fluctuations, in a statistical tie with Brazil. Du Bois, Tan, and Mintz, *World of Soy*, 5.

21   Oliveira and Schneider, "Politics of Flexible Soybeans," 4.

22   "China's Rice, Soybean Imports Top the World in 2017," *People's Daily Online*, 1 February 2018.

23   Oliveira and Schneider, "Politics of Flexible Soybeans," 4.

24   Schneider, "Wasting the Rural," 2.

25   For more on China's industrial meat regime, see Schneider, "Wasting the Rural." For soybean's transformation from agricultural commodity in the service of a diverse array of processed soyfoods to an industrial commodity for an industrial meat sector, see Oliveira and Schneider, "The Politics of Flexible Soybeans."

26   Oliveira and Schneider, "Politics of Flexible Soybeans."11.

27   CCTV English translation. *A Bite of China*, episode 3, "Inspiration for Change."

28   See, for example, Mei Chin, "Magic of Dou Jiang."

29   Kathy Chen, "New Craze Seizes China's Consumers."

30   Wiley, *Re-imagining Milk.*

31   The 2016 dietary pagoda is a revision of the 2007 food pagoda. Chinese Nutrition Society, *Food Guide Pagoda for Chinese Residents.*

32   For more detailed comments and comparisons of Chinese, Japanese, and American dietary recommendations, see Wang et al., "Dietary Guidelines for Chinese Residents (2016)."

33   Quoted in Wiley, "Milk for 'Growth'," 18; originally appeared as "Wen Jiabao: Rang mei yige Zhongguo haizi meitian dou neng he shang yi jin nai," *SINA*, 11 December 2006, http://news.sina.com.cn/c/h/2006-12-11/022311751790.shtml.

34   Eric Meyer, "China and Its Coming Great Milk Battle."

Bibliography

Adachi, Kinnosuke. *Manchuria: A Survey.* New York: R. M. McBride & Co., 1925.

Adolph, William H. (Dou Weilian 竇維廉). "Chinese Foodstuffs: Composition and Nutritive Value." *Transactions of the Science Society of China* (1926): 11–32.

———. "A 4000-Year Experiment." *Scientific American* 143, no. 6 (December 1930): 425–28.

———. "The Protein Problem of China." *Science* 100, no. 2584 (1944): 1–4.

———. "A Study of North China Dietaries." *Journal of Home Economics* 17 (1924): 1–7.

———. "Sushi de Zhongguo." *Kexue huabao* 3, no. 1 (1945): 9.

———. "Vegetarian China." *Scientific American* 159, no. 3 (September 1938): 133–35.

Adolph, William H., and S. C. Chen. "Bone Building Properties of Soybean Diets." *Chinese Journal of Physiology* 6 (1932): 59–62.

Adolph, William H., and Wei-Hsin Hsu. "Fuel Values of Every-Day Chinese Foods." *China Medical Journal* (1924): 1041–45.

Aibo. "Ying'er yinshi de wenti." *Weishengbao* 2, no. 16 (1930): 15.

Amelung, Iwo. "*The Complete Compilation of New Knowledge,* Xinxue beizuan 新學備纂 (1902): Its Classification Scheme and Its Sources." In *Chinese Encyclopaedias of New Global Knowledge: Changing Ways of Thought (1870–1930),* edited by Milena Dolzelová-Velingerová and Rudolf G. Wagner, 85–102. Heidelberg: Springer, 2014.

Ames, Robert T. "Meaning as Imaging: Prologomena to a Confucian Epistemology." In *Culture and Modernity,* edited by Eliot Deatsch, 227–44. Honolulu: University of Hawai'i Press, 1991.

Anagnost, Ann. "The Corporeal Politics of Quality (*Suzhi*)." *Public Culture* 16 (2004): 189–208.

Anderson, E. N. *Food and Environment in Early and Medieval China.* Philadelphia: University of Pennsylvania Press, 2014.

Anderson, E. N., and Marja L. Anderson. "Modern China: South." In *Food in Chinese Culture: Anthropological and Historical Perspectives,* edited by K. C. Chang, 317–82. New Haven, CT: Yale University Press, 1977.

Andrews, Bridie. *The Making of Modern Chinese Medicine, 1850–1960*. Vancouver: University of British Columbia Press, 2014.

Andrews, Bridie, and Mary Brown Bullock, eds. *Medical Transitions in Twentieth-Century China*. Bloomington: Indiana University Press, 2014.

Anonymous. "State Medicine for China." *National Medical Journal of China* 14, no. 2 (1928): 119–20.

Apple, Rima D. *Mothers and Medicine: A Social History of Infant Feeding, 1890–1950*. Madison: University of Wisconsin Press, 1987.

Appleton, Vivia. "Growth of Chinese Children in Hawaii and in China." *American Journal of Physical Anthropology* 10, no. 2 (1927): 237–52.

———. "Growth of Kwangtung Chinese in Hawaii." *American Journal of Physical Anthropology* 9, no. 3 (1928): 473–500.

Arkush, R. David. *Fei Xiaotong and Sociology in Revolutionary China*. Cambridge, MA: Council on East Asian Studies, Harvard University Press, 1981.

Arnold, David. "The 'Discovery' of Malnutrition and Diet in Colonial India." *Indian Economic and Social History Review* 31, no. 1 (1994): 1–26.

———, ed. *Warm Climates and Western Medicine: The Emergence of Tropical Medicine, 1500–1900*. Amsterdam: Rodopi, 1996.

Auden, W. H., and Christopher Isherwood. *Journey to a War*. New York: Random House, 1939.

Bai, Limin. *Shaping the Ideal Child: Children and Their Primers in Late Imperial China*. Hong Kong: Chinese University Press, 2005.

Bailey, Paul. "Cultural Connections in a New Global Space: Li Shizeng and the Chinese Francophone Project in the Early Twentieth Century." In *Print, Profit, and Perception: Ideas, Information, and Knowledge in Chinese Societies, 1895–1949*, edited by Pei-yin Lin and Weipin Tsai, 17–39. Leiden: Brill, 2014.

———. *Gender and Education in China: Gender Discourses and Women's Schooling in the Early Twentieth Century*. London: Routledge, 2007.

———. *Reform the People: Changing Attitudes towards Popular Education in Early Twentieth-Century China*. Vancouver: University of British Columbia Press, 1990.

———. "The Sino-French Connection: The Chinese Worker-Student Movement in France, 1902–1928." In *China and the West: Ideas and Activists*, edited by David S. G. Goodman, 72–103. Manchester, UK: Manchester University Press, 1990.

Baldwin, Bird T. *The Physical Growth of Children from Birth to Maturity*. Iowa City: University of Iowa Press, 1921.

Barlow, Tani E. "Advertising Ephemera and the Angel of History." *Positions: East Asia Cultures Critique* 20, no. 1 (2012): 111–58.

———. "Buying In: Advertising and the Sexy Modern Girl Icon in Shanghai in the 1920s and 1930s." In *The Modern Girl Around the World: Consumption, Modernity, and Globalization*, edited by Alys Eve Weinbaum, Lynn M. Thomas, Priti

Ramamurthy, Uta G. Poiger, Madeleine Yue Dong, and Tani E. Barlow, 288–316. Durham, NC: Duke University Press, 2008.

———. "Debates over Colonial Modernity in East Asia and Another Alternative." *Cultural Studies* 26, no. 5 (September 2012): 617–44.

Barnes, Nicole. "Protecting the National Body: Gender and Public Health in Southwest during the War with Japan, 1937–1945." PhD diss., University of California, Irvine, 2012.

Barona, Josep L. *From Hunger to Malnutrition: The Political Economy of Scientific Knowledge in Europe, 1918–1960.* Brussels: PIE Peter Lang, 2012.

———. *The Problem of Nutrition: Experimental Science, Public Health, and Economy in Europe, 1914–1945.* Brussels: BEL Peter Lang, 2010.

Bays, Daniel H. *A New History of Christianity in China.* Malden, MA: Wiley-Blackwell, 2012.

Benedict, Francis. "Nutritive Requirements of the Body." *American Journal of Physiology* 16, no. 4 (1906): 409–37.

"Bensheng shangqing: huangdou zhangjia." *Hubei shangwubao* 25 (1899): 10–11.

Bergère, Marie-Claire. *Shanghai: China's Gateway to Modernity.* Stanford, CA: Stanford University Press, 2009.

Bickers, Robert. "Walter H. Medhurst (1796–1857)." In *Oxford Dictionary of National Biography.* Oxford: Oxford University Press, 2004; online ed., 2011. https://doi-org.proxy.library.emory.edu/10.1093/ref:odnb/18494.

Blin, Henri. "Le soja ou fève de Mandchourie: Productions et utilisations." *La Nature* (Paris) 38, no. 1 (1910): 141–42.

Blum, Jeremy. "*A Bite of China*: Patriotic, Nostalgic Food Porn Back for Second Season." *South China Morning Post*, 6 May 2014.

Brantley, Cynthia. "Kikiyu-Maasai Nutrition and Colonial Science: The Orr and Gilks Study in the Late 1920s Revisited." *International Journal of African Historical Studies* 30 (1997): 49–86.

Bray, Francesca. "Agricultural Illustrations: Blueprints or Icon?" In *Graphics and Text in the Production of Technical Knowledge in China: The Warp and the Weft,* edited by Francesca Bray, Vera Dorofeeva-Lichtmann, and George Métailié, 521–68. Leiden: Brill, 2007.

———. *Agriculture.* Part 2 of *Science and Civilization in China,* vol. 6, *Biology and Biological Technology,* by Joseph Needham. Cambridge: Cambridge University Press, 1984.

———. "Introduction: The Powers of *Tu.*" In *Graphics and Text in the Production of Technical Knowledge in China: The Warp and the Weft,* edited by Francesca Bray, Vera Dorofeeva-Lichtmann, and George Métailié, 1–82. Leiden: Brill, 2007.

———. *Technology, Gender, and History in Imperial China: Great Transformations Reconsidered.* London: Routledge, 2013.

———. "Towards a Critical History of Non-Western Technology." In *China and Historical Capitalism: Genealogies of Knowledge*, edited by Gregory Blue and Timothy Brook, 158–209. Cambridge: Cambridge University Press, 2002.

Bray, Francesca, Peter A. Coclanis, Edda L. Fields-Black, and Dagmar Schäfer, eds. *Rice: Global Networks and New Histories*. New York: Cambridge University Press, 2015.

Brock, William H. *Justus von Liebig: The Chemical Gatekeeper*. Cambridge: Cambridge University Press, 1997.

Brown, Shannon R. "Cakes and Oil: Technology Transfer and Chinese Soybean Processing, 1860–1895." *Comparative Studies of Society and History* 23, no. 3 (1981): 449–63.

"Bulletin agricole et horticole: Le congrès international de laiterie." *La gazette du Village* 42, no. 2 (8 January 1905): 719.

Bullock, Mary Brown. *An American Transplant: The Rockefeller Foundation and Peking Union Medical College*. Berkeley: University of California Press, 1980.

Cang Shui. "Tebie diaocha: Huangdou yu douyou doubing zhi shuchu gaikuang." *Yinhang zhoubao* 3, no. 23 (1919): 34–37.

Carpenter, Kenneth J. *Protein and Energy: A Study of Changing Ideas in Nutrition*. Cambridge: Cambridge University Press, 1994.

Chadarevian, Soraya de, and Harmke Kamminga, eds. *Molecularizing Biology and Medicine: New Practices and Alliances, 1910s–1970s*. Amsterdam: Harwood Academic Publishers, 1998.

Chan, Harry. "Wet Grinding of Soybean Curtails Value." *China Press*, 17 August 1941.

Chang, K. C., ed. *Food in Chinese Culture: Anthropological and Historical Perspectives*. New Haven, CT: Yale University Press, 1977.

Chaou, Jean de. "Une curieuse plante." In Société d'Horticulture and d'Agriculture, *Bulletin Trimestriel 1907 Juillet, Août, Septembre*, no. 47. Paris: Limoges, 1907.

Chen Bangxian. "Ertong yingyang wenti." *Shenzhou yiyao xuebao* 2, no. 9 (1934): 11–18.

Chen Chun. "Yingyangsu yu ertong jianquan fayu zhi guanxi." *Nü feng* 28, no. 5 (1939): 16.

Chen Hong, trans. "Nongchan zhizaoxue." *Nongxuebao* 115 (1900): 11–60.

———. "Nongchan zhizaoxue." *Nongxuebao* 116 (1900): 11–58.

———. "Nongchan zhizaoxue." *Nongxuebao* 117 (1900): 11–49, 51–55.

Chen Hsiu-ching. "Qingmo shangzhan xia de shanghai 'Wunonghui': Luo Zhenyu nongshang wei zhongxin de shentao (1896–1911)." *Huangpu xuebao* 55, no. 2 (2008): 85–103.

Chen, Janet Y. *Guilty of Indigence: The Urban Poor in China, 1900–1953*. Princeton, NJ: Princeton University Press, 2012.

Chen, Kathy. "New Craze Seizes China's Consumers: A Glass of Milk." *Wall Street Journal*, 28 February 2013.

Chen, Shiwei. "Government and Academy in Republican China: History of Academia Sinica, 1927–1949." PhD diss., Harvard University, 1998.

Chen Weiguo, ed. *Xizhen Lao Shanghai gupiao jian cang lu*. Shanghai: Shanghai Yundong Chubanshe, 2007.

Chen Xiaoqing, dir. *A Bite of China*. Season 1, episode "Inspiration for China." Aired May 2012. http://english.cntv.cn/special/a_bite_of_china/homepage/index .shtml.

Chi, Ta-chih, and Su Der-long. "Delousing in Refugee Camps." *Chinese Medical Journal* 53 (1938): 271–77.

Chiang, Yung-chen. *Social Engineering and the Social Sciences in China, 1919–1949*. Cambridge: Cambridge University Press, 2001.

Chin, Mei. "The Magic of Dou Jiang: Salty Soy Milk Soup Is Better Than It Sounds." *Lucky Peach*. http://luckypeach.com/the-magic-of-dou-jiang (accessed July 2017).

China Press. "Dr. H. C. Hou Lectures on Diet Before Local Public Health Club." 23 December 1936.

———. "Pure Fruit Drinks Co. Swamped with Orders for New Vito-Milk." 17 June 1941.

"China's Rice, Soybean Imports Top the World in 2017." *People's Daily Online*, 1 February 2018.

Chinese Nutrition Society. *The Food Guide Pagoda for Chinese Residents*. www.cnsoc .org/content/details_208_20713.html (accessed July 2016).

Chou Chun-Yen. "Xiongbu yu pingbu: Jindai Zhongguo buru guannian de bianqian (1900–1949)." *Jindai Zhongguo funüshi yanjiu* 18 (2010): 1–52.

Chow, Jason. "CCTV's 'Bite of China' Takes Off, and Steam Pots, Pigs' Feet Benefit Too." *Wall Street Journal* blog, 11 June 2012.

Christian Science Monitor. "Paris and the Bean." 24 January 1911.

Cong, Xiaoping. *Teachers' Schools and the Making of the Modern Chinese Nation-State, 1897–1937*. Vancouver: University of British Columbia Press, 2007.

Cullather, Nick. "The Foreign Policy of the Calorie." *American Historical Review* 112, no. 2 (April 2007): 337–64.

———. *The Hungry World: America's Cold War against Poverty in Asia*. Cambridge, MA: Harvard University Press, 2010.

Culp, Robert. *Articulating Citizenship: Civic Education and Student Politics in Southeastern China, 1912–1940*. Cambridge, MA: Harvard University Asia Center, 2007.

———. "Mass Production of Knowledge and the Industrialization of Mental Labor: The Rise of the Petty Intellectual." In *Knowledge Acts in Modern China: Ideas, Institutions, and Identities*, edited by Robert Culp, Eddy U, and Wen-hsin Yeh, 207–41. Berkeley: Institute of East Asian Studies, University of California, Berkeley, 2016.

Daston, Lorraine, ed. *Biographies of Scientific Objects*. Chicago: University of Chicago Press, 2000.

Dikötter, Frank. *The Discourse of Race in Modern China*. Stanford, CA: Stanford University Press, 1992.

Dillon, Nara. "The Politics of Philanthropy: Social Networks and Refugee Relief in Shanghai, 1932–1949." In *At the Crossroads of Empires: Middlemen, Social Networks, and State-Building in Republican Shanghai*, edited by Nara Dillon and Jean C. Oi, 179–205. Stanford, CA: Stanford University Press, 2008.

Doodha, N. B. "Organization of Refugee Camps as Worked Out by the Visiting Committee." *China Quarterly* 3, no. 1 (Winter 1937–1938): 88–94.

"Doujiang ke dai rennai." *Xing hua* 32 (1935): 18–19.

"Doujiang zhi fenxi." *Nankai daxue yingyong huaxue yanjiusuo baogaoshu* 1 (1933): 21–22.

"Douru, huashengru, yumi mian yu niurufen yingyang jiazhi zhi bijiao." *Nankai daxue yingyong huaxue yanjiusuo baogaoshu* 3 (1935): 71–76.

"Douru yu niuru zhi bijiao." *Zhongxi yixue bao* 8 (1910): 8.

Du, S., Bu Lu, F. Zhai, and B. M. Popkin. "A New Stage of Nutrition Transition in China." *Public Health Nutrition* 5 (2002): 169–74.

Du Bois, Christine M., Chee-Beng Tan, and Sidney W. Mintz, eds. *The World of Soy*. Urbana: University of Illinois Press, 2008.

DuPuis, E. Melanie. *Dangerous Digestion: The Politics of American Dietary Advice*. Berkeley: University of California Press, 2015.

———. *Nature's Perfect Food: How Milk Became America's Drink*. New York: New York University Press, 2002.

Duus, Peter. "Economic Dimensions of Meiji Imperialism: The Case of Korea, 1895–1910." In *The Japanese Colonial Empire, 1895–1945*, edited by Ramon H. Myers and Mark R. Peattie, 128–71. Princeton, NJ: Princeton University Press, 1984.

———. *The Japanese Informal Empire in China, 1895–1937*. Princeton, NJ: Princeton University Press, 1989.

Earle, H. G. "Basal Metabolism of Chinese and Westerners." *Chinese Journal of Physiology* 1 (1928): 59–92.

Edwards, Louise. *Gender, Politics, and Democracy: Women's Suffrage in China*. Stanford, CA: Stanford University Press, 2008.

Ehara, Ayako. "The Changes of Terms about Food in Household Textbooks: The Term about Nutrition" [in Japanese]. *Journal of Home Economics of Japan* 43, no. 6 (1992): 533–42.

Eliott, Mark C. *The Manchu Way: The Eight Banners and Ethnic Identity in Late Imperial China*. Stanford, CA: Stanford University Press, 2001.

Elman, Benjamin. "From Pre-modern Chinese Natural Studies to Modern Science in China." In *Mapping Meanings: The Field of New Learning in Late Qing China*, edited by Michael Lackner and Natascha Vittinghoff, 25–74. Leiden: Brill, 2004.

———. *On Their Own Terms: Science in China, 1550–1900*. Cambridge, MA: Harvard University Press, 2005.

———. "Toward a History of Modern Science in Republican China." In *Science and Technology in Modern China, 1880s–1940s*, edited by Jing Tsu and Benjamin Elman, 15–38. Leiden: Brill, 2014.

Embrey, Hartley. "The Investigation of Chinese Foods." *China Medical Journal* 35 (1921): 420–47.

Embrey, Hartley, and Tsan Ch'ing Wang. "Analyses of Some Chinese Foods." *China Medical Journal* 35 (1921): 247–57.

Engelhardt, Ute. "Dietetics in Tang China and the First Extant Works of *Materia Dietetica*." In *Innovation in Chinese Medicine*, edited by Elisabeth Hsu, 173–91. Cambridge: Cambridge University Press, 2001.

"Exposition de la Meunerie et Salon de l'Alimentation." *Gazette du Village* 46, no. 1 (3 January 1909): 760.

Fan, Fa-ti. "How Did the Chinese Become Native? Science and the Search for National Origins in the May Fourth Era." In *Beyond the May Fourth Paradigm: In Search of Chinese Modernity*, edited by Kai-wing Chow, Tze-ki Hon, Hung-yok Ip, and Don C. Price, 183–208. Lanham, MD: Lexington Books, 2008.

Fan, T., T. Wu, and F. T. Chu. "Metabolic Studies on the Roasted Soybean Meal as an Infant Food." *Chinese Medical Journal* 56 (1940): 53–67.

Farquhar, Judith. *Appetites: Food and Sex in Post-socialist China.* Durham, NC: Duke University Press, 2002.

Farquhar, Judith, and Qicheng Zhang. *Ten Thousand Things: Nurturing Life in Contemporary Beijing.* New York: Zone Books, 2012.

Faulkner, Frank T. *Infant and Child Nutrition Worldwide: Issues and Perspectives.* Boca Raton, FL: CRC Press, 1991.

Fédération Internationale de Laiterie, Comité Français. *2e Congrès International de Laiterie Paris, 16–19 Octobre 1905: Compt-rendu des séances, Excursions, Liste des Congressistes.* Paris: Condé-sur-l'Escaut, Impr. F. Descamps, [1905].

Fernsebner, Susan R. "A People's Playthings: Toys, Childhood, and Chinese identity, 1909–1933." *Postcolonial Studies* 6, no. 3 (2003): 269–93.

Fildes, Valerie A. *Breasts, Bottles, and Babies: A History of Infant Feeding.* Edinburgh: Edinburgh University Press, 1986.

Finnane, Antonia. "Food and Place: Zhu Ziqing's Essay 'Speaking of Yangzhou' (*Shuo Yangzhou*, 1934)." In *Yangzhou, a Place in Literature: The Local in Chinese Cultural History*, edited by Roland Altenburger, Margaret B. Wan, and Vibeke Børdahl, 308–20. Honolulu: University of Hawai'i Press, 2015.

Fomon, Samuel J. "Infant Feeding in the 20th Century: Formula and Beikost." *Journal of Nutrition* 131 (2001): 409S–420S.

Fortune, Robert. *A Residence among the Chinese: Inland, on the Coast, and at Sea. Being a Narrative of Scenes and Adventures during a Third Visit to China, from 1853 to 1856.* London: John Murray, 1857.

———. *Three Years' Wandering in the Northern Provinces of China, Including a Visit to the Tea, Silk, and Cotton Countries, with an Account of the Agriculture of the Chinese, New Plants, etc.* 2nd ed. London: John Murray, 1847.

Franco, Jennifer, Jun Borras, Pietje Vervest, S. Ryan Isakson, and Les Levidow. "Towards Understanding the Politics of Flex Crops and Commodities: Implications for Research and Policy Advocacy." *Think Piece Series on Flex Crops and Commodities* (Transnational Institute Agrarian Justice Program), no. 1 (June 2014).

Friedenwald, Julius, and John Ruhräh. *Diet in Health and Disease.* London: W. B. Saunders, 1905.

Fu, Jia-Chen. "Measuring Up: Anthropometrics and the Chinese Body in Republican Period China." *Bulletin of the History of Medicine* 90, no. 4 (December 2016): 643–71.

Fuller, Frank, Jikun Huang, Hengyun Ma, and Scott Rozele. "Got Milk? The Rapid Rise of China's Dairy Sector and Its Future Prospects." *Food Policy* 31 (2006): 201–15.

Gamble, Sidney D. *How Chinese Families Live in Peiping.* New York: Funk & Wagnalls, 1933.

———. *Peking: A Social Survey.* New York: George H. Doran, 1921.

Ge Chunlin. "Zhongxuesheng shanshi yingyang chubu yanjiu." *Kexue* 20, no. 7 (July 1936): 564–74.

Gerth, Karl. *As China Goes, So Goes the World: How Chinese Consumers Are Transforming the World.* New York: Hill and Wang, 2010.

Glosser, Susan. *Chinese Visions of Family and State, 1915–1953.* Berkeley: University of California, 2003.

———. "Milk for Health, Milk for Profit: Shanghai's Chinese Dairy Industry under Japanese Occupation." In *Inventing Nanjing Road: Commercial Culture in Shanghai, 1900–1945*, edited by Sherman Cochran, 207–33. Ithaca, NY: East Asia Program, Cornell University, 2000.

Goodman, Bryna, and Wendy Larson, eds. *Gender in Motion.* London: Rowman and Littlefield, 2005.

Goossaert, Vincent, and David A. Palmer. *The Religious Question in Modern China.* Chicago: University of Chicago Press, 2011.

Gottschang, Thomas R. "Economic Change, Disasters, and Migration: The Historical Case of Manchuria." *Economic Development and Cultural Change* 35, no. 3 (April 1987): 461–90.

Gottschang, Thomas R., and Diana Lary. *Swallows and Settlers: The Great Migration from North China to Manchuria.* Ann Arbor: Center for Chinese Studies, University of Michigan, 2000.

Gould, B. W., and J. V. Hector. "An Assessment of the Current Structure of Food Demand in Urban China." *Agricultural Economics* 34 (2006): 1–16.

Gratzer, Walter. *Terrors of the Table: The Curious History of Nutrition*. Oxford: Oxford University Press, 2005.

"Guowai yaowen: Bali doufu gongsi gaikuang." *Shiye zazhi* 37 (1920): 142–44.

Guy, Ruth A., and K. S. Yeh. "Soybean Milk as a Food for Young Infants." *Chinese Medical Journal* 54, no. 1 (1938): 1–30.

———. "Peking Diets." *Chinese Medical Journal* 54, no. 3 (September 1938): 201–22.

Halpern, S. A. *American Pediatrics: The Social Dynamics of Professionalism, 1880–1980*. Berkeley: University of California Press, 1988.

Hammond, John, and Hsia Sheng. "The Development and Diet of Chinese Children." *American Journal of Diseases of Children* 29, no. 6 (1925): 729–42.

Han, Bingbin. "*A Bite of China* to Return with Worldview." *China Daily* (US ed.), 4 May 2015.

Hanson, Marta. *Speaking of Epidemics in Chinese Medicine: Disease and Geographic Imagination in Late Imperial China*. Oxford: Routledge, 2011.

Hayford, Charles. "Chinese and American Characteristics: Arthur H. Smith and the Respectable Middle Class View of China." In *Christianity in China: Early Protestant Missionary Writings*, edited by Suzanne Wilson Barnett and John K. Fairbank, 153–74. Cambridge, MA: Committee on American-East Asian Relations of the Department of History in Collaboration with the Council on East Asian Studies, Harvard University Press, 1985.

———. "The Several Worlds of Lin Yutang's Gastronomy." In *The Cross-Cultural Legacy of Lin Yutang: Critical Perspectives*, edited by Qian Suoqiao, 232–51. Berkeley: Institute of East Asian Studies, University of California, 2015.

———. *To the People: James Yen and Village China*. New York: Columbia University Press, 1990.

He, Yuna, Xiaoguang Yang, Juan Xia, Liyun Zhao, and Yuexin Yang. "Consumption of Meat and Dairy Products in China: A Review." *Proceedings of the Nutrition Society* 75 (2016): 385–91.

Hegsted, D. Mark. "Relevance of Animal Studies to Human Disease." *Cancer Research* 35 (November 1975): 3537–39.

Henriot, Christian. "Rice, Power and People: The Politics of Food Supply in Wartime Shanghai (1937–1945)." *Twentieth-Century China* 26, no. 1 (November 2000): 41–84.

———. "Shanghai and the Experience of War: The Fate of Refugees." *European Journal of East Asian Studies* 5, no. 2 (2006): 215–45.

Hitier, H. "Société Nationale d'Agriculture de France: Le soja." *Journal d'agriculture pratique* 74, no. 1 (1910): 24–25.

Holt, L. Emmett. *Standards for Growth and Nutrition*. New York: Child Health Organization, 1918.

Hommel, Rudolf. *China at Work*. New York: John Day, 1937.

Hon, Tze-ki. "Zhang Zhidong's Proposal for Reform: A New Reading." In *Rethinking the 1898 Reform Period: Political and Cultural Change in Late Qing China*, edited by Rebecca Karl and Peter Zarrow, 77–98. Cambridge, MA: Harvard University Asia Center, Harvard University, 2002.

Horkheimer, Max, and Theodor W. Adorno. *Dialectic of Enlightenment*. New York: Continuum, 1987.

Hoshino, Tokuji. *Economic History of Manchuria Compiled in Commemoration of the Decennial of the Bank of Chosen*. Seoul: [The Bank], 1921.

Hou, Xiangchuan (H. C. Hou). "Dietary Principles in Ancient Chinese Medicine." *Chinese Medical Journal* 53 (1938): 347–52.

———. *Meeting of Members of the Commission and Other Nutrition Experts: Note on Chinese Dietary Standards and Some Dietary Problems among War Refugees*. Geneva: League of Nations Health Organization, 1939.

———. *Nutritional Studies in Shanghai*. Chinese Medical Association, Special Report Series no. 12. Shanghai: Henry Lester Institute of Medical Research, 1939.

———. *Yingyang quefabing gangyao ji tupu*. Beijing: Renmin Weisheng Chubanshe, 1957.

Howell, David L. *Capitalism From Within: Economy, Society, and the State in a Japanese Fishery*. Berkeley: University of California Press, 1995.

———. "Proto-industrial Origins of Japanese Capitalism." *Journal of Asian Studies* 51, no. 2 (May 1992): 269–86.

Hsiao, Hsin-huang Michael. "From Europe to North America: The Development of Sociology in Twentieth Century China." In *China and the West: Ideas and Activists*, edited by David S. G. Goodman, 130–46. Manchester, UK: Manchester University Press, 1990.

Hsiung, Ping-chen. *A Tender Voyage: Children and Childhood in Late Imperial China*. Stanford, CA: Stanford University Press, 2005.

———. "To Nurse the Young: Breastfeeding and Infant Feeding in Late Imperial China." *Journal of Family History* 20 (September 1995): 217–38.

Hu Chengdian. "Dadou zhi zhizaopin ji qi gongyong." *Hunan sheng nonghui bao* 1, no. 9 (1917): 50–54.

Hu, Danian. *China and Albert Einstein: The Reception of the Physicist and His Theory in China, 1917–1979*. Cambridge, MA: Harvard University Press, 2005.

Huang, H. T. "Early Uses of Soybean in Chinese History." In *The World of Soy*, edited by Christine M. Du Bois, Chee-Beng Tan, and Sidney W. Mintz, 45–55. Urbana: University of Illinois Press, 2008.

———. *Fermentations and Food Science*. Part 5 of *Science and Civilization in China*, vol. 6, *Biology and Biological Technology*, by Joseph Needham. Cambridge: Cambridge University Press, 2000.

Huang, J. K. and R. Scott. "Market Development and Food Demand in Rural China." *China Economic Review* 9 (1998): 25–45.

Huang, Max K. W. "Medical Advertising and Cultural Translation: The Case of *Shenbao* in Early Twentieth-Century China." In *Print, Profit, and Perception: Ideas, Information, and Knowledge in Chinese Societies, 1895–1949*, edited by Pei-yin Lin and Weipin Tsai, 114–47. Leiden: Brill, 2014.

Huang, Philip C. C. "Development or Involution in Eighteenth-Century Britain and China? A Review of Kenneth Pomeranz's 'The Great Divergence: China, Europe, and the Making of the Modern World Economy.'" *Journal of Asian Studies* 61, no. 2 (2002): 501–38.

Huang Shirong. "Da dou de gongyong." In *Wei tui ju suibi* (1908). Reprinted in *Wenhui quanshu*. Jiading: Huang Shi, 1916.

Huff, Joyce L. "Corporeal Economies: Work and Waste in Nineteenth-Century Constructions of Alimentation." In *Cultures of the Abdomen: Diet, Digestion, and Fat in the Modern World*, edited by Christopher E. Forth and Ana Carden-Coyne, 31–49. New York: Palgrave-Macmillan, 2005.

Huters, Ted. "Culture, Capital, and Temptations of the Imagined Market: The Case of the Commercial Press." In *Beyond the May Fourth Paradigm: In Search of Chinese Modernity*, edited by Kai-wing Chow et al., 27–50. Lanham, MD: Lexington Books, 2008.

Hymowitz, Theodore. "Dorsett-Morse Soybean Collection Trip to East Asia: 50 Year Retrospective." *Economic Botany* 38, no. 4 (October–Dececember 1984): 378–88.

Isett, Christopher. *State, Peasant, and Merchant in Qing Manchuria, 1644–1862*. Stanford, CA: Stanford University Press, 2007.

———. "Sugar Manufacture and the Agrarian Economy of Nineteenth-Century Taiwan." *Modern China* 21, no. 2 (April 1995): 233–59.

Jacko, Tamara. "Cultivating Citizens: *Suzhi* (Quality) Discourse in the PRC." *Positions: East Asia Cultures Critique* 17, no. 3 (2009): 523–35.

Ji Hongkun. "Ding Fubao he Zhongguo jindai yingyang weisheng kexue." *Yangzhou daxue pengren xuebao* 25, no. 2 (2008): 34–36.

———. "Jindai yixue he yingyangxue dongchao yu Oumei chuanjiaoshi de zuoyong." *Yangzhou daxue pengren xuebao* 25, no. 1 (2008): 44–47.

———. "Zheng Zhenwen he tade yingyang huaxue." *Yangzhou daxue pengren xuebao* 25, no. 3 (2008): 42–45.

Jia Ruzhong, Wei Huimin, and Liu Guiyu. "Ertong jie jinian de qingxing ji banfa." *Shida yuekan* 13 (1934): 187–255.

Jiang Faxian. "Ying'er buyang wenti." *Jian yu mei* 11 (1948): 20–21.

Jin Mingyuan. "'Shengnong bencao jing' shiyao tantao." In *Bainian Daoxue jinghua jicheng diwuji daoyi yangsheng juansi*, edited by Zhan Shichuang, 347–50. Chengdu: Bashu shushe, 2014.

"Jinsan nianjian shuru zhi Yingguo zhi dadou lei." *Huashang lianhehui bao* 13 (1910): 97–98.

"Jishi: sanduo douruchang faxing doufujiang." *Wujiang* 30 (1922): 1.

Johnson, Tina Phillips. *Delivering the Nation: Modern Childbirth in Republican China.* Lanham, MD: Lexington Books, 2011.

Johnson, Tina Phillips, and Yi-Li Wu. "Maternal and Child Health in Nineteenth- to Twenty-first-Century China." In *Medical Transitions in Twentieth-Century China,* edited by Bridie Andrews and Mary Brown Bullock, 51–68. Bloomington: Indiana University Press, 2014.

Jones, Andrew F. *Developmental Fairy Tales: Evolutionary Thinking and Modern Chinese Culture.* Cambridge, MA: Harvard University Press, 2011.

Judge, Joan. "Meng Mu Meets the Modern: Female Exemplars in Late-Qing Textbooks for Girls and Women." *Jindai Zhongguo funü shi yanjiu* 8 (June 2000): 133–77.

———. *Republican Lens: Gender, Visuality, and Experience in the Early Chinese Periodical Press.* Berkeley: University of California Press, 2016.

Kamminga, Harmke, and Andrew Cunningham, eds. *The Science and Culture of Nutrition, 1840–1940.* Amsterdam: Rodopi, 1995.

Kawai Taizo. *Nyugyu oyobi seinyu shinsho.* Tokyo: Bokuchiku Zasshisha, Meiji 25 [1892].

Kearney, John. "Food Consumption Trends and Drivers." *Philosophical Transaction: Biological Sciences* 365, no. 1554 (September 2010): 2793–807.

Kirby, William. "Technocratic Organization and Technological Development in China: The National Experience and Legacy, 1928–1953." In *Science and Technology in Post-Mao China,* edited by Denis Fred Simon and Merle Goldman, 23–44. Cambridge, MA: Council on East Asian Studies, Harvard University, 1989.

Klein, Jakob A. "Buddhist Vegetarian Restaurants and the Changing Meanings of Meat in Urban China." *Ethnos* 82, no. 2 (2017): 252–76.

Kleinman, Arthur. "What is Specific to Western Medicine." In *Companion Encyclopedia of the History of Medicine,* vol. 1, edited by W. F. Bynum and Roy Porter, 15–23. London: Routledge, 2004.

Kohn, Livia, ed. *Daoist Body Cultivation: Traditional Models and Contemporary Practices.* Magdalena: Three Pine Press, 2006.

———. *The Taoist Experience: An Anthology.* Albany: State University of New York Press, 1993.

———. *Taoist Meditation and Longevity Techniques.* Ann Arbor: Center for Chinese Studies, University of Michigan, 1989.

Kriedte, Peter, Hans Medick, and Jürgen Schlumbohm. *Industrialization Before Industrialization.* Cambridge: Cambridge University Press, 1981.

Kwok, D. W. Y. *Scientism in Chinese Thought, 1900–1950.* New Haven, CT: Yale University Press, 1965.

Lackner, Michael, and Natascha Vittinghoff, eds. *Mapping Meanings: The Field of New Learning in Late Qing China.* Leiden: Brill, 2004.

Lackner, Michael, Iwo Amelung, and Joachim Kurtz, eds. *New Terms for New Ideas: Western Knowledge and Lexical Change in Late Imperial China*. Leiden: Brill, 2001.

LaFeber, Walter. *The Cambridge History of American Foreign Relations, Volume II: The American Search for Opportunity, 1865–1913*. Cambridge: Cambridge University Press, 1995.

Lai, David Chuenyan. *Chinatowns: Towns within Cities in Canada*. Vancouver: University of British Columbia Press, 1988.

Lam, Tong. *A Passion for Facts: Social Surveys and the Construction of the Chinese Nation-State, 1900–1949*. Berkeley: University of California Press, 2011.

Laoshao nian. "Ying'er buru wenti." *Zhongguo kangjian yuebao* 1, no. 4 (1933): 55.

Lary, Diana. *The Chinese People at War: Human Suffering and Social Transformation, 1937–1945*. New York: Cambridge University Press, 2010.

Laudan, Rachel. *Cuisine and Empire: Cooking in World History*. Berkeley: University of California Press, 2013.

———. "Power Cuisines, Dietary Determinism, and Nutritional Crisis: The Origins of the Globalization of the Western Diet." Presented at the Interactions: Regional Studies, Global Processes, and Historical Analysis conference, Washington, DC, 28 February–3 March 2001. http://webdoc.sub.gwdg.de/ebook/p/2005/history_cooperative/www.historycooperative.org/proceedings/interactions/laudan.html.

Laughlin, Charles A. *The Literature of Leisure and Chinese Modernity*. Honolulu: University of Hawai'i Press, 2008.

Le Figaro. "A Travers Paris." 27 December 1902.

League of Nations. *Nutrition. Final Report of the Mixed Committee of the League of Nations on the Relation of Nutrition of Health, Agriculture, and Economic Policy*. [Geneva]: League of Nations, [1937].

———. *The Problem of Nutrition*. Vol. 2, *Report on the Physiological Bases of Nutrition*. Geneva: League of Nations, 1936.

Lean, Eugenia. "Proofreading Science: Editing and Experimentation in Manuals by a 1930s Industrialist." In *Science and Technology in Modern China, 1880s–1940s*, edited by Jing Tsu and Benjamin A. Elman, 185–208. Leiden: Brill, 2014.

Lee, Leo Ou-fan. *Shanghai Modern: The Flowering of a New Urban Culture in China, 1930–1945*. Cambridge, MA: Harvard University Press, 1999.

Lee, Seung-joon. *Gourmets in the Land of Famine: The Culture and Politics of Rice Consumption in Modern Canton, 1900–1937*. Stanford, CA: Stanford University Press, 2011.

———. "The Patriot's Scientific Diet: Nutrition Science and Dietary Reform Campaigns in China, 1910s–1950s." *Modern Asian Studies* 49, no. 6 (November 2015): 1808–39.

———. "Taste in Numbers: Science and the Food Problem in Republican Guangzhou, 1927–1937." *Twentieth-Century China* 35, no. 2 (April 2010): 81–103.

Lei, Sean Hsiang-lin. *Neither Donkey nor Horse: Medicine in the Struggle over China's Modernity.* Chicago: University of Chicago Press, 2014.

———. "When Chinese Medicine Encountered the State, 1910–1949." PhD diss., University of Chicago, 1999.

Lemarié, Charles. "Les sojas du Japan." *Bulletin Economique de l'Indochine* (Hanoi) 13, no. 85 (1910): 493–98.

Leung, Angela Ki Che. "To Build or to Transform Vegetarian China?" In *Moral Foods,* edited by Angela Ki Che Leung and Melissa Caldwell. Honolulu: University of Hawai'i Press, forthcoming.

Levenstein, Harvey A. *Paradox of Plenty: A Social History of Eating in Modern America.* New York: Oxford University Press, 1993.

———. *Revolution at the Table: The Transformation of the American Diet.* Berkeley: University of California Press, 2003.

Li, Jinghan. *Dingxian shehui gaikuang diaocha.* Shanghai: Shanghai Shudian, 1992. First published in 1933 by Zhonghua Pingmin Jiaoyu Cujinhui (Peiping).

Li, Lillian M. *Fighting Famine in North China: State, Market, and Environmental Decline, 1690s–1990s.* Stanford, CA: Stanford University Press, 2007.

Li, Shang-jen. "Eating Well in China: Diet and Hygiene in Nineteenth-Century Treaty Ports." In *Health and Hygiene in Chinese East Asia: Policies and Publics in the Long Twentieth Century,* edited by Angela Ki Che Leung and Charlotte Furth, 109–31. Durham, NC: Duke University Press, 2010.

Li Shangyue. "Dadou zhi gailiang." *Fengtian quanye bao* (1910): 6.

Li Shizeng (Li Yuying). *Da Dou: Le soja.* Paris: Société Biologique de l'Extrême Orient, 1910.

———. "Dadou shipin zhi gongyong." *Tongwenbao* 417 (1910): 5–7.

———. "Ershi'er sui chuyou sihai." In *Li Shizeng xiansheng wenji xiace.* Taipei: Zhongguo Guomindang Zhongyang Weiyuanhui Dangshi Weiyuanhui, Zhongyang Wenwu Gongyingshe, 1980.

———. "Le soja." *L'agriculture pratique des pays chauds (Bulletin du Jardin Colonial)* 11, no. 2 (September 1911): 178.

———. *Li Shizeng xiansheng jinianji.* Taipei: s.n., 1974.

———. "Lun dadou gongyi wei Zhongguo zhizi zhi techang." *Dixue zazhi* 1, no. 4 (1910): 6–11.

———. "Vegetable Milk and Its Derivatives." British Patent 30275. Filed 30 December 1910 and accepted 29 February 1912.

———. "Xinzhishi: lun dadou gongyi wei Zhongguo zhizao zhi techang." *Dongfang zazhi* 7, no. 7 (1910): 29–38.

Li Suizhi. "Xueling ertong yu yingyang wenti." *Hangzhou shizhengfu jiaoyu zhoukan* 159–160 (1934): 107–8.

Li Xizhen, "Jieshao yige Zhongguo ertong zhi shenchang tizhong biao." *Zhejiang jiaoyuxinzheng zhoukan* 4, no. 24 (1933): 3–5.

Li Yongfang. "Qingmo nonghui shulun." *Studies in Qing History* 1, no. 1 (February 2006): 1–16.

Li Yuanxin, ed. *World Chinese Biographies*. Shanghai: Globe Publishing Co., 1944.

Li Zhongping. "Cong jindai niuru guanggao kan Zhongguo de xiandaixing—yi 1927–1937 nian *Shenbao* wei zhongxin de kaocha." *Anhui daxue xuebao (Zhexue shehui kexue ban)* 3 (2010): 106–13.

Lin Yutang. *My Country and My People*. London: William Heinemann, 1936.

Lin Ziyang. "Huaren shenchang tizhong zhi tongji." *Guoli Beiping daxue yixueyuan ershi zhounian jiniankan* (July 1934): 153–58.

Liu, Lydia. *Translingual Practice: Literature, National Culture, and Translated Modernity, China, 1900–1937*. Stanford, CA: Stanford University Press, 1995.

Liu, Xun. *Daoist Modern: Innovation, Lay Practice, and the Community of Inner Alchemy in Republican Shanghai*. Cambridge, MA: Harvard University Asia Center, 2009.

Lo, Vivienne. "Pleasure, Prohibition, and Pain: Food and Medicine in Traditional China." In *Of Tripod and Palate: Food, Politics, and Religion in Traditional China*, edited by Roel Sterckx, 163–85. New York: Palgrave Macmillan, 2005.

Long Bojian. "Gailiang Zhongguo shanshi fangfa." *Yiyao xue* 11, no. 11 (1934): 50–52.

Lu, Gwei-djen and Joseph Needham. "A Contribution to the History of Chinese Dietetics." *Isis* 42, no. 1 (1951): 13–20.

Lu Yongchun. "Yingyang de wenti." *Qinghua zhoukan* 33, no. 7/8 (1930): 549–50.

Lü Shunzhang. *Qingmo Zhong Ri jiaoyu wenhua jiaoliu zhi yanjiu*. Beijing: Shangwu Yinshuguan, 2012.

"Lun Zhongguo shanshi you gailiang zhi biyao." *Yixue zazhi* 67 (1932): 11, 14–17.

Luo Dengyi. "Jinshi yingyang huaxueshang danbaizhi yanjiu zhi fazhan." *Ziranjie* 4, no. 9 (1929): 791–808.

———. "Shanshi biaozhun lun." *Ziran Jie* 6, no. 1 (1931): 30–45.

———. "Shanshi zhidao lun." *Dongfang zazhi* 28, no. 3 (1931): 75–85.

———. "Shushi lun." *Dongfang zazhi* 28, no. 23 (1931): 51–59.

———. "Zhongguo shiwu lun." *Ziranjie* 4, no. 10 (1929): 879–911.

Ma Weizhong and Dong Junjue. *Chen Sanli nianpu*. Suzhou: Suzhou Daxue Chubanshe, 2010.

Mao Renren. "Lun Zhongguo shanshi you gailiang zhi biyao." *Zhongguo yixue yuekan* 1, no. 2 (1928): 1–7.

Mar, P. G. "Physical Measurements of Cantonese School Boys in Shanghai." In *Nutritional Studies in Shanghai*, 47–58. Shanghai: Henry Lester Institute for Medical Research, 1939.

Markel, Howard. "For the Welfare of Children: The Origins of the Relationship between US Public Health Workers and Pediatricians." In *Formative Years: Children's Health in the United States, 1880–2000*, edited by Alexandra Minna Stern and Howard Markel, 47–65. Ann Arbor: University of Michigan Press, 2002.

Masini, Federico. *The Formation of Modern Chinese Lexicon and Its Evolution Toward a National Language: The Period from 1840 to 1898.* Berkeley: Project on Linguistic Analysis, University of California, 1993.

Matsusaka, Yoshihisa Tak. *The Making of Japanese Manchuria.* Cambridge, MA: Harvard University Asia Center, Harvard University Press, 2001.

Maynard, L. A. "Wilbur O. Atwater, a Biographical Sketch." *Journal of Nutrition* 78 (1962): 3–9.

McCollum, Elmer V. *The Newer Knowledge of Nutrition: The Use of Food for the Preservation of Vitality and Health.* New York: Macmillan, 1918.

———. *The Newer Knowledge of Nutrition: The Use of Food for the Preservation of Vitality and Health.* 2nd ed. New York: Macmillan, 1922.

———. "Who Discovered Vitamins?" *Science* 118, no. 3073 (20 November 1953): 632.

McIsaac, Isabel. "Practical Points on Private Nursing: Convenient Diet-lists for Private Duty Nurses." *American Journal of Nursing* 1, no. 2 (November 1900): 119–29.

McKeown, Adam. *Melancholy Order: Asian Migration and the Globalization of Borders.* New York: Columbia University Press, 2008.

Medhurst, Walter H. *China: Its State and Prospects with Especial Reference to the Spread of the Gospel: Containing Allusions to the Antiquity, Extent, Population, Civilization, Literature, and Religion of the Chinese.* Boston: Crocker & Brewster, 1838.

Mendenhall, Dorothy Reed. *Milk: The Indispensable Food for Children.* Publication 163. Washington, DC: Government Printing Office, 1918.

Meng, Tianpei, and Sidney Gamble. "Prices, Wages and Standards of Living in Peking, 1900–1924." *Chinese Social and Political Science Review* (July 1926) (special supplement).

Merkel-Hess, Kate. *The Rural Modern: Reconstructing the Self and State in Republican China.* Chicago: University of Chicago Press, 2016.

Meyer, Eric. "China and Its Coming Great Milk Battle." *Forbes,* 30 October 2014.

Milles, Dietrich. "Working Capacity and Calorie Consumption: The History of Rational Physical Economy." In *The Science and Culture of Nutrition, 1840–1940,* edited by Harmke Kamminga and Andrew Cunningham, 75–96. Amsterdam: Rodopi, 1995.

Min, Shi, Jun-fei Bai, James Seale Jr., and Thomas Wahl. "Demographics, Societal Aging, and Meat Consumption in China." *Journal of Integrative Agriculture* 14, no. 6 (2015): 995–1007.

Ming. "Xinfa zhi doujiang." *Jiaoyu duanbo* (1934): 51.

Mitchell, Timothy. *Rule of Experts: Egypt, Techno-Politics, Modernity.* Berkeley: University of California Press, 2002.

Mitter, Rana. "Classifying Citizens in Nationalist China during World War II, 1937–1941." *Modern Asian Studies* 45, no. 2 (2011): 243–75.

———. "Writing War: Autobiography, Modernity and Wartime Narrative in Nationalist China, 1937–1946." *Transactions of the Royal Historical Society* 18 (2008): 187–210.

Mittler, Barbara. *A Newspaper for China? Power, Identity, and Chang in Shanghai's News Media, 1872–1912.* Cambridge, MA: Harvard University Asia Center, 2004.

Morris, Andrew D. *Marrow of the Nation: A History of Sport and Physical Culture in Republican China.* Berkeley: University of California Press, 2004.

Mudry, Jessica. *Measured Meals: Nutrition in America.* Albany: State University of New York Press, 2009.

Murphy, Rachel. "Turning Peasants into Modern Chinese Citizens: 'Population Quality' Discourse, Demographic Transition, and Primary Education." *China Quarterly* 117 (2004): 1–20.

Muzumdar, Sucheta. *Sugar and Society in China: Peasants, Technology, and the World Market.* Cambridge, MA: Harvard University Asia Center, 1998.

Nagler, Etha M. "The Problem of Food and Shelter for Refugees in Shanghai." *China Quarterly* 3, no. 1 (Winter 1937–38): 69–70.

Nakayama, Izumi. "Nutritional and Moral Responsibilities: Motherhood and Breast Milk in Modern Japan." In *Moral Foods*, edited by Angela Ki Che Leung and Melissa Caldwell. Honolulu: University of Hawai'i Press, forthcoming.

Neushul, Peter, and Zuoyue Wang. "Between the Devil and the Deep Sea: C. K. Tseng, Mariculture, and the Politics of Science in Modern China." *Isis* 91 (2000): 59–88.

"News and Notes." *Chinese Medical Journal* 53 (1938): 302–3.

"News and Notes." *Chinese Medical Journal* 53, no. 4 (1938): 397–98.

"Ni youmeiyou liuxin dao ni haizi de shanshi?" *Jiating yu funü* 3, no. 6 (1940): 224–27.

Ni Zhangqi (T. G. Ni). "Height-Weight Measurements of Shanghai School Children." In *Nutritional Studies in Shanghai*, 59–74. Shanghai: Henry Lester Institute for Medical Research, 1939.

Nitti, Francesco. "Food and Labor-Power of Nations." *Economic Journal* 6, no. 21 (1896): 30–63.

"Niuzhuang dadou doubing shangqing: Yi *Zhongwai shangye xinbao*." *Hubei shangwubao* 30 (1899): 10.

Norse, David, and Xiaotang Ju. "Environmental Costs of China's Food Security." *Agriculture, Ecosystems and Environment* 209 (1 November 2015): 5–14.

North-China Herald. "Beancake for Youngsters." 31 August 1938.

———. "A Chinese Factory in France." 3 February 1911.

———. "An Efficient Refugee Camp." 31 January 1940.

———. "A Franco-Chinese Industry." 15 April 1911.

———. "Health Department Annual Report: Acting Commissioner's Introduction, Vital Statistics, and Communicable Diseases." 9 March 1938.

———. "Japan's Foreign Policy." 3 February 1911.

———. "Peak Reached in Refugees." 1 September 1937.

———. "13,000 Order Vito-Milk." 18 June 1941.

Oliveira, Gustavo de L. T., and Mindi Schneider. "The Politics of Flexible Soybeans: China, Brazil, and Global Agroindustrial Restructuring." *Journal of Peasant Studies* (2015): 1–28.

Paxson, Heather. "Rethinking Food and Its Eaters: Opening the Black Boxes of Safety and Nutrition." In *The Handbook of Food and Anthropology*, edited by Jakob A. Klein and James L. Watson, 268–88. London: Bloomsbury, 2016.

Piper, C. V., and W. J. Morse. *The Soybean: History, Varieties, and Field Studies.* Farmers' Bulletin No. 1520. Washington, DC: US Department of Agriculture, 1910, revised 1949.

———. *The Soybean, with Special Reference to Its Utilization for Oil, Cake, and Other Products.* Bulletin No. 439. Washington, DC: US Department of Agriculture, 1916.

Platt, B. S. "An Approach to the Problems of Infant Nutrition in China." *Chinese Medical Journal* 50 (April 1936): 415–16.

———. "The Soya Bean in Human Nutrition." *Chemistry and Industry* 32 (1956): 834–37.

Platt, B. S., and S. Y. Gin. "Chinese Methods of Infant Feeding and Nursing." *Archives of Disease in Childhood* 13, no. 76 (1938): 343–54.

Pletcher, David M. *The Diplomacy of Involvement: American Economic Expansion Across the Pacific, 1784–1900.* Columbia: University of Missouri, 2001.

Plum, M. Colette. "Orphans in the Family: Family Reform and Children's Citizenship during the Anti-Japanese War, 1937–45." In *Beyond Suffering: Recounting War in Modern China*, edited by James A. Flath and Norman Smith, 186–208. Vancouver: University of British Columbia Press, 2011.

Pollard, David. "Zhu Ziqing (1898–1948)." In *The Chinese Essay*, translated and edited by David Pollard, 216–25. London: Hurst and Company, 2000.

Pomeranz, Kenneth. *The Great Divergence: China Europe, and the Making of the Modern World Economy.* Princeton, NJ: Princeton University, 2000.

Popkin, Barry M. "Synthesis and Implications: China's Nutrition Transition in the Context of Changes Across Other Low and Middle Income Countries." *Obesity Reviews* 15, no. 1 (January 2014): 60–67.

Prodöhl, Ines. "'A Miracle Bean': How Soy Conquered the West, 1909–1950." *Bulletin of the German Historical Institute* 46 (Spring 2010): 111–29.

———. "Versatile and Cheap: A Global History of Soy in the First Half of the Twentieth Century." *Journal of Global History* 8, no. 3 (2013): 461–82.

Qiao Shumin. "Feichang shiqi zhong zhi yingyang wenti." *Kexue shijie* 5, no. 10 (1936): 862–69.

Reardon-Anderson, James. *Reluctant Pioneers: China's Expansion Northward, 1644–1937.* Stanford, CA: Stanford University Press, 2005.

———. *The Study of Change: Chemistry in China, 1840–1949.* Cambridge: Cambridge University Press, 1991.

Reinders, Eric. "Blessed Are the Meat Eaters: Christian Antivegetarianism and the Missionary Encounter with Chinese Buddhism." *Positions: East Asia Cultures Critique* 12, no. 2 (2004): 509–37.

Reynolds, Douglas. *China 1898–1912: The Xinzheng Revolution and Japan.* Cambridge, MA: Council on East Asian Studies, Harvard University Press, 1993.

Ristaino, Marcia R. *The Jacquinot Safe Zone: Wartime Refugees in Shanghai.* Stanford, CA: Stanford University Press, 2008.

Roberts, J. A. G. *China to Chinatown: Chinese Food in the West.* London: Reaktion Books, 2002.

Rogaski, Ruth. *Hygienic Modernity: Meanings of Health and Disease in Treaty-Port China.* Berkeley: University of California Press, 2004.

Rohrer, Finlo. "China Drinks Its Milk." *BBC News*, 7 August 2007.

Rose, Sarah. *For All the Tea in China: Espionage, Empire, and the Secret Formula for the World's Favorite Drink.* London: Hutchinson, 2009.

Sabban, Françoise. "Court Cuisine in Fourteenth-Century Imperial China: Some Culinary Aspects of Hu Sihui's Yinshan Zhengyao." *Food and Foodways* 1, no. 2 (1986): 161–70.

———. "Session 4: To Each His Own Milk, Questions and Responses with Françoise Sabban." Presented at Cultures des Laits du Monde, 8th International Symposium, 6–7 May 2010, Muséum national d'Histoire naturelle, Paris.

———. "The Taste for Milk in Modern China (1865–1937)." In *Food Consumption in Global Perspective: Essays in the Anthropology of Food in Honor of Jack Goody,* edited by Jakob A. Klein and Anne Murcott, 182–208. New York: Palgrave Macmillan, 2014.

"Sanru zhi gongyong yu jinji: douru, niuru, maru." *Yiyao changshi bao* 2 (1930): 3.

Schneider, Helen. *Keeping the Nation's House: Domestic Management and the Making of Modern China.* Vancouver: University of British Columbia Press, 2011.

Schneider, Laurence. *Biology and Revolution in Twentieth-Century China.* Oxford: Rowman & Littlefield, 2003.

Schneider, Mindi. "Developing the Meat Grab." *Journal of Peasant Studies* 41, no. 4 (2014): 613–33.

———. "Wasting the Rural: Meat, Manure, and the Politics of Agro-Industrialization in Contemporary China." *Geoforum* (2015). http://dx.doi.org/10.1016/j.geoforum.2015.12.001.

Schlegel, G. "The Chinese Bean-Curd and Soy and the Soya-Bread of Mr. Lecerf." *T'oung pao* 5, no. 2 (1894): 135–46.

Schwartz, Benjamin. *In the Search of Wealth and Power: Yen Fu and the West.* Cambridge, MA: Belknap Press of Harvard University Press, 1964.

Scrinis, Gyorgy. *Nutritionism: The Science and Politics of Dietary Advice*. New York: Columbia University Press, 2013.

Sengupta, Jayanta. "Nation on a Platter: The Culture and Politics of Foods and Cuisine in Colonial Bengal." *Modern Asian Studies* 44, no. 1 (2010): 81–98.

Sengupta, Pallav. "The Laboratory Rat: Relating Its Age with Humans." *International Journal of Preventive Medicine* 4, no. 6 (2013): 624–30.

Shanghai Times. "New World Camp Made Habitable with Sanitation Improved." 23 September 1937.

"Shangqing: bensheng, huangdou xiaochang." *Shangwubao* 11 (1900): 1.

Shao Qiu. "Zai tan ying'er buru wenti." *Fangzhou* 5 (1935): 6–10.

Shao Wenshan. "Tantan ying'er weisheng de jijian zhongyao wenti." *Yiyao pinglun* 55 (1933): 54–55.

Shapin, Steven. *Never Pure: Historical Studies of Science as If It Was Produced by People with Bodies, Situated in Time, Space, Culture, and Society, and Struggling for Credibility and Authority*. Baltimore: Johns Hopkins University Press, 2010.

Shaw, Norman. *Soya Bean of Manchuria*. Shanghai: Statistical Department of the Inspectorate General of Customs, 1911.

Shen, Grace Yen. "Murky Waters: Thoughts on Desire, Utility, and the 'Sea of Modern Science.'" *Isis* 98, no. 3 (2007): 584–96.

———. "Taking to the Field: Geological Fieldwork and National Identity in Republican China." *Osiris* 24, no. 1 (2009): 231–52.

———. *Unearthing the Nation: Modern Geology and Nationalism in Republican China*. Chicago: University of Chicago Press, 2014.

Shen Hong, trans. "Niuru xinshu xia." *Nongxue bao* 21–27 (1898).

Shen Tong. *Yingyang xinlun*. [Chongqing]: Zhongguo Wenhua Fuwu She, 1944.

Shenbao. "Doufu he doufujiang." 5 January 1939.

———. "Lun jiating jiaoyu." 8 January 1922.

———. "Xiao'er tianran de buru zhi jiazhi." 17 May 1923.

———. "Ying'er tiaoyang fa." 17 March 1921.

———. "Yu er fa." 23 December 1917.

———. "Yu er fa (zai) (xu)." 25 December 1917.

Sheng Keyou. "Ertong yingyang wenti." *Anhui jiaoyu budao xunkan* 2, no. 24–25 (1937): 29–32.

Sheng Yin. "Manzhou dadou zhi xinshichang." *Tongwen bao* 416 (1910): 7.

"Shi weisheng shiwusuo faming doujiang buying." *Guangji yikan* 10, no. 10 (1933): 92–93.

Shi Youwei. *Hanyu wailaici*. Beijing: Shangwu Yinshuguan, 2013.

Shijie She. *Lü Ou jianyu yundong*. Tours: Lü Ou Zazhishe, [1916].

Shurtleff, William, and Akiko Aoyagi. "History of Soymilk and Dairy-Like Soymilk Products." 2004. www.soyinfocenter.com/HSS/soymilk3.php.

———. *Li Yu-ying (Li Shizeng)—History of His Work with Soyfoods and Soybeans in France, and His Political Career in China and Taiwan (1881–1973): Extensively Annotated Bibliography and Sourcebook.* Lafeyette, CA: Soyinfo Center, 2011.

Siddal, A. C. and Y. T. Chiu. "A Feeding Experiment with Soybean Milk." *Lingnan Science Journal* 10, no. 4 (1931): 387–57.

Sigley, Gary. "Suzhi, the Body, and the Fortunes of Technoscientific Reasoning in Contemporary China." *Positions: East Asia Cultures Critique* 17, no. 3 (2009): 537–66.

SINA. "Wen Jiabao: Rang mei yige Zhongguo haizi meitian dou neng he shang yi jin nai." 11 December 2006. http://news.sina.com.cn/c/h/2006-12-11/022311751790.shtml.

Sivin, Nathan. *Traditional Medicine in Contemporary China: A Partial Translation of "Revised Outline of Chinese Medicine" (1972) with an Introductory Study on Change in Present-Day and Early Medicine.* Ann Arbor: Center for Chinese Studies, University of Michigan, 1987.

Smith, Arthur H. *Chinese Characteristics.* Shanghai: North-China Herald Office, 1890.

———. *Chinese Characteristics.* Edinburgh and London: Oliphant, Anderson, and Ferrier, 1897.

Smith, Hilary. "Foot *Qi*: History of a Chinese Medical Disorder." PhD diss., University of Pennsylvania, 2008.

———. "Good Food, Bad Bodies, Milk Culture and Lactose Intolerance." In *Moral Foods*, edited by Angela Ki Che Leung and Melissa Caldwell. Honolulu: University of Hawai'i Press, forthcoming.

State Historical Society of Missouri. *The Missouri Historical Review October 1920–July 1921.* Columbia: State Historical Society of Missouri, 1921.

"State Medicine for China." *The National Medical Journal of China* 14, no. 2 (1928): 119–20.

Sterckx, Roel. "Food and Philosophy in Early China." In *Of Tripod and Palate: Food, Politics, and Religion in Traditional China*, edited by Roel Sterckx, 34–61. New York: Palgrave Macmillan, 2005.

———, ed. *Of Tripod and Palate: Food, Politics, and Religion in Traditional China.* New York: Palgrave Macmillan, 2005.

Stevenson, Paul H. "Collected Anthropometric Data on the Chinese." *China Medical Journal* 39, no. 10 (October 1925): 855–98.

Stoddard, John L. *China.* Chicago: Belford, Middlebrook, 1897.

Su Fei. "Dou ji douru." *Beiping nongbao* 11, no. 6 (3 March 1934).

Su Zufei. *Ertong yingyang.* Shanghai: Yamei Gufen Youxian Gongsi, 1935.

Swislocki, Mark. *Culinary Nostalgia: Regional Food Culture and the Urban Experience in Shanghai.* Stanford, CA: Stanford University Press, 2009.

———. "Feast and Famine in Republican Shanghai: Urban Food Culture, Nutrition, and the State." PhD diss., Stanford University, 2001.

———. "Nutritional Governmentality: Food and the Politics of Health in Late Imperial and Republican China," *Radical History Review* 110 (Spring 2011): 9–35.

Sze, Szeming. "Medical Care for Shanghai Refugees." *China Quarterly* 3, no. 1 (Winter 1937–1938): 77.

Tao, L. K (Tao Menghe). *Livelihood in Peking: An Analysis of the Budgets of Sixty Families.* Beijing: Social Research Department, China Foundation, 1928.

Thompson, Malcolm. "Foucault, Fields of Governability, and the Population-Family-Economy Nexus in China." *History and Theory* 51 (February 2012): 42–62.

Tillman, Margaret Mih. "Precocious Politics: Preschool Education and Child Protection in China." PhD diss., University of California at Berkeley, 2013.

The Times. "The Soya Bean." 19 July 1910.

Tsing, Anna. "Worlding the Matsutake Diaspora: Or Can Actor-Network Theory Experiment with Holism?" In *Experiments in Holism: Theory and Practice in Contemporary Anthropology,* edited by Ton Otto and Nils Bubrandt, 47–66. Malden, MA: Wiley-Blackwell, 2010.

Tso, Ernest (Zhu Shenzhi). "A Comparison of the Nutritive Properties of Soybean 'Milk' and Cow's Milk." *Chinese Journal of Physiology* 3, no. 4 (1929): 353–62.

———. "The Development of an Infant Fed Eight Months on a Soybean Milk Diet." *Chinese Journal of Physiology* 2, no. 1 (1928): 33–40.

———. "Yong douru bu ying'er zhi chengji." *Weisheng yuekan* 4 (1928): 5–11.

Tso, Ernest, and K. C. Chang. "A Soluble Soybean Milk Powder and Its Adaptation to Infant Feeding." *Chinese Journal of Physiology* 3, no. 2 (1931): 199–203.

Tso, Ernest, M. Yee, and T. T. Chen. "The Nitrogen, Calcium, and Phosphorous Metabolism in Infant Fed on Soybean Milk." *Chinese Journal of Physiology* 2 (1928): 409–14.

Tsu, Jing. *Failure, Nationalism, and Literature: The Makings of Modern Chinese Identity, 1895–1937.* Stanford, CA: Stanford University Press, 2005.

Tsu, Jing, and Benjamin A. Elman, eds. *Science and Technology in Modern China, 1880s–1940s.* Leiden: Brill, 2014.

Tung, Chen-lung. "Physical Measurements in Chinese." *Chinese Journal of Physiology* 1 (1928): 107–18.

Unschuld, Paul U. *Medicine in China: A History of Pharmaceutics.* Berkeley: University of California Press, 1986.

US Department of Agriculture. *The International Dairy Federation and International Dairy Congresses.* Washington DC: US Department of Agriculture, Bureau of Animal Industry, 1904.

"The Use of 'Soy Bean' as a Food in Diabetes." *Lancet* (24 December 1910): 1844–45.

Valenze, Deborah. *Milk: A Local and Global History.* New Haven, CT: Yale University Press, 2011.

Vernon, James. *Hunger: A Modern History*. Cambridge, MA: Belknap Press of Harvard University Press, 2007.

Vittinghoff, Natascha. "Social Actors in the Field of Learning in Nineteenth Century China." In *Mapping Meanings: The Field of New Learning in Late Qing China*, edited by Michael Lackner and Natascha Vittinghoff, 75–118. Leiden: Brill, 2004.

Wakeman, Frederic, Jr. "Occupied Shanghai: The Struggle between Chinese and Western Medicine. In *China at War: Regions of China, 1937–1945*, edited by Stephen R. Mackinnon, Diana Lary, and Ezra F. Vogel, 265–87. Stanford, CA: Stanford University Press, 2007.

Waley-Cohen, Joanna. "The Quest for Perfect Balance: Taste and Gastronomy in Imperial China." In *Food: The History of Taste*, edited by Paul Freedman, 99–134. Berkeley: University of California Press, 2007.

Wan, Xin. "Sushi shu yu hunshi shu qiguan liang du zhi bijiao." *Zhonghua yixue zazhi* 20, no. 4 (1934): 521–22.

Wang, C. C. "Basal Metabolism of American-born Chinese Girls and of American Girls of the Same Age." *American Journal of Diseases of Children* 48, no. 5 (1934): 1041–49.

Wang, C. C., and Jean E. Hawks. "Basal Metabolism of Twenty-One Chinese Children Reared or Born and Reared in the United States." *American Journal of Diseases of Children* 44, no. 1 (1932): 69–80.

Wang, Hsien-chun. "Revising the Niuzhuang Oil Mill (1868–1870): Transferring Western Technology into China." *Enterprise and Society* 14, no. 4 (2013): 749–68.

Wang, Jimin. "Zhongguo yinghai tige zhi di'er ci baogao." *Zhonghua yixue zazhi* 11 (1925).

Wang, Shan-shan, Sovichea Lay, Hai-ning Yu, and Sheng-rong Shen. "Dietary Guidelines for Chinese Residents (2016): Comments and Comparisons." *Journal of Zhejiang University: Science B (Biomedicine and Biotechnology)* 17, no. 9 (2016): 649–56.

Wang, Susie. "Buyu Zhongguo: Jindai Zhongguo de niuru xiaofei—ershi shiji er, sanling niandai Shanghai wei zhongxin de kaocha." *Journal of Chinese Dietary Culture* 7, no. 1 (2011): 207–39.

Wang, Yangzong. "1850 niandai zhi 1910 nian Zhongguo yu Riben zhi jian kexue shuji de jiaoliu shulue." *Tozai gakujutsu kenkyu kiyo* (Kansai University) 33 (March 2000): 144–45.

Wang, Yejian. "Jindai Zhongguo nongye de chengzhang ji qi weiji." *Zhongyang yanjiuyuan jindaishi yanjiusuo jikan* 7 (1976): 355–70.

Wang, Zuoyue. "Saving China through Science: The Science Society of China, Scientific Nationalism, and Civil Society in Republican China." *Osiris*, 2nd series, 17 (2002): 291–322.

Watson, James L. "Meat: A Cultural Biography in (South) China." In *Food Consumption in Global Perspective: Essays in the Anthropology of Food in Honor of Jack Goody*, edited by J. A. Klein and A. Murcott, 25–44. Basingstoke, UK: Palgrave Macmillan, 2014.

Watt, John R. *Public Medicine in Wartime China: Biomedicine, State Medicine, and the Rise of China's National Medical Colleges, 1931–1945*. Boston: Rosenberg Institute for East Asian Studies, Suffolk University, 2012.

Wen, Shuang. "Mediated Imaginations: Chinese-Arab Connections in the Late Nineteenth and Early Twentieth Centuries." PhD diss., Georgetown University, 2015.

Wen Zhongjie, "Huang douru zhi yanjiu." *Kexue congkan* 3 (1930): 1–19.

Wiley, Andrea S. "Cow's Milk as Children's Food: Insights from India and the United States." In *The Handbook of Food and Anthropology*, edited by Jakob A. Klein and James L. Watson, 227–48. London: Bloomsbury, 2016.

———. "Milk for 'Growth': Global and Local Meanings of Milk Consumption in China, India, and the United States." *Food and Foodways* 19, no. 1–2 (2011): 11–33.

———. *Re-imagining Milk*. New York: Routledge, 2011.

Will, Pierre-Étienne. *Bureaucracy and Famine in Eighteenth-Century China*, translated by Elborg Foster. Stanford, CA: Stanford University Press, 1990.

Will, Pierre-Étienne, and R. Bin Wong, with James Lee. *Nourish the People: The State Civilian Granary System in China, 1650–1850*. Ann Arbor: Center for Chinese Studies, University of Michigan, 1991.

Williams, Faith M., and Carle C. Zimmerman. "Studies of Family Living in the United States and Other Countries: Analysis of Material and Method." In *United States Department of Agriculture Miscellaneous Publication No. 223*, 59–55. Washington DC (December 1935).

Wilson, James Harrison. *China, Travels and Investigations in the "Middle Kingdom": A Study of Its Civilization and Possibilities with a Glance at Japan*. New York: D. Appleton, 1887.

Wilson, S. D. "A Study of Chinese Foods." *China Medical Journal* 34 (1920): 503–8.

Wolff, David. "Bean There: Toward a Soy-Based History of Northeast Asia," *South Atlantic Quarterly* 99, no. 1 (2000): 241–52.

Wong, Lawrence Wang-chi. "Beyond *Xin Da Ya*: Translation Problems in the Late Qing." In *Mapping Meanings: The Field of New Learning in Late Qing China*, edited by Michael Lackner and Natasha Vittinghoff, 239–64. Leiden: Brill, 2004.

Worboys, Michael. "The Discovery of Colonial Malnutrition Between the Wars." In *Imperial Medicine and Indigenous Societies*, edited by David Arnold, 208–25. Manchester, UK: Manchester University Press, 1988.

Wray, William D. "Japan's Big-Three Service Enterprises in China, 1896–1926." In *The Japanese Informal Empire in China, 1895–1937*, edited by Peter Duus, Ramon H. Myers, and Mark R. Peattie, 31–64. Princeton, NJ: Princeton University Press, 1989.

Wu, Daisy Yen, comp. and ed. *Hsien Wu, 1893–1959: In Loving Memory*. Boston: n.a., 1959.

Wu, Shellen. *Empires of Coal: Fueling China's Entry into the Modern World Order, 1860–1920*. Stanford, CA: Stanford University Press, 2015.

Wu, Shengqing. *Modern Archaics: Continuity and Innovation in the Chinese Lyric Tradition, 1900–1947*. Cambridge, MA: Harvard University Asia Center, 2013.

Wu Xian (Wu Hsien). "Chinese Diet in the Light of Modern Knowledge of Nutrition." *Chinese Social and Political Science Review* 11 (1927): 56–81.

———. "Danbaizhilei zhi shengli de jiazhi." *Kexue* 11, no. 8 (1936): 1049–54.

———. "Vegetarianism," *Journal of Oriental Medicine* 11, no. 1 (July 1929): 1–11.

———. "Woguoren zhi chifan wenti." *Duli pinglun* 2 (May 1932): 15–19.

———. "Zhongguo shiwu zhi xiandai yingyang zhishi." *Xieyi tongsu yuekan* 4, no. 3 (1927): 2–15.

———. "Zhongguo shiwu zhi xiandai yingyang zhishi." *Yixue zhoukan ji* 1 (1928): 85–97.

Wu Xian and Daisy Yen Wu. "Growth of Rats on Vegetarian Diets." *Chinese Journal of Physiology* 2, no. 2 (1928): 173–93.

———. "Study of Dietaries in Peking." *Chinese Journal of Physiology* 1 (1928): 142–43.

Wu Xian and Tung-Tou Chen. "Growth and Reproduction of Rats on Vegetarian Diets." *Chinese Journal of Physiology* 3, no. 2 (1929): 157–70.

Wu Xiang. "Guoren shengli shuizhun zhi yanjiu." *Xueshu huikan* 1, no. 2 (December 1944): 32–84.

Xie Baoling. "Ertong yingyang wenti." *Jiankang jiaoyu* 2, no. 3 (1937): 1.

Xiong Yuezhi. *Xixue dongjian yu wan Qing shehui*. Shanghai: Shanghai Renmin Chubanshe, 1994.

Xu, Guoqi. *Strangers on the Western Front*. Cambridge, MA: Harvard University Press, 2011.

Xu Pengcheng, "Yingyang de shengli jichu." *Kexue* 21, no. 1 (January 1937): 50–57.

Xu Shijin and Wu Liguo. "Shanghai shi xueling ertong shenchang tizhong zhi cubu yanjiu." *Zhongghua yixue zazhi* 18, no. 6 (1932): 977–87.

Xu Yizhe. "Ertong shiwu yingyang wenti." *Ertong yu jiaoshi* 19 (1935): 974–77.

Xue, Yong. "A 'Fertilizer Revolution'?: A Critical Response to Pomeranz's Theory of 'Geographic Luck.'" *Modern China* 33, no. 2 (April 2007): 41–71.

Yang, Chia-Ling, and Roderick Whitfield, eds. *Lost Generation: Luo Zhenyu, Qing Loyalists and the Formation of Modern Chinese Culture*. London: Saffron Books, 2012.

Yang, Gonghuan, Yu Wang, Yixin Zhang, George F. Gao, Xiaofeng Liang, Maigeng Zhou, Xia Wan, et al. "Rapid Health Transition in China 1990–2010: Findings from the Global Burden of Disease Study 2010." *Lancet* 381, no. 9882 (8–14 June 2013): 1987–2015.

Yang, Robert N. "Julean Arnold and American Economic Perspectives of China, 1902–1946." MA thesis, San Jose State University, 1994.

ibliography

Yang, Ximeng, and Tao Menghe. *A Study of the Standard of Living of the Working Families in Shanghai.* Beiping: Social Research Institute, 1930.

Yeh, Wen-hsin. *Shanghai Splendor: A Cultural History, 1843–1945.* Berkeley: University of California Press, 2008.

Yi, Feng. "Élites locales et solidarité: L'aide aux réfugiés à Shanghai (1937–1940)." *Études chinoises* 15, no. 1–2 (1996): 71–106.

Yi Ren. "Bali doufu gongsi yu liufa qingong jianxue." *Shixue jikan* 2 (1993): 35.

"Yijie xiaoxi: jingshi weisheng shiwusuo faming doujiang buying." *Guangji yikan* 10, no. 10 (1935): 6.

"Yingyang bu liang." *Xuexiao yu jiating* 6 (1934): 28.

Yip, Ka-che. *Health and National Reconstruction in Nationalist China: The Development of Modern Health Services, 1928–1937.* Ann Arbor, MI: Association for Asian Studies, 1995.

"Yishi xinwen: neiguo zhi bu: Shanghai: Shengsheng doujiang zhi fada." *Yixue shijie* 28 (1913): 59.

"Yong douru bu yinghai zhi chengji." *Weisheng gongbao* 2 (1929): 5.

Yoon, Seungjoo. "Literati-Journalists of the *Chinese Progress (Shiwubao)* in Discord, 1896–1898." In *Rethinking the 1898 Reform Period: Political and Cultural Change in Late Qing China,* edited by Rebecca E. Karl and Peter Zarrow, 48–76. Cambridge, MA: Harvard University Asia Center, 2002.

Yu, Xiaohua. "Meat Consumption in China and Its Impact on International Food Security: Status Quo, Trends, and Policies." *Journal of Integrative Agriculture* 14, no. 6 (2015): 989–94.

Yü, Yingshih. "Han." In *Food in Chinese Culture: Anthropological and Historical Perspectives,* edited by K. C. Chang, 53–84. New Haven, CT: Yale University Press, 1977.

Yue, Meng. "Hybrid Science versus Modernity: The Practice of the Jiangnan Arsenal, 1864–1897." *East Asian Science, Technology, and Medicine* 16 (1999): 13–52.

Yun Daiying. "Weisheng zhi ying'er burufa." *Dongfang zazhi* 16, no. 3 (1919): 180–83.

"Zawen: doujiang shangshi." *Qinghua zhoukan* 322 (1924): 24.

Zhai, Fengying, Huijun Wang, Shufa Da, Yuna He, Zhihong Wang, Keyou Ge, and Barry M. Popkin. "Prospective Study on Nutrition Transition in China." *Nutrition Reviews* 67 (suppl. 1) (2009): S56–S61.

Zhang Bufan, trans. "Bu ru'er rengong yingyangfa." *Dongfang zazhi* 14, no. 12 (1917): 4.

Zhang Jian. *Kexue shetuan zai jindai Zhongguo de mingyun: yi Zhongguo kexueshe wei zhongxin.* Jinan: Shandong Jiaoyu Chubanshe, 2005.

Zhao Yunshan and Wang Zhangsu. "Buli cun liufa gongyi xuexiao." In *Geming huiyi lu,* edited by Renmin Chubanshe, vol. 20, 101–8. Beijing: Renmin Chubanshe, 1980–86.

Zheng Ji. "Qingnian zeye wenti taolun." *Xuesheng zazhi* 12, no. 7 (1925): 29–31.

———. "Shiwu yu jiankang." *Kexue* 18, no. 12 (1934): 1557–61.

————. "Zhongguoren de shanshi wenti." *Kexue shijie* 3, no. 10 (1934): 885–87.

————. "Zhongguoren zhi yingyang gaikuang." *Kexue* 23, no. 1 (January 1939): 25–34.

Zheng Ji, Tao Hong, and Zhu Zhanggeng. "Nanjing dongji shanshi diaocha," *Kexue* 19, no. 11 (November 1935): 1753–58.

Zhou, Gang. *Placing the Modern Chinese Vernacular in Transnational Literature.* New York: Palgrave Macmillan, 2011.

Zhou Yunfen. "Ruyou'er zhi fayu ji qi yingyangfa." *Xinyiyao kan* 129–130 (1943): 27–9.

Zhu Chuanyu, comp. *Li Shizeng zhuanji ziliao.* Vol. 1. Taipei: Tianyi Chubanshe, 1979.

Zhu Zhenjun. "Shanghai ren zhi shanshi." *Kexue* 18, no. 9 (1934): 1174–92.

Zhu Ziqing. "Dongtian." *Zhu Ziqing sanwen xuan.* Nanjing: Yilin Chubanshe, 2016.

Zhu Zuoting. *Xiaoxue ertong yingyang zhi yanjiu.* Shanghai: Zhongxuesheng Shuju, 1935.

"Zuo douru de fazi." *Guanhua zhuyin zimu bao* 100 (1920): 20–22.

INDEX

bean milk cooperative, 160
bean residue cakes (*douzha bing*), 130, 139, 154, 159, 163, 167, 169
beancake, 22–24, 28, 32, 199n21
Beiping Health Demonstration Station, 106
Benedict, Francis G., 83, 212n62
Beneficial Soybean Milk Company (Youyi Douru Gongsi), 112–13, 114–15, 119, 120, 218n2
"Benevolent Cause," 33
Bing Zhi, 73
biochemistry. *See* chemistry; Hou Xiangchuan; Luo Dengyi; Wu Xian; Zheng Ji
biomedicine, 130, 138, 143, 149, 220–21n4
A Bite of China (documentary series), 182–84, 185, 187–88, 198n37, 227n7
body: analogy with race and national strength, 72–73; concept of, in nutrition science, 8; correspondences with five flavors, 45; as microcosm of cosmos, 44; and qi, 7, 44, 112; as steam engine, 9; weakness of, 48–49, 71, 73–74, 95
Book of Changes (Yijing), 4
Book of Odes (Shijing), 21
botanic gardens, 27, 201n46
boycotts of foreign goods, 37
Bray, Francesca, 22, 182–83, 228n9
Brazil, 187, 228n20
bread-and-beef diet, 71
breastfeeding, 91–92, 103–4, 105. *See also* infant feeding
British East India Company, 52
Buck, J. Lossing, 81, 155, 175
Buddhism, and Chinese diet, 84–85
Bullock, Mary, 47

bunao (brain nourishing), 119, 120, 219n20
Burgess, John, 57–58

C

cabbage, 53, 59, 85, 101, 213n70
calcium, 8, 121, 150, 184, 210n7; added to soybean milk, 4, 141–42, 145, 162, 170–71, 223n58, 225n22; in Glycine logo, 128
calories: caloric intake since 1970s, 186; in late nineteenth-century nutrition science, 61, 77; and nutritional adequacy, 210n7; from proteins, 85; standards for, 80; total daily intake, 80, 88, 99
Cantonese, measurement studies of, 76, 211n32
Cantonese Refugees' Relief Committee (Shanghai), 136, 221n24
Cantonese Residents Association (Shanghai), 134, 221n24
Cao Jiao, 74
carbohydrates, 22, 63, 88, 99, 113, 227n47. *See also* dietary trinity
casein, 34, 35, 215n35
cat, consumption of, 50, 206n30
Chahar, 132
Chan, Dr. Harry (Chen Daming), 121–22, 126, 220n41. *See also* Glycine Soybean Compound
Chan Tong Ork, 121
"character of calculability" (Mitchell), 144, 223n54
chemistry: and agricultural products, 32; biochemistry, 61, 111, 178, 205n4; and nutrition science, 47–48, 61–62, 64, 78, 80, 87, 165, 175; and the soybean, 5, 16, 108, 114
Chen, C. C., 158

Chen Bangjian, 97
Chen Peilan, 156
Chen Sanli, "Playfully Composed while Drinking *Doujiang*," 4–5, 14, 195n7
Chen Yingning, 113–14
Chengdu, China Nutritional Aid Council branch in, 158, 163
Chi, Dr. T. C., 137
Chiang Kai-shek, 129
child psychology, 95, 215n22
children: categorization of, for nutritional assistance, 159–60; and Chinese nutrition science, 95–98; and developmentalist thinking, 90; distribution of soybean milk to, 4, 130, 138–39, 141*fig.*, 150*fig.*, 151, 159–61, 163, 179; in experimental trials, 168; growth and development of, 95–98, 103; and health of nation, 90, 94–95, 97–98; milk drinking and, 90, 92–93; need for proteins in diet, 96–97; as refugees in Shanghai, 121, 129–30, 145–46, 179; size and weight of, 90, 124; as target of soybean milk advertisements, 111, 120, 124, 127. *See also* infant feeding; infant mortality; Refugee Children's Nutritional Aid Committee
children's magazines, 95
China Chemical Works, Ltd., 166
China Child Welfare, 138, 148, 157, 164, 168, 175, 222–23n41
China Commercial Bean Curd Milk Company, 218n2
China Cotton Manufacturing Company, 166, 166–67, 168
China Health and Nutrition Survey (2002), 186
China Nutritional Aid Council (Zhonghua Yingyang Cujinhui): branches in southwest provinces,

158, 163, 174; business ventures, 168–70, 174; Chengdu branch, 158, 163; Chongqing branch, 163, 174; clinical studies, 162–63; distribution centers, 161, 162, 163; endorsement of soybean milk products, 170–72; funding for, 164; Guangxi branch, 163, 226n29; Hou Xiangchuan and, 151–52, 165, 169, 170, 174; Jiangxi branch, 163; Kunming branch, 154, 158, 159–61, 163, 165, 226n29; membership and officers, 143, 148, 165; move to Chongqing, 174; name of, 225n13, 226n30; Nellie Lee and, 151–52, 161–62, 173, 174; nutritional activism and outreach, 131, 151, 159, 161, 162–64, 166, 180; payment scheme, 161–62; postcard produced by, 177–78, 178*fig.*, 189; relations with SMC Public Health Department, 171–72; replacements for Nellie Lee, 175; research and production projects in Shanghai, 166–68; restaurants and food shops, 163; Shanghai committee, 159, 164–69; soybean milk formulas of, 159, 163, 168, 169, 225n22; target recipients, 159–60
China Quarterly, photographs of refugee relief work, 129, 131*fig.*, 150*fig.*, 152
Chinese Business News (Huashang lianhebao), 32
Chinese cuisine, 198n37. *See also A Bite of China*; culinary knowledge
Chinese diet: and agricultural labor, 70; Chinese interest in, 57–58; and Chinese national character, 56–57; and Chinese weakness, 48–49, 71, 73–74, 76, 95; compared with Japan and India, 59–60; contrasted with Scottish farm laborers, 52; as

adequacy, 86; proteins and, 70, 79–80; of rats and humans, 213n76; soybean milk and, 88, 90, 105–6. *See also* height and weight; infant feeding; nutrition

Guangda Milk Technology Park, 189

Guangxi, China Nutritional Aid Council branch in, 163, 226n29

guomin zhi mu (mothers of citizens), 101–2, 216n59

Guy, Ruth, 80

H

Hammond, John, 99–100, 216n48

Hankou, 32

Hao Tong, 80

Hartley, Robert Milham, 91–92

Harvard University; Medical School, 42; School of Public Health, 93

height and weight, 74, 75–76, 84, 85–86, 99, 124, 146, 216n47. *See also* growth

Henningsen Produce Company, 166

Henriot, Christian, 134

Henry Lester Institute of Medical Research (Shanghai), 46, 75, 76, 102, 105, 226n32

Ho, Florence Pen, 156

home economics, 139, 156, 175, 197n28

Hopkins, Sir Frederick Gowland, 78, 92

Hospital for Refugee Children (Shanghai), 139

Hou Xiangchuan (H. C. Hou): endorsement of soybean milk products, 170–71, 175; on milk, 121; recipe for soybean milk, 145, 168, 169, 223n58; as second-generation medical scientist, 47; soybean advocacy, 114, 173, 179; views on Chinese diet, 12, 46, 184; work on nutritional standards for refugees,

143–46, 164–65; work with China Nutritional Aid Council, 151–52, 165, 169–70, 174; work with Refugee Children's Committee, 139, 154, 165, 226n32

Hu Sihui, *Yinshan zhengyao* (Propriety and Essentials of Food and Drink), 46, 205n18

Huaming (Shandong), diet of, 82

Huang, Dr. T. F., 158, 165

Huang, H. T., 16, 21

Huang Shirong, 38

Hubei Agricultural Office, 31

Hubei Business News (Hubei shangwubao), 32

human body. *See* body

hunger and malnutrition, 149–50, 224n70. *See also* Chinese diet: inadequacy of; famine; malnutrition

hunting, 84

hygiene, 41, 53, 115, 136, 185, 196–97n23

I

illnesses of civilization (*wenming bing*), 73

Imperial Maritime Customs, 23, 28, 63, 199–200n23

Imperial University (Beijing), 30

Independent Thought (Duli pinglun), 84

infant feeding: breastfeeding, 91–92, 103–4, 105; changing understandings of, 219n27; with Glycine Soybean Compound, 124; milk and, 92, 101–2, 139, 217n81; of refugees, 139–40; with soybean milk, 103, 105–7, 120, 140

infant mortality, 75–76, 79, 86, 92, 93, 107

inner alchemy, 113

Institute of Social Research, 58

International Dairy Congress, 35, 36
iron, 114, 121, 162, 210n7

J

jail inmates, 167
Japan: agricultural research, 31–32;
    Chinese students in, 29, 202n60;
    cultivation of soybeans, 26;
    invasion of Shanghai, 4, 120–21,
    122, 133; and Manchurian soybean
    trade, 24–26, 27, 28, 32, 39; as model
    for modernization, 29; Nationalist
    attack on naval fleets, 129;
    occupation of Manchuria, 19, 26,
    132; possession of Shandong, 72;
    puppet government in Shanghai,
    174; relations with Russia, 19, 27,
    201n43; residents in China, 132–33;
    soy food products of, 26
Ji Hongkun, 7
jiang (fermented soybean paste), 22
Jiangxi, China Nutritional Aid Council
    branch in, 163
Jiangxi Provincial Medical College,
    163
Jiangxi Provincial War Orphanage
    Number Two, 163
jiangyou (soy sauce), 18, 22, 26, 31–32
Jin Baoshan (P. Z. King), 148–49
Jin Shuchu (Sohtsu G. King), 64,
    209n89
jing (sexual potency), 112; jing qi shen,
    112–13; jingqi, 115–16
Jiujiang, 32
Jones, Andrew F., 95
Jordan, J. H., 126, 170
Journal of Chinese and Western Medicines
    (Zhongxi yixuebao), "A Comparison
    of Soybean Milk and Cow's Milk,"
    38–39

journals: agricultural, 30–31; medical,
    38–39, 106, 146, 196n20; popular, 4,
    69, 95, 146, 214n14; scientific, 8, 73,
    107, 146, 196n14; women's, 71, 106, 146
Judge, Joan, 181

K

kagaku (knowledge classified by field),
    29
Kawai, Taizo, New Treatise on Cow's Milk
    and Its Products, 31
Kellogg, Dr. John Harvey, 83
kexue (knowledge classified by field), 29
kidneys, 63
King, P. Z. (Jin Baoshan), 148–49
Korea, as market for US goods, 52
Ku, Emperor, 74
Kunming, China Nutritional Aid
    Council branch in, 154, 158, 159–61,
    163, 165, 226n29
Kwang Chi Medical Journal (Guangji
    yikan), 106

L

labor: agricultural, 52, 70; and food
    supply, 60–61, 82, 83, 98, 212n62;
    white and coolie, 207n61
Ladies' Journal (Funü zazhi), 94
Lam, Tong, 57, 58, 60–61, 208n78
Land of Famine, 3, 150
League of Nations: cross-national
    studies of nutrition, 94, 214n17;
    definition of protective foods,
    80–81; guidelines and standards,
    80, 171; nutrition report of 1936,
    94, 121
Lee, Nellie: career of, 155; education in
    United States, 139, 155, 156, 175–76;
    move from Shanghai to

Chongqing, 153–54; nutritional activism during wartime, 156–58; soybean advocacy, 12, 179; work with China Nutritional Aid Council, 151–52, 161–62, 173, 174; work with Refugee Children's Committee, 139–40, 155, 156

Li, Dr. Ting'an, 140

Li, Shang-Jen, 62

Li Hongzhang, 29, 52, 206n42

Li Jinghan, 57, 70, 81, 209nn5,6

Li Liweng (Li Yu), 49

Li Shizeng (Li Yuying): advocacy of soybean, 18, 179, 187; *Da Dou*, 204n99; food products produced by, 36, 38; patents for soy products, 35, 203n82; presentation to International Dairy Congress, 35, 36; and refashioning of *doujiang*, 90; soybean foods factory in France, 20, 33–34, 34*fig.*, 38, 39, 123, 199n6, 204n101; soybean research and writing, 34, 36–38, 204n99; "vegetable milk," 34–35, 203n82; views on vegetarianism, 185, 211n43

Liao Valley (Manchuria), 26

Liebig, Justus von, 78

Lim, Dr. Robert, 165

Lin Yutang, *My Country and My People*, 49, 183

lipoxidase, 22

Lister Institute (London), 77

Liu Xun, 114

London Missionary Society, 50, 63

London School of Economics, 58

London School of Tropical Medicine, 63

longevity, 111, 112, 115, 119

Lu Gwei-djen, "A Contribution to the History of Chinese Dietetics," 6, 195n8

Lu Xun, 57

Luo Dengyi, 69, 78, 179, 209n3

Luo Zhenyu, 30–31, 202nn62,65,67

M

Maasai, 94

Mackay, J. A., 157

Macleod, Dr. Florence L., 175

maifan (wheat granules), 21

malnutrition: in children, 98, 106, 130, 139, 140, 146, 154, 159; Chinese diet and, 65, 70; and hunger, 149–50, 224n70; soybean milk and, 4, 14, 106, 132

Manchuria: Han migration to, 25–26; Japanese occupation of, 19, 26, 132; Japan's interest in, 24, 33; population of, 200n33; as preserve of Manchu heritage, 25; region of, defined, 200n28; and Russian expansion, 25; as source of soy, 23, 26, 32–33, 187, 199n21; and soybean trade, 23–24, 26–28, 32–33, 39, 202–3n72

Manson, Patrick, 63

Mar, P. G. (Peter), 76, 226n32

Marco Polo Incident (1937), 132–33

Maritime Customs Services, 23, 28, 63, 199–200n23

Mawangdui (Hunan), 22

May Fourth Movement, 66

Maynard, Leonard A., 175

McCollum, Elmer V.: animal feeding experiments, 79; on Asian diets, 103; *Newer Knowledge of Nutrition*, 77, 93–94, 211n36, 217n68; popularization of milk, 93, 107, 214n14; study of milk and vitamins, 81, 92, 93

measurement studies, 75–76, 99–100, 146, 211n32

meat: Chinese consumption of, 53, 59, 63, 65, 186, 187, 208n73, 209n6; and Chinese labor in United States, 207n61; economics of raising, 100; industrial meat regime, 187; price of, during wartime, 153; as progress, 186; as a protective food in Asian diets, 81; in Western diets, 63, 71. *See also* animal-derived proteins

Medhurst, Walter H., 49, 51

medical scientists, second generation of, 47. *See also* Hou Xiangchuan; Shen Tong; Zheng Ji

Mencius, 74, 147

milk: advertisements for, 94; associated with race and cultural advancement, 93, 102, 107, 179, 214n13; associated with wealth and power, 89–90, 94, 121; and child growth and development, 88, 90, 92, 105, 139–40; in Chinese diet, 53, 59, 188–89; connection to Central Asian nomads, 89; in culinary treatises, 89; European and American conception of, 89, 92; as medicine or tonic, 89; powdered, 80, 102, 106, 124, 213n71; as protective food, 80–81, 90, 94, 107, 110; scientific study of, 91; as universal nourishment, 91–92, 107; in upper-class diet of Tang period, 213–14n1. *See also* breastfeeding; cow's milk; soybean milk

Milles, Dietrich, 82

millet, 45, 51, 55, 59, 65, 70, 99; in five grains, 16, 21, 43, 45, 198n42; used in animal feeding experiments, 85

minerals, 80, 86, 94, 210n7, 212n48. *See also* calcium

Ministry of Education (Qing), 30

missionaries, 7–8, 49, 50–52, 54–55, 63, 207n51. *See also* Smith, Arthur

Mitchell, Timothy, 144, 223n54

Mittler, Barbara, 116

Modern Parents, 95

modernity, 15, 110, 111, 174, 179

mortality rates, 75, 98, 210n27; infant, 75–76, 79, 86, 92, 93, 107

motherhood, 101–2, 216n59

Mount Holyoke College, 155, 156

Mr. Science and Mr. Democracy, 66

Mudry, Jessica, 8

Mulder, Gerrit Jan, 78, 214n4

mung beans, 42; drink made by fermenting, 97, 215n35

Municipal Government of Greater Shanghai, 16

museums, 29, 177

mutton, 45, 46, 53, 59, 100, 208n73

N

Nanjing Biological Research Center (Nanjing Shengwu Yanjiusuo), 48, 80

Nanjing soybean milk program, 106

National Central University, 73, 76

national characteristics, 57, 74

National Child Welfare Association of China (Zhonghua Ciyou Xiehui), 95, 215n25

National Children's Day, 95, 215n25

national deficiency, 47, 72–73, 74, 86

National Goods Movement (Guohuo Yundong), 104

National Health Administration, 149

National Nanjing University, 47

national salvation, 143, 149

nationalism, 12, 111, 148

Nationalist government, 148, 150, 160
native-place associations, 133–34, 148,
    221n24, 222n30
natto (fermented beans), 26
Natural World (Ziranjie), 69
Needham, Joseph, "A Contribution to
    the History of Chinese Dietetics," 6,
    195n8
New Culture Movement, 66, 95
New World refugee camp, 136
New York Association for Improving
    the Condition of the Poor, 91–92
New York cigarettes, 111
newspapers, 3, 4, 19, 29, 41, 71, 122,
    202n65. See also *Shenbao*
1911 revolution, 72
nitrogen, 35, 77, 212n48; nitrogen
    fixing, 22, 27, 34
Niuzhuang, 32, 202n72. *See also*
    Manchuria
Nongbaoguan (Agriculture Journal
    Publishing House), 30
Nongxuebao (Agricultural News), 30–32,
    202n67
Nongxueshe (Society for Learning
    Agriculture), 30
North-China Herald, 19–20, 133
Nourishing Life Soybean Milk Com-
    pany (Shengsheng Douru Gongsi),
    113, 115, 119, 120
"nourishing the people" (*yangmin*), 12,
    132, 147
nuclear family, 94, 116–17, 127
nutrition: in ancient China, 84; during
    childhood, 73, 96–98, 103, 105–6,
    130, 139, 146; Chinese word for, 10;
    milk and, 31, 88, 91–92, 94, 105, 107;
    and national strength, 12–13, 73–74,
    90, 94–95, 98; of refugees, 139–40;
    soybean as, 3–5, 67–68, 87–88;
    standards and guidelines, 80, 82,

142–43, 158, 165, 210n7; term for,
    11–12, 197n28; vegetarian diet and,
    71, 79, 85–86. *See also* China
    Nutritional Aid Council; Chinese
    diet; growth; malnutrition;
    nutrition science; nutritional
    activism; Refugee Children's
    Nutritional Aid Committee;
    soybean milk
nutrition science: accountability in,
    42, 43, 48, 66, 179; antecedents of, 7;
    chemistry and, 7–8, 47–48, 62, 64,
    78, 80, 87, 165, 175; and Chinese
    medicine, 46; in Chongqing, 153;
    concept of body in, 8–9; and
    concept of Chinese diet, 12–13, 42,
    44, 46–47, 63–65, 67–68, 86;
    domestication of, 8–9, 184;
    emphasis on children, 95–98;
    histories of, 6–7; hunger and
    malnutrition in, 149–50; late
    nineteenth-century, 61–62, 64, 77;
    as scientific discipline, 5, 7–8, 11;
    study of soybeans, 5, 13, 34, 68, 88,
    105–6; and traditional ways of
    thinking about food, 9, 47; univer-
    sality of, 64; and Western learning,
    7–8, 10. *See also* Chinese diet; Wu
    Xian; Zheng Ji
nutritional activism: in China and the
    West, 5–6; of China Nutritional Aid
    Council, 131, 151, 159, 162–63, 166;
    compared with Qing famine relief,
    148; malnutrition and hunger in, 14,
    149–50; Refugee Children's Commit-
    tee and, 138, 151; and refugee work,
    130–31; role of science in, 144, 146,
    149–50; in southwest, 159; soybean
    advocacy, 12, 18, 114, 157–58, 173, 179,
    187; women and, 156
"nutritionism" (Scrinis), 8

distribution of soybean milk, 130, 138–39; funding and membership, 138, 148; and nutritional activism, 131–32, 144, 148, 151; plans to expand to southwest, 146; research of Hou Xiangchuan, 143–46; selection of soybean as nutritional supplement, 141–42; and Shanghai committee of China Nutritional Aid Council, 164–65; targets for assistance, 158, 159. *See also* China Nutritional Aid Council

refugee relief, 17, 121, 129–30, 133–37, 164–65, 221n15, 222n30. *See also* refugee camps; Refugee Children's Nutritional Aid Committee

Refugee Relief Committee (Nanmin Jiuji Weiyuanhui), 221n15

Rehe, 132

restaurants, 15, 43, 134, 163, 206n31

rheumatic fever, 63

rice, 15–16, 70, 100; in five grains, 16, 21, 198n42

ritual, food and, 44

Roberts, J. A. G., 49

Robertson, Robert C., 136

Ruan Qiyu, 106

Russia, 19, 25, 27, 201n43

Russo-Japanese War of 1905, 27, 201n43

S

St. John's University, 154; medical school, 46

sanitation, 137–38, 149. *See also* hygiene

Schmidt, Carl, 91

Schneider, Helen, 156

School for Poor Children (Beijing), 99

Schwartz, Benjamin, 74

science: agricultural, 30–31; Chinese intellectuals and, 66–67, 197n25; and imperialism, 9–10; Japan and, 10–11, 29–30, 197n23; journals, 8, 73, 107, 146, 196n14; and nutritional activism, 144, 146, 149–50; organizations, 197n25; practice of, 197n25; Qing dynasty, 10–11, 197n25; terms for, 29. *See also* chemistry; nutrition science

Science (Kexue), 73, 146

Science Collectanea (Kexue congkan), 107

Scotland, farm laborer's diet in, 52

Scrinis, Gyorgy, 8

sea transport, 23–24

seasons, 70, 113, 118, 119

Second Sino-Japanese War, 143, 154

self-strengthening, 29, 206n42

Seventh-Day Adventists, 83

Shandong, 72, 82

Shandong University, 80

Shanghai: China Nutritional Aid Council committee in, 159, 164–69; dairy industry in, 102; foreign concessions, 129, 133, 154, 174, 220n1; Japanese attack and occupation, 121–22, 133, 146; municipal government, 16; newspapers, 3, 19, 122, 202n65; refugees in, 129–30, 133–37; soybean milk factories, 109, 112–18, 218n2; Ward Road Jail, 167; Western medicine in, 138. *See also* refugee camps; Refugee Children's Nutritional Aid Committee; refugee relief; Shanghai International Red Cross; Shanghai Municipal Council

Shanghai International Red Cross, 133–35, 138, 144, 221n15, 222nn29,32; Refugee Health Committee, 165

Shanghai International Relief Committee, 143, 165, 221n15

Shanghai Municipal Council: defined, 199n2; Food, Dairies, and Markets Division, 109; jail authorities, 167; and *North-China Herald*, 19; and refugee relief, 133, 134, 135–36, 222n30. *See also* Shanghai Municipal Council Public Health Department

Shanghai Municipal Council Public Health Department: and endorsement of Vito-Milk, 170–71, 227n47; inspectors and analysts, 126, 133, 220n41; and refugee diet, 143; and refugee health, 136–37, 222nn29,30; rejection of Welly's license application, 172

Shanghai Nanmin Ertong Yingyang Weiyuanhui. *See* Refugee Children's Nutritional Aid Committee

Shanghai Times, 136

Shanghai United Epidemiology Committee, 137, 222n32

Shanghai Wing On Bakery, 139

Shanhaiguan customs office, 23

Shantung Christian University (Cheeloo University), 65

Shejianshang de Zhongguo (A bite of China; documentary series), 182–84, 185, 187–88, 198n37, 227n7

Shen, Grace, 8

Shen Hong, 31–32, 202n67

Shen Nong, 74, 100

Shen Tong, 46–47, 121

Shenbao: article on health benefits of tofu, 3, 184, 185; advertisements for soybean milk, 172, 172*fig.*; milk advertisements, 94

Sheng, Hsia, 99–100, 216n48

Sherman, Henry C., 62, 79, 212n49; Diet No. 13, 213n71

shi (fermented soy relish), 22

shijin (interdictions), 46

Shijing (Book of odes), 21

Shiwubao (Current affairs), 202n65

Shouxing (god of longevity), 115, 116*fig.*

"Sick Man of Asia," 40, 98

Sikhs, consumption of milk, 94

silk, 33, 37–38

Sino-Japanese War of 1895, 26, 29

Slonaker, James R., 79

Smith, Arthur, 54–55, 207n51; *Chinese Characteristics*, 55, 207nn49,54; on Chinese diet, 55–57

Smith, Edgar Fahs, 65

soap, 14, 21, 27, 33, 39, 201n43

social relationships, food and, 44

social surveys, 57–60, 58–61, 66–67, 208nn66,78; rural and urban, 60–61

Société d'Agriculture de France, 35

society and modernity, 111. *See also* modernity

Society for Cautious Diet and Hygiene, 41

Society for Learning Agriculture (Nongxueshe), 30

South Manchurian Railway, 27

Southwestern University (National Southwest Associated University), 225n16; bean milk cooperative, 160

soy oil, 22, 23, 28, 32, 33, 187

soy proteins, 17, 22, 34, 88

soy relish, 22

soy sauce, 17, 22, 26, 31–32

soybean consciousness, 18, 174, 179–80. *See also* nutritional activism

"Soybean Family Driving Madame Cow into the Museum," 177–78, 178*fig.*, 189

soybean meal, 101

soybean milk: advertisements for, 9, 112–20, 123–27; affordability of, 106, 107, 108, 124, 125; for brain-nourishing, 119, 120, 219n20; characterized as cooling, 115; commercialization of, 168–72, 175; consumed by elderly, 120, 128; as cow's milk substitute, 34–35, 39, 91, 103, 106–7, 108, 120, 121, 123, 141–42, 157, 179, 188; distribution in interior, 157; distribution to refugee children, 130, 131*fig.*, 138–40, 141*fig.*, 151, 159; flavored, 119; formulas for, 145, 159, 163, 166, 168, 171, 225n22; fortified with calcium and vitamins, 4, 141–42, 145, 162, 170–71, 223n58, 225n22; for infant feeding, 88, 103, 105–7, 108, 120, 217–18n83; invention and reinvention of, 5–6, 17; and longevity, 111, 112; manufacturers in Shanghai, 109, 112–18, 218n2; marketing of, 110–11; nutritional value of, 4, 5, 18, 36, 88, 105–6, 141–42, 163; packaging of, 111–12, 118, 119–20; popularity of, 17; powder, 168; sanitary properties of, 107, 108; scientific, 109–10, 118, 181–82, 188; vitamins in, 141, 170–71, 227n47; as worldwide staple item, 188. See also *doujiang*; Hou Xiangchuan; Li Shizeng; Tso, Ernest

soybean paste, 22

soybean residue cakes (*douzha bing*), 130, 139, 154, 159, 163, 167, 169

soybean trade: Chinese imports, 187; dominated by Japan, 32; Manchurian, 24–26, 27, 28, 32, 39, 199n21; after Russo-Japanese War, 27–28; and perceptions of soybeans, 39; sea transport, 24, 200n24

soybeans: advocacy of, 12, 18, 114, 157–58, 173, 179, 187; in ancient China, 16–17, 43; as animal feed, 28, 35, 187; in China today, 15, 186–87; in Chinese cuisine, 142, 183–84, 198n37; and Chinese frugality, 56,

179; and Chineseness, 14–15, 186–88; cultivation of, 21, 22–23, 43; digestibility of, 17, 21–22, 105, 106–7, 118, 183; European use of, 33; extraction of oil from, 22, 200n24; as famine crop, 22, 28; as fertilizer, 23, 24–26, 28; as flex crop, 186; as food for diabetics, 27, 201n48; food products produced from, 21, 36, 38; global diffusion of, 17, 188; and industrial modernity, 17–18, 20, 32, 33, 39, 174, 179; as inferior grain, 21; and Japanese-Russian imperial competition, 201n43; meanings and temporalities of, 17–18, 39; nutritional research, 5, 13, 34, 105–6; nutritional value, 3–5, 67–68, 87–88, 183; in postcard produced by China Nutritional Aid Council, 177–78, 178*fig.*; producers of, 186–87, 228n20; wet ground and roasted, 105, 118. See also beancake; soybean milk; soybean residue cakes; soybean trade

spices, 48

sports, 73

Stoddard, John L., *China* travelogue, 50, 206n30

students, as target for soybean milk distribution, 160

Su Shi (Su Dongpo), 4, 49

Su Zufei, 106

sugar, 23, 24

Sun Company, 168–69

Sun Simiao, 45

Sun Yat-sen, 41, 211n43; "The Problem of Food," 204n1

sweet potatoes, 51, 53, 70

swill milk, 91–92

Swislocki, Mark, 9, 196n20, 224n70

Sze, Dr. Sao-ke Alfred, 165

Sze Szeming, 160, 165–66
Szent-Györgyi, Albert, 78

227n47; vitamin D, 8, 171, 227n47; vitamin C, 78
Vito-Milk: Green Spot, 125–26; Pure Fruit Drinks, 170–71
Voit, Carl von, 82, 212n58

W

Wakeman, Frederic, Jr., 222n40
Wang Guowei, 31, 202n67
Wang, Tsan Ch'ing, 62
Wang Zhen, 22
Ward Road Jail, 167
warlordism, 72
"we are what we eat," 8
wealth and power (*fuqiang*), 29, 74–75, 87, 186; milk and, 89–90, 94, 121
Webb, Sidney, 58
weisheng, 196–97n23. *See also* hygiene
Welly Soya Milk (Weili Dounai), 171–72
Wen Jiaobao, 189
Wen Shuang, 17
Wen Wang, Emperor, 74
Wen Zhongjie, 107
West China Union University, 158
Western learning, 7–8, 10, 28–30
Western medicine, 130, 138, 143, 149, 220–21n4
wet nurses, 104, 125
wheat, 21, 53, 59, 65, 99, 100, 101; in five grains, 16, 21, 198n42; used in animal feeding experiments, 80, 85; used in soybean milk, 114
Will, Pierre-Etienne, 147
Williams, S. W., *The Middle Kingdom*, 50
Wilson, D. S., 61
Wilson, James Harrison, 52–54
women's education, 155–56
women's magazines, 71, 106, 146

Woods, C. D., 61
Worboys, Michael, 64, 149
World Health Organization, 166
World of Soy (Du Bois, Tan, and Mintz), 17
World War I, 72
Wu, Daisy Yen, 62, 65, 79, 85, 212n49
Wu, Shellen, 11
Wu Tingfang, 211n43; Society for Cautious Diet and Hygiene, 41
wu wei (five flavors/sapors), 45, 205n14
Wu Xian (Wu Hsien): and adequacy of Chinese diet, 12, 42, 63–65, 67, 70, 179; and China Nutritional Aid Council, 165; on Chinese weakness, 74; desire for accountability, 66; influence on Luo Dengyi, 69; lecture on Chinese diet, 41, 79, 205n4, 208n79, 209n92; marriages of, 62; on milk, 121; nutrition textbook *Yingyang gailun*, 210n27; on protein needs of children, 96–97; rat experiments with vegetarian diet, 79–80, 85–86; research on nutrition, 42, 62, 65–66, 85, 208n79; study abroad, 11, 41–42, 206n21; view of nutrition and national progress, 11, 83–84, 101, 184; view of soybean as protein source, 88, 179, 185
Wu Xiang, 76
wugu (five staple grains), 16, 21, 43, 198n42

X

xiao baicai, 85–86, 213n70
xiao jiating (nuclear family), 94, 116–17, 127
Xingzheng Reforms, 30
Xu Guangxi, *Complete Treatise on the Administration of Agriculture*, 24
Xu Shou, 8, 10

CPSIA information can be obtained
at www.ICGtesting.com
Printed in the USA
FSHW010056100120
65945FS